2023-2024 NAPLEX® Practice Questions

5th Edition

RxPharmacist, LLC
ISBN: 9798375431628

COPYRIGHT

FOREWORD

We understand how it feels being a pharmacy student or professional looking forward to an exciting journey in getting licensed! Let's be honest, this is probably one of the most stressful times in your life, studying hard for the NAPLEX® with the fear of not passing…

After passing the NAPLEX®, we realized that practicing with more questions would have really boosted our confidence when taking the exam. The goal of this practice question exam book is to help students and fellow pharmacist colleagues in their studies with the most up-to-date material and questions mimicking the actual exam.

Hope this guide serves you well! Best of luck!

Table of Contents

Exam Overview

We would highly recommend to first review the NAPLEX®/MPJE® Registration Bulletin which can be found at: http://www.nabp.net/programs/examination/naplex/registration-bulletin

The NAPLEX® consists of **250 test questions** and the test time is a maximum of **6 hours** total. Of the 250 test questions, 200 are used to calculate your score and the other 50 are dispersed throughout the exam so you won't know which ones are not counted toward your score. The NABP online registration and cost is **$575** per exam attempt. You may take the exam **up to 5 attempts**, but you must wait **45 days** between attempts.

Be sure to answer EVERY SINGLE QUESTION. Remember that this exam is taken on a computer - you CANNOT return to the previous question to change your answer and you CANNOT skip any questions. Try to be cognizant of the amount of time you spend on each question and answer every single question with your first gut instinct.

On January 18, 2021, there were updates to the NAPLEX® in terms of scoring and competency statements. Now exam results will read as "Pass" or "Fail" without a numerical score. Additionally, new graduates (you!) MUST have your school of pharmacy send an official transcript to NABP so you can take the NAPLEX® and/or MPJE®.

The main things you need to know is the exam is broken down to 6 main areas (used to be just 2):
   Area 1 - Obtain, Interpret, or Assess Data, Medical, or Patient Information (~18% of the exam)
- Know the significance of the chief complaint, medication history, lifestyle habits, risk factors, and other such information that you would typically gather from a patient or their chart.
   Area 2 – Identify Drug Characteristics (~14% of the exam)
- Know the brand/generic names, classes, mechanisms of actions, and boxed warnings of drugs.
   Area 3 – Develop or Manage Treatment Plans (~35% of the exam)
- Know the dosing, adverse effects, drug interactions, PK/PD, and treatment goals of drugs. Pharmacists are the drug experts! Also know non-pharm therapy like lifestyle changes or CAM (Complementary and Alternative Medicine).
   Area 4 – Perform Calculations (~14% of the exam)
- Know how to calculate things like dose conversions, rates of administration, and quantities to dispense or compound.
   Area 5 – Compound, Dispense, or Administer Drugs, or Manage Delivery Systems (~11% of the exam)
- Know techniques/procedures/equipment needed for sterile and non-sterile compounding, as well as drug administration techniques.
   Area 6 – Develop or Manage Practice or Medication-Use Systems to Ensure Safety and Quality (~7% of the exam)
- Know how to practice as a pharmacist alongside other professions, and about vulnerable/special populations.

Types of Exam Questions

Multiple-Choice Questions (potentially up to a third of the questions)
Which of the following is a known side effect of Lisinopril?
   a) Dry Cough
   b) Uncontrollable bleeding
   c) Dry eyes
   d) Yellow discharge from ears

   Answer: A

Multiple-Response Questions (potentially up to a third of the questions)
What counselling information should a pharmacist provide to a patient taking fexofenadine? (Select **ALL** that apply.)

   a) Do not exceed the recommended dose
   b) Avoid grapefruit and grapefruit juice
   c) Avoid if sensitive to any ingredients of the product
   d) Avoid live vaccinations

   Answer: A, B, C

> You can't use your personal calculator, need to use Pearson Vue's on-screen calculator during the exam

Constructed-Response Questions (Calculation questions, required to use computer calculator)

What is the loading dose, in grams, of a medication for an 82 kg patient if the volume of distribution is 0.43 L/kg and the desired plasma level is 40 mg/L?

(Answer must be numeric; round the answer to the nearest **tenths**.)

1.41

Ordered-Response Questions (Very few of these type of questions)

List the compounding garbing in order. (ALL options must be used)
Left-click mouse to highlight, drag, and order the answer options.

Unordered Options	Ordered Response (Answer)
Don facial mask	Don shoe covers
Don shoe covers	Don head cover
Don sterile gloves	Don facial mask
Don head cover	Don sterile gloves

Hot Spot Questions (one of the previous contributors to this book only got 1 question like this…)

Using the diagram below, identify where in the HIV life-cycle transcription and translation occurs. (Select the **text** response and left click the mouse. To change your answer, move the cursor, select alternate **text** response, and click).

Picture referenced from: AIDSinfo (NIH): HIV Overview, The HIV Life Cycle http://aidsinfo.nih.gov/education-materials/fact-sheets/19/73/the-hiv-life-cycle

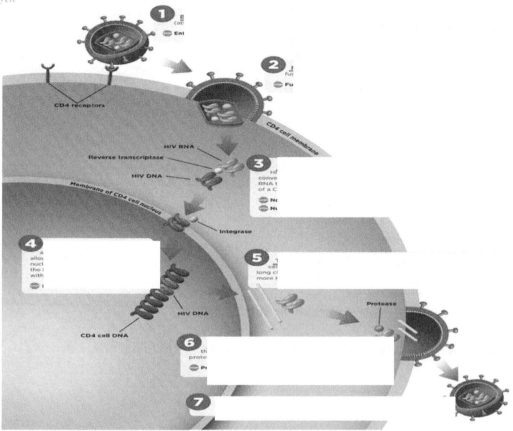

Answer: Step #5 Transcription and Translation

How do I register to take the NAPLEX?

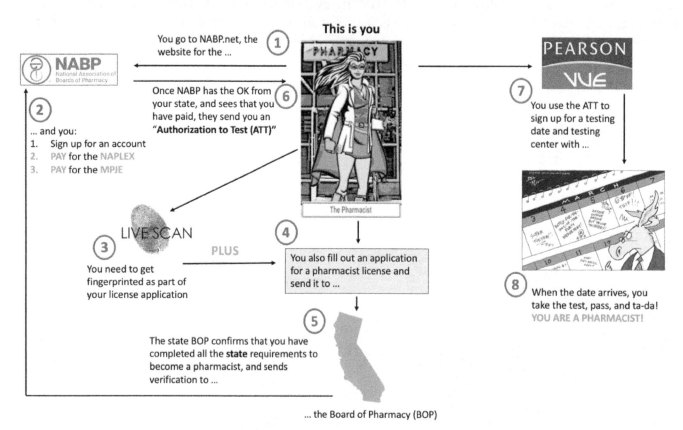

So now that we had a quick overview of the NAPLEX® exam we will get straight to the practice questions! Ready? Set? Go!

Calculation Practice Questions

There are 175 calculation questions split into 4 sections. Time is limited on the real exam, so it's important to practice answering questions like these quickly! We recommend timing yourself in order to practice answering questions at a quick pace.

Section 1: 50 questions, Time: 60 minutes

1. What is the final concentration (expressed as a ratio strength) of a solution if 8 capsules (54 mg each) are dissolved in 1 pint of simple syrup? (Round the answer to the nearest **whole number**.)

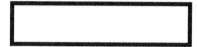

2. You receive the following hyperalimentation solution:

Amino Acids 8.5%	500 mL	Amino Acids 8.5%
Dextrose 70%	500 mL	Dextrose 70%
Sodium Chloride	25 mEq	NaCl 4 mEq/mL
Potassium Chloride	18 mEq	KCl 2 mEq/mL
Magnesium Sulfate	10 mEq	Magnesium Sulfate 4.08 mEq/mL
Calcium Gluconate	15 mEq	Calcium Gluconate 0.465 mEq/mL
Potassium Phosphate	17 mmol	Potassium Phosphate 3 mmol/mL
Multi-Vitamins 12	10 mL	MVI-12 10 mL vial
Trace Elements	3 mL	Trace Elements 3 mL vial

    What is the total volume of the final hyperalimentation solution? (Round the answer to the nearest **whole number**.)

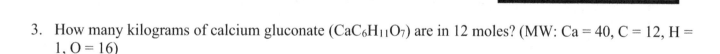

3. How many kilograms of calcium gluconate ($CaC_6H_{11}O_7$) are in 12 moles? (MW: Ca = 40, C = 12, H = 1, O = 16)

    a) 0.24
    b) 2.34
    c) 2.82
    d) 2820
    e) 2400

4. How many mL of a drug solution should be measured to obtain 36 grams of the solution if the specific gravity is 0.92?

    a) 0.03
    b) 39
    c) 33
    d) 36
    e) 29

5. A mother of a 6-month-old infant requests assistance with an over the counter fever product - acetaminophen 80 mg/0.8 mL. Her child weighs 15 pounds and the recommended dose of acetaminophen for fever in infants is 10-15 mg/kg every 6 to 8 hours. Which of the following would be appropriate instructions for her to follow?

    a) Give 3.3 mL by mouth every 6 to 8 hours
    b) Give 1.5 mL by mouth every 6 to 8 hours
    c) Give 0.5 mL by mouth every 6 to 8 hours
    d) Give 2 mL by mouth every 6 to 8 hours
    e) Give 0.8 mL by mouth every 6 to 8 hours

6. A postmenopausal woman consumes 600 mg of calcium carbonate with breakfast and dinner. How many mEq is she receiving daily? (MW: Ca = 40, C = 12, O = 16) (Round the answer to the nearest **whole number**.)

7. How much sodium chloride (in mg) is needed to make the solution below isotonic? (Round the answer to the nearest **whole number**.)

		E value
Drug X	0.004% w/v	0.92
Drug Y	1.2%	0.36
Purified water qs 30 mL		

8. An order is received for a new patient admitted to the hospital. The loading dose is 5 mg/kg ideal body weight. The maintenance dose is 2 mg/kg ideal body weight per hour. The patient is a 56-year-old female weighing 157 lbs. She is 5' 7" tall. Calculate the maintenance dose for this patient. How much drug (in grams) will this patient receive over a 48-hour period?

    a) 6851 grams
    b) 5.91 grams
    c) 6.9 grams
    d) 122 grams
    e) 5866 grams

9. How much, in liters, of a 12% w/v solution can be made if you have 500 mL of a 25% solution and 2 liters of a 3% solution?

    a) 0.2 L
    b) 1.2 L
    c) 3.3 L
    d) 205 mL
    e) 1222 mL

2023-2024 NAPLEX® Practice Questions | RxPharmacist, LLC © 2023

10. A medication order is received for prednisolone 60 mg/m^2/day in 3 divided doses for 2 weeks followed by 45 mg/m^2/day in 2 divided doses for 2 weeks followed by 30 mg/m^2 once daily for 2 weeks followed by 20 mg/m^2 every other day for 2 weeks. Prednisolone is available as a 125 mg/5 mL solution. The patient is a 63-year-old man weighing 246 lbs and standing 5' 11" tall. What is the morning dose, in mg, of prednisolone during the second phase of the taper? (Round the answer to the nearest **whole number**.)

11. A pharmacist compounding 8 ounces of ointment needs to add 56 grams of a solution (density = 0.62), which contains the active ingredient. What volume, in L, of solution is needed?

   a) 0.01
   b) 0.09
   c) 0.72
   d) 90
   e) 720

12. How many grams of a 4.6% w/w ointment can you prepare with 1 kg of a 10.7% w/w ointment and 500 g of a 2.9% w/w ointment?

   a) 391
   b) 639
   c) 1794
   d) 2294
   e) 4588

13. A 57-year-old, 142 lb woman presented to the Emergency Department with a fever of 102.7°F for 3 days. She has an open ulceration on her left leg determined to be cellulitis. She is admitted to the hospital to receive IV antibiotics. A culture determines sensitivity to cephalosporins. Cefazolin at a dose of 1.5 g IV every 8 hours for 3 days is started. The physician orders the cefazolin (1g/50mL) to be infused at 2g/hr. On the 4th day, the patient is released from the hospital and is prescribed cephalexin 500 mg, 4 times daily for 7 days.

   How many bags of IV antibiotics are needed over the 3 days? (Round the answer to the nearest **whole number**.)

14. A medication order is received for gentamicin 1.7 mg/kg IV every 8 hours in 50 mL NS. The patient is a 56-year-old female weighing 145 lb and standing 5' 4" tall. Gentamicin is available in a 2 mL single use vial (40 mg/mL). How many mg of gentamicin will the patient receive daily?

   a) 43
   b) 94
   c) 128
   d) 302
   e) 337

15. A pharmacist compounding 6 ounces of ointment needs 26 grams of coal tar solution (specific gravity 0.84). What volume, in mL, of solution is needed?

    a) 0.03
    b) 22
    c) 31
    d) 131
    e) 53

16. If 250 mL of a 20% (v/v) solution is diluted to 2000 mL, what will be the final percent strength (v/v)? (Round the answer to the nearest **tenths**.)

17. How many milligrams of sodium citrate ($Na_3C_6H_5O_7$) are in 3 moles? (MW: Na = 23, C = 12, H = 1, O = 16) (Round the answer to the nearest **whole number**.)

18. A male patient is 6' 4" tall and weighs 258 pounds. He presents to the outpatient infusion center today to receive "Drug x" in a dose of 17.5 mcg/kg. Calculate, in milligrams, the dose of "Drug x" he will receive.

    a) 0.002
    b) 2.05
    c) 4.5
    d) 2053
    e) 4115

19. A 31-year-old, 5' 3", 156 lb woman presented to the emergency department with severe dysphagia and has been receiving hemodialysis twice a week. She is admitted to the hospital for dehydration. She is to receive fluid replacement for dehydration 4 times daily and total parenteral nutrition every 3 days for caloric needs. She is released from the hospital on day 6 and will be re-evaluated on an outpatient basis for nutritional needs.

    How many mL of a 50% dextrose solution is needed for this patient? Assume amino acids = 0.75 g/kg body weight and provides 4 kcal/g; lipids = 30% of total daily calories and provide 9 kcal/g; and dextrose = 3.4 kcal/g. Assume a stress factor adjustment of 1.2 due to hemodialysis. (Round the answer to the nearest **whole number**.)

    Male = 66 + (13.7 × W) + (5 × H) - (6.8 × A)
    Female = 655 + (9.6 × W) + (1.8 × H) - (4.7 × A)
    A = age in years, W = weight in kg, H = height in cm

20. A 49-year-old, 220 lb man, presented to the emergency department with a pulse ox reading of 89, blood pressure of 180/92, and a pulse of 126. He is administered O2 via nasal cannula and 1 liter of normal saline over 3 hours. He has a history of diabetes and hypertension. He is admitted to the hospital on observational status to monitor his vital signs. Once admitted, he is given Cipro®, 400 mg/200 mL, every 12 hours, infused at 500 mg/hr.

    What is the flow rate (mL/hr) of the normal saline?

    a) 450
    b) 250
    c) 336
    d) 332
    e) 333

21. How many milliliters of methyl salicylate (100% (v/v)) should be used in compounding the following prescription?

    Methyl salicylate 8% (v/v); Liniment base ad 300 mL
    Sig: For external use

    a) 23 mL
    b) 24 mL
    c) 200 mL
    d) 19 mL
    e) 240 mL

22. If a prescription is written for an elixir that contains 50 mcg of a specific active ingredient in 1 mL, what would be the equivalent amount of active ingredient if the total amount to be dispensed is 3 mL?

    a) 151 mg
    b) 15 mg
    c) 1.5 mg
    d) 0.15 mg
    e) 1510 mg

23. A pharmacist receives a prescription for lactulose 4 tablespoonsful 3 times daily. How much lactulose, in liters, would be dispensed for a 30-day supply?

    a) 5.2
    b) 5.3
    c) 5.4
    d) 5400
    e) 540

24. A 34-year-old, 178-lb male hiker presents with a rash covering his legs and feet. He is given 0.75 mg/kg dose of IM Depo-Medrol® (40 mg/mL) for immediate relief of urticaria and rash. He is also prescribed a topical calamine compound and a prednisone taper to be taken over 5 days.

Calamine	100 mg
Phenol	600 mg
Zinc Oxide	300 mg

How many grams of phenol is needed to make 2 oz of the calamine mixture?

a) 33
b) 350
c) 38
d) 34
e) 340

25. A nutritional supplement contains:

Protein	6.9 g/100 mL
Fat	3.2 g/100 mL
Carbohydrate	15 g/100 mL

What is the total number of calories received from 8 ounces of the supplement? (Round the answer to the nearest **whole number**.)

26. A medication order is received for gentamicin 1.7 mg/kg IV every 8 hours in 50 mL NS. The patient is a 56-year-old female weighing 165 lb and standing 5' 8" tall. Gentamicin is available in a 2 mL single use vial (40 mg/mL). If the infusion is administered over 30 minutes and the administration set delivers 20 drops per mL, how many drops per minute will the patient receive? (Round the answer to the nearest **whole number**.)

27. A 34-year-old, 178 lbs. male hiker presents with a rash covering his legs and feet. He is given 0.75 mg/kg dose of IM Depo-Medrol® (40 mg/mL) for immediate relief of urticaria and rash. He is also prescribed a topical calamine compound and a prednisone taper to be taken over 5 days.

Calamine	100 mg
Phenol	600 mg
Zinc Oxide	300 mg

What is the Depo-Medrol® concentration expressed as a ratio strength?

a) 1:26 (w/v)
b) 25:1 (w/v)
c) 1:41 (w/v)
d) 1:25 (w/v)
e) 40:1 (w/v)

28. An asthmatic patient had been stabilized on IV aminophylline 40 mg/hr with therapeutic theophylline level. The patient is now to be discharged from the hospital. What daily oral dose of Theo-24® (a sustained theophylline product with assumed bioavailability of 100%) should he receive?

    a) 800 mg/day
    b) 850 mg/day
    c) 900 mg/day
    d) 750 mg/day
    e) 700 mg/day

29. Drug X (380 mg) is dissolved in 120 mL of purified water. What is the resulting concentration, expressed as a ratio?

    a) 1:333
    b) 1:33
    c) 1:316
    d) 1:335
    e) 1:361

30. A 70 kg patient is to receive dopamine infused intravenously at 10 micrograms/kg/minute. The hospital currently has premixed 250-mL bags containing 400 mg of dopamine in each bag. The nurse asks you to confirm the patient's IV infusion rate.

    What infusion rate is correct in this case?

    a) 24.25 mL/hr
    b) 25.25 mL/hr
    c) 26.25 mL/hr
    d) 27.25 mL/hr
    e) 25 mL/hr

31. What is the final concentration if 37.5 grams of a 12.2% w/w ointment are mixed with 62.5 grams of a 17.6% w/w ointment? (Round the answer to the nearest **tenths**.)

32. How many mEq of potassium are in a 100 mL solution containing 0.5 g of KCl (MW: K = 39; Cl = 35.5)? (Round the answer to the nearest **whole number**.)

33. What is the concentration, in mOsm/L if 500 mg of potassium chloride is dissolved in 250 mL of normal saline? (MW: K = 39, Cl = 35.5, Na = 23) (Round the answer to the nearest **whole number**.)

34. How many millimoles of dietary potassium does a person consume if he ingests ¼ of a pear (680 mg potassium)? (MW: K = 39, Cl = 35.5) (Round the answer to the nearest **tenths**.)

35. If 25 liters of Drug Z weighs 55,020 grams, what is its density?

    a) 2.2 g/mL
    b) 2.5 g/mL
    c) 2.8 g/mL
    d) 3.0 g/mL
    e) 2.0 g/mL

36. You received a prescription order of an elixir containing 100 ppm of an active ingredient. Which of the following would represent an equivalent amount of the active ingredient?

    a) 1 g in 1,000 mL
    b) 1 g in 10,000 mL
    c) 1 g in 100 mL
    d) 1 g in 1 mL
    e) 1 g in 10 mL

37. How many calories would be provided to a patient who receives 1 liter of D5W?

    a) 180 kcal
    b) 190 kcal
    c) 170 kcal
    d) 200 kcal
    e) 150 kcal

38. A 59-year-old, 156 lb female presents to her physician with hot flashes. Her provider prescribes estrogen/progesterone sublingual drops. The directions are "Place 1 drop under the tongue daily."

Estrogen	0.5 g
Progesterone	0.8 g
Saccharin	100 mg
Silica gel	200 mg
Cherry flavor	10 gtt
Almond Oil	10 ml

How many milligrams/days of progesterone is the patient receiving per dose if the dropper delivers 15 gtt/mL? (Round the answer to the nearest **tenths**.)

39. A 24-year-old male comes into the pharmacy with the following prescription for his upper respiratory infection:

>   Ciprofloxacin suspension 500 mg/5 mL Q12H #100 mL
>   Sig: 1 tsp BID stat

How many days will this patient's therapy last?

   a) 5 days
   b) 10 days
   c) 15 days
   d) 3 days
   e) 7 days

40. A man is brought to the ED unresponsive and has a strong smell of alcohol on his breath. He begins to become slightly responsive and the staff is notified by the patient he is an alcoholic. The ED physician orders a "banana bag," aka rally pack, to be administered over 6 hours.

>   "Banana Bag" (aka rally pack)
>   1 L normal saline
>   thiamine (100 mg/mL, 2 mL) 100 mg
>   folic acid (5 mg/mL, 10 mL) 1 mg
>   MVI (1 mL vial) 1 vial
>   magnesium sulfate (0.5 g/mL, 2 mL) 3 g

How much magnesium sulfate (mL) is needed to make the patient's bag plus an additional 4 bags?

   a) 33 mL
   b) 30 mL
   c) 35 mL
   d) 40 mL
   e) 29 mL

41. A patient is using a drug solution containing 10 mg of clindamycin per mL in a 30 mL package. What is the strength of clindamycin in the solution used by the patient? (Round the answer to the nearest **whole number**.)

42. A patient needs to change his regular human insulin product from the U-100 formulation to the U-500 formulation. If he has been taking 0.4 mL of the initial formulation with good control, how much (mL) of the new formulation would you advise him to take? (Round the answer to the nearest **hundredths**.

43. A pharmacist compounding 2 ounces of ointment needs 5 grams of Drug X solution (specific gravity 0.43). What volume, in mL, of solution is needed? (Round the answer to the nearest **tenths**.)

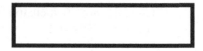

44. How many millimoles of dietary potassium does a patient consume if she ingests 3 servings of soup (240 mg potassium per serving)? (MW: K = 39, Cl = 35.5)

    a) 11.5
    b) 15.5
    c) 18
    d) 18.5
    e) 19

45. A 47-year-old, 6' 1", 198 lb man presented to the emergency department with COPD exacerbation. He is admitted to the hospital for pneumonia as confirmed on a chest x-ray. He receives temporary nutritional replenishment via TPN due to esophageal cancer. He is to receive fluid replacement for dehydration 4 times daily and total parenteral nutrition every 3 days for caloric needs. The patient is released from the hospital on day 8 and will be re-evaluated on an outpatient basis for nutritional needs.

Calculate the resting metabolic energy according to the Harris-Benedict equation. Assume amino acids = 0.75 g/kg body weight and provides 4 kcal/g; lipids = 30% of total daily calories and provide 9 kcal/g; and dextrose = 3.4 kcal/g.

Male = 66 + (13.7 × W) + (5 × H) - (6.8 × A)
Female = 655 + (9.6 × W) + (1.8 × H) - (4.7 × A)
A = age in years, W = weight in kg, H = height in cm

    a) 1907 kcal
    b) 2107 kcal
    c) 2000 kcal
    d) 2300 kcal
    e) 1800 kcal

46. How many kilograms of potassium chloride are in 5 moles? (MW: K = 39, Cl = 35.5)

    a) 0.30
    b) 0.37
    c) 0.20
    d) 0.25
    e) 0.40

47. A 57-year-old, 142 lb woman presented to the emergency department with a fever of 102.7°F for 3 days. She has an open ulceration on her left leg determined to be cellulitis. She is admitted to the hospital to receive IV antibiotics. A culture determines sensitivity to cephalosporins. Cefazolin is started at a dose of 1.5 g IV every 8 hours for 3 days. The physician orders the cefazolin (1 g/50 mL) be infused at 2 g/hr. On the 4th day, the patient is released from the hospital and is prescribed cephalexin 500 mg 4 times daily for 7 days.

At what flow rate (gtt/min) is the antibiotic to be infused if the drop factor is 18 gtt/mL? (Round the answer to the nearest **whole number**.)

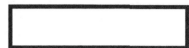

48. How many kilograms of ferrous gluconate ($C_{12}H_{22}FeO_{14}$) are in 3 moles? (MW: Fe = 56, C = 12, H = 1, O = 16)

   a) 1.3
   b) 1338
   c) 1200
   d) 1.2
   e) 446

49. What is the total volume, in mL, of a 2.7% solution that can be made by diluting one ounce of a 10.7% solution?

   a) 119
   b) 150
   c) 100
   d) 89
   e) 41

50. How many milligrams is 154 nanograms?

   a) 0.000154
   b) 0.00154
   c) 0.0154
   d) 0.154
   e) 1.54

Section 2: 50 questions, Time: 60 minutes

1.

PATIENT PROFILE						
Patient Name: Winston Paine				Address: 21 Rivershore, Daytona Beach, FL		
Age: 55	Sex: M		Race: W	Height: 5'9"	Weight: 300 lb	
Allergies: NKDA				Diagnoses: CKD		
MEDICATIONS						
Date	Rx#	Prescriber	Drug	Quantity	Sig	Refills
02/1/21	4308	Dr. Strange, MD	Ferric Citrate 1 g tab	30	1 tab PO TID x 2 weeks	1
ADDITIONAL INFO						
Date	Urine Protein	Creatinine Clearance (CrCl)	Serum Phosphate	BP	HR	Temp
12/01/20	2+	35 mL/min	4.6	130/80	67	99°F

How many milligrams of ferric ion (Fe^{3+}, 55.85 g/mol) are provided by each 1-gram ferric citrate (MW = 265.93 g/mol)?

a) 200 mg
b) 230 mg
c) 210 mg
d) 250 mg
e) 266 mg

2. In the metric system, "mega" is how many times bigger than "kilo"? (Round the answer to the nearest **whole number**.)

```

```

3. You receive the following hyperalimentation solution:

Amino Acids 8.5%	500 mL	Amino Acids 8.5%
Dextrose 70%	500 mL	Dextrose 70%
Sodium Chloride	25 mEq	NaCl 4 mEq/mL
Potassium Chloride	18 mEq	KCl 2 mEq/mL
Magnesium Sulfate	10 mEq	Magnesium Sulfate 4.08 mEq/mL
Calcium Gluconate	15 mEq	Calcium Gluconate 0.465 mEq/mL
Potassium Phosphate	17 mmol	Potassium Phosphate 3 mmol/mL
Multi-Vitamins 12	10 mL	MVI-12 10 mL vial
Trace Elements	3 mL	Trace Elements 3 mL vial

What is the volume of calcium gluconate needed in the final solution?

a) 32.36 mL
b) 30.36 mL
c) 35.26 mL
d) 34 mL
e) 31.26 mL

4. How much sodium chloride (in g) is needed to make the solution below isotonic? (Round the answer to the nearest **tenths**.)

		E value
Drug Z	0.05% w/v	0.82
Drug X	2.7%	0.07
Purified water qs 60 mL		

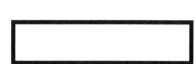

5. A pharmacist receives a prescription for lactulose 2 tbsp TID. How much lactulose, in liters, would be dispensed for a 30-day supply?

   a) 2
   b) 2700
   c) 27
   d) 2.7
   e) 270

6. A pharmacist receives the following order for a hyperalimentation solution:

Amino Acids 8.5%	500 mL	Amino Acids 8.5%
Dextrose 70%	500 mL	Dextrose 70%
Sodium Chloride	25 mEq	NaCl 4 mEq/mL
Potassium Chloride	18 mEq	KCl 2 mEq/mL
Magnesium Sulfate	10 mEq	Magnesium Sulfate 4.08 mEq/mL
Calcium Gluconate	15 mEq	Calcium Gluconate 0.465 mEq/mL
Potassium Phosphate	17 mmol	Potassium Phosphate 3 mmol/mL
Multi-Vitamins 12	10 mL	MVI-12 10 mL vial
Trace Elements	3 mL	Trace Elements 3 mL vial

What is the volume of potassium chloride needed in the final solution?

   a) 6.7 mL
   b) 7 mL
   c) 5.6 mL
   d) 8 mL
   e) 9 mL

7. A pharmacist compounding 4 ounces of ointment needs 15 grams of coal tar solution (specific gravity 0.84). What volume (in mL) of solution is needed? (Round the answer to the nearest **whole number**.)

8. A 49-year-old, 186 lb male housepainter is admitted to the hospital for severe dehydration. He is given a 500 mL bolus of normal saline, followed by 1000 mL of normal saline with 30 mg propranolol for tachycardia in a 50 mL piggyback. The piggyback runs over 1 hour and the additional 1000 mL normal saline runs for an additional 7.5 hours.

    What is the ratio strength and corresponding percentage strength of the propranolol solution?

    a) 1: 333 (w/v), 0.3%
    b) 1:1,666 (w/v), 0.06%
    c) 1:3,333 (w/v), 0.03%
    d) 1:6,666 (w/v), 0.06%
    e) 1:3,333 (w/v), 0.3%

9. How much sodium chloride (in mg) is needed to make the solution below isotonic? (Round the answer to the nearest **whole number**.)

		E value
Drug A	0.5% w/v	0.54
Drug B	2%	0.26
Purified water qs 180 mL		

    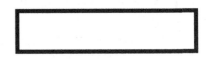

10. The pharmacy received a TPN order for 1.5 mEq of magnesium in 100 mL of IV fluid. The valence of Mg is +2 and molecular weight is 24. What would be the corresponding strength of magnesium?

    a) 460 mg/L
    b) 560 mg/L
    c) 180 mg/L
    d) 360 mg/L
    e) 300 mg/L

11. What is the volume of magnesium sulfate needed in the final solution?

Amino Acids 8.5%	500 mL	Amino Acids 8.5%
Dextrose 70%	500 mL	Dextrose 70%
Sodium Chloride	25 mEq	NaCl 4 mEq/mL
Potassium Chloride	18 mEq	KCl 2 mEq/mL
Magnesium Sulfate	10 mEq	Magnesium Sulfate 4.08 mEq/mL
Calcium Gluconate	15 mEq	Calcium Gluconate 0.465 mEq/mL
Potassium Phosphate	17 mmol	Potassium Phosphate 3 mmol/mL
Multi-Vitamins 12	10 mL	MVI-12 10 mL vial
Trace Elements	3 mL	Trace Elements 3 mL vial

    a) 3 mL
    b) 2.45 mL
    c) 4 mL
    d) 6 mL
    e) 5 mL

12. How many milligrams of sodium bicarbonate ($NaHCO_3$) are in 7 moles?
    (MW: Na = 23, C = 12, H = 1, O = 16)

    a) 588 mg
    b) 600 mg
    c) 600,000 mg
    d) 588,000 mg
    e) 84 mg

13. How much of a 7% w/v solution can be made if you have 360 mL of a 12.5% solution and 2 liters of a 3% solution? (Round the answer to the nearest **whole number**.)

14.

PATIENT PROFILE					
Patient Name: Mika Rose			Address: 3659 Longfellow Road, Perry, FL		
Age: 35	Sex: M	Race: W	Height: 4' 9"		Weight: 158.4 lb
Allergies: NKDA			Diagnoses: Uveitis		
MEDICATIONS					
Date	**Rx#**	**Prescriber**	**Drug**	**Quantity**	**Sig**	**Refills**
1/01/21	46-01	Dr. Stone, MD	Homatropine 5% Opth. Drops	5 mL	1 gtt o.d. TID	0
1/10/21	46-02	Dr. Stone, MD	Prednisolone Acetate 1% Opth. Drops	5 mL	2 gtt o.d. QID	1

The homatropine ophthalmic solution must be compounded as a preservative-free product using homatropine hydrobromide, USP (E = 0.17). According to the USP XXI, solubilization of homatropine requires Sorensen's Modified Phosphate Buffer. If it is recommended that a buffer comprises at least 1/3 of the solution volume, what is the minimum volume of Sorensen's Modified Phosphate Buffer (pH 7.4) that is required to prepare this product? (Round the answer to the nearest **tenths**.)

15. A hospital pharmacist received an order for piperacillin/tazobactam sodium 3.375 g IV every 6 hours in 100 mL normal saline infused over 30 minutes. If the administration set delivers 15 drops of solution per mL, how many drops per minute must be regulated to deliver the medication as prescribed?

    a) 50 drops/minute
    b) 60 drops/minute
    c) 55 drops/minute
    d) 45 drops/minute
    e) 58 drops/minute

16.

PATIENT PROFILE						
Patient Name: Miles Morales			Address: 56 Carol Road, Jacksonville, FL			
Age: 69	Sex: M		Race: AA	Height: 5'8"	Weight: 185 lb	
Allergies: Penicillin			Diagnoses: HTN, Type 2 DM, COPD			
MEDICATIONS						
Date	Rx#	Prescriber	Drug	Quantity	Sig	Refills
2/10/21	77-1	Dr. Strange, MD	Metformin 500 mg	30	1 tablet PO daily	4
2/10/21	77-2	Dr. Strange, MD	Lisinopril 5 mg	30	1 tablet PO BID	5

What is the patient's BMI?

a) 22
b) 25
c) 28
d) 20
e) 30

17. A patient gives you a prescription for a prednisone taper: prednisone 30 mg daily x 5 days, then decrease by 5 mg every 3 days until taper ends. How many prednisone 5 mg tablets will be dispensed to fill this prescription? (Round the answer to the nearest **whole number**.)

18. A female patient is 5' 5" tall and weighs 140 lb. She presents to the outpatient infusion center today to receive Herceptin® 6 mg/kg. Calculate, in grams, the dose of Herceptin® she will receive?

a) 0.38 g
b) 0.40 g
c) 360 g
d) 381.6 g
e) 63.6 g

19. What would be the equivalent ratio strength of a 10% w/v solution?

a) 1:10
b) 1:100
c) 1: 1,000
d) 1:11
e) 1:1

20. You receive the following order:

Amino Acids 8.5%	500 mL	Amino Acids 8.5%
Dextrose 70%	500 mL	Dextrose 70%
Sodium Chloride	20 mEq	NaCl 4 mEq/mL
Potassium Chloride	15 mEq	KCl 2 mEq/mL
Magnesium Sulfate	8 mEq	Magnesium Sulfate 4.08 mEq/mL
Calcium Gluconate	12 mEq	Calcium Gluconate 0.465 mEq/mL
Potassium Phosphate	23 mmol	Potassium Phosphate 3 mmol/mL
Multi-Vitamins 12	10 mL	MVI-12 10 mL vial

How many kcal/day would this patient receive if the flow rate of the TPN is 150mL/hr? Assume 4 kcal/g provided by amino acids, 3.4 kcal/g provided by parenteral dextrose, and 9 kcal/g provided by lipids. (Round the answer to the nearest **whole number**.)

21. You received the following order for a 120 lb patient:

Amino Acids 8.5%	1.5 g/kg	Amino Acids 8.5%, 1000 mL bottle
Dextrose 70%	5 g/kg	Dextrose 70%, 500 mL bottle
Sodium Chloride	10 mEq	NaCl 4 mEq/mL
Potassium Chloride	20 mEq	KCl 2 mEq/mL
Magnesium Sulfate	8 mEq	Magnesium Sulfate 4.08 mEq/mL
Calcium Gluconate	10 mEq	Calcium Gluconate 0.465 mEq/mL
Potassium Phosphate	20 mmol	Potassium Phosphate 3 mmol/mL
Multi-Vitamins 12	10 mL	MVI-12 10 mL vial

What volume of 70% dextrose solution is needed to prepare this hyperalimentation solution? (Round the answer to the nearest **whole number**.)

22. A pharmacist compounding 46 ounces of ointment needs 24 grams of drug N solution (specific gravity 0.62). What volume, in L, of solution is needed?

a) 0.03 L
b) 0.3 L
c) 0.4 L
d) 0.44 L
e) 0.04 L

23.

PATIENT PROFILE					
Patient Name: Edalyn Clawthorne			Address: 227 Boiling Isles, Houston, TX		
Age: 67	Sex: F	Race: W	Height: 5'4"	Weight: 185 lb	
Allergies: Quinolones			Diagnoses: psoriasis, dermatitis		
MEDICATIONS					
Date	Rx#	Prescriber	Drug	Quantity	Sig	Refills
3/26/21	778	Dr. King, MD	Triamcinolone acetonide 0.025%	60 g	Apply to AA QID PRN	4
3/26/21	779	Dr. King, MD	Crude Coal tar gel	33 g	Apply to AA at hs	5

How many mL of triamcinolone acetonide suspension 40 mg/mL would be needed to compound Rx#778? (Round the answer to the nearest **hundredths**.)

24.

PATIENT PROFILE					
Patient Name: Stanford Pines			Address: 618 Mystery St, Gravity Falls, Oregon		
Age: 10	Sex: M	Race: W	Height: 4'4"	Weight: 33.3 kg	
Allergies: Lipitor			Diagnoses: moderate asthma		
MEDICATIONS					
Date	Rx#	Prescriber	Drug	Quantity	Sig	Refills
6/18/21	888	Dr. Bill, MD	Advair® 250/50 mcg	1 Diskus	Inhale 1 puff PO BID	1
6/18/21	889	Dr. Bill, MD	Singulair® 10 mg	30	Take 1 tablet PO HS	2

Stanford goes to see Dr. Bill c/o sore throat, cough, and rhinorrhea. Patient has a fever of 101.3°F. Dr. Bill diagnoses him with an URI and states he will call in a prescription for amoxicillin to the local pharmacy. While you are on duty at the pharmacy, Dr. Bill calls in amoxicillin and wants you to calculate the dose. He wants the patient to receive 30 mg/kg/day PO divided every 12 hours for 10 days. What do you dispense?

   a) Amoxicillin 250 mg/5 mL sig 5 teaspoonfuls PO Q12hr x 10 days
   b) Amoxicillin 250 mg/5 mL sig 3 teaspoonfuls PO Q12hr x 10 days
   c) Amoxicillin 250 mg/5 mL sig 2 teaspoonfuls PO Q12hr x 10 days
   d) Amoxicillin 250 mg/5 mL sig 4 teaspoonfuls PO Q12hr x 10 days
   e) Amoxicillin 250 mg/5 mL sig 1 teaspoonfuls PO Q12hr x 10 days

25. If 785 mL of alcohol weighs 775 g, what is its density? (Round the answer to the nearest **hundredths**.)

26. What is the osmolarity of a solution, in mOsm/L, if 750 mg of potassium chloride injection is added to 500 mL of normal saline? (Molecular weight: K+ 39, Cl- 35.5, Na+ 23)

    a) 348
    b) 337
    c) 300
    d) 174
    e) 340

27.

PATIENT PROFILE						
Patient Name: Bugs Bunny			Address: 6 Looney Tunes Way, Hollywood, CA			
Age: 31	Sex: M	Race: W	Height: 5'3"		Weight: 180 lbs	
Allergies: sulfa drugs			Diagnosis: bipolar disorder, allergies			
MEDICATIONS						
Date	Rx#	Prescriber	Drug	Quantity	Sig	Refills
1/13/21	888	Dr. Acme, MD	ProAir HFA	1 inhaler (200 puffs)	Inhale 2 puffs PO QID PRN	2

During allergy season, if the patient uses Rx #888 as prescribed to the max, for how many days will each prescription last? (Round the answer to the nearest **whole number**.)

28. Which of the following dextrose solutions is isotonic ($E_{dextrose} = 0.18$)?

    a) 2.5% dextrose in water
    b) 50% dextrose in water
    c) 5% dextrose in water
    d) 10% dextrose in water
    e) 20% dextrose in water

29.

PATIENT PROFILE						
Patient Name: Trucy Wright			Address: 5 Bashful Way, Cleveland, OH			
Age: 41	Sex: F	Race: AA	Height: 5'6"		Weight: 132 lbs	
Allergies: lisinopril			Diagnosis: ESRD, HTN			
MEDICATIONS						
Date	Rx#	Prescriber	Drug	Quantity	Sig	Refills
6/1/21	999	Dr. Fey, MD	Valcyte® 450 mg	60	Take 1 tablet PO BID	2
6/1/21	997	Dr. Fey, MD	Propranolol 25 mg	30	Take 1 tablet PO daily	2

This patient's serum creatinine at 6 months post-transplant was measured at 1.9 mg/dL. Using the Cockcroft-Gault equation, what is the best estimate of this patient's creatinine clearance? (Round the answer to the nearest **whole number**.)

30.

PATIENT PROFILE						
Patient Name: Artemis Luna			Address: 17 N Washington Square, Salem, MA			
Age: 21	Sex: F		Race: W	Height: 5'6"	Weight: 132 lbs	
Allergies: Lopressor			Diagnoses: allergies			
MEDICATIONS						
Date	Rx#	Prescriber	Drug	Quantity	Sig	Refills
4/5/21	967	Dr. Blodd, MD	Protonix® Injection	40 mg in 100 mL NS	IV infusion over 15 minutes daily	0
4/5/21	968	Dr. Blodd, MD	Quetiapine 10 mg	30	Take 1 tablet PO daily	1

Protonix (pantoprazole) Injection® is available as a 40 mg per vial solution. What is an appropriate infusion rate for the drug product if an IV administration set calibrated to 20 drops/mL is used?

a) 100 drops/minute
b) 150 drops/minute
c) 200 drops/minute
d) 10 drops/minute
e) 20 drops/minute

31.

PATIENT PROFILE						
Patient Name: Jojo Siwa			Address: 67 Famous Way, Hollywood, CA			
Age: 7	Sex: F		Race: W	Height: 3'3"	Weight: 39 lbs	
Allergies: Sulfa drugs			Diagnoses: depression, ADHD			
MEDICATIONS						
Date	Rx#	Prescriber	Drug	Quantity	Sig	Refills
12/29	567	Dr. Kim, MD	Vyvanse® 30 mg	30	1 tablet PO QAM	1

Dr. Harrison calls and wants you to dispense Omnicef® 250 mg/5 mL and wants you to calculate the dose giving 14 mg/kg q 24 hours for 10 days. Calculate an appropriate dosing volume of Omnicef® suspension for this patient.

a) 7.5 mL PO daily for 10 days
b) 6 mL PO daily for 10 days
c) 4 mL PO daily for 10 days
d) 5 mL PO daily for 10 days
e) 8 mL PO daily for 10 days

32. How much sodium chloride (in g) is needed to make the solution below isotonic? (Round the answer to the nearest **hundredths**.)

		E value
Drug A	0.75% w/v	0.52
Drug B	3% w/v	0.13
Purified water qs 480 mL		

33. A 59-year-old, 136 lb female nurse presents to her family physician with hot flashes and fatigue. Her provider prescribes a compound for estrogen/progesterone sublingual drops. The directions for this compound are "Place 1 drop under the tongue once daily."

       Estrogen 0.5 g
       Progesterone 0.8 g
       Saccharin 100 mg
       Silica Gel 200 mg
       Cherry Flavor 10 gtt
       Almond Oil a.d. 10 mL

How many milliliters of cherry flavor is needed to prepare 45 mL of the estrogen/progesterone compound with a drop factor of 15 gtt/mL? (Round the answer to the nearest **whole number**.)

34. A 49-year-old, 186 lb male housepainter is admitted to the hospital for severe dehydration. He is given a 500 mL bolus of normal saline, followed by 1000 mL of normal saline with 30 mg propranolol for tachycardia in a 50 mL piggyback. The piggyback runs over 1 hour and the additional 1000 mL normal saline runs for an additional 7.5 hours.

What is the flow rate (mL/min) of the second normal saline bag over its 8.5-hour administration period if the drop factor is 15 gtt/mL? (Round the answer to the nearest **whole number**.)

35. You receive the following order:

Amino Acids 8.5%	1.5 g/kg	Amino Acids 8.5%, 1000 mL bottle
Dextrose 70%	5 g/kg	Dextrose 70%, 500 mL bottle
Sodium Chloride	10 mEq	NaCl 4 mEq/mL
Potassium Chloride	20 mEq	KCl 2 mEq/mL
Magnesium Sulfate	8 mEq	Magnesium Sulfate 4.08 mEq/mL
Calcium Gluconate	12 mEq	Calcium Gluconate 0.465 mEq/mL
Potassium Phosphate	20 mmol	Potassium Phosphate 3 mmol/mL
Multi-Vitamins 12	10 mL	MVI-12 10 mL vial

What is the volume of calcium gluconate needed in the final solution?

   a) 30 mL
   b) 28 mL
   c) 26 mL
   d) 20 mL
   e) 22 mL

36. A nutritional supplement contains:

> Protein 8.3 g/100 mL
> Fat   3.6 g/100 mL
> Carb   15 g/100 mL

What number of calories are received from fat in 4 ounces of the supplement?

a) 35 kcal
b) 33 kcal
c) 44 kcal
d) 30 kcal
e) 39 kcal

37. A 35-year-old, 5' 5", 136 lb woman presented to the emergency department with severe dysphagia and has been receiving hemodialysis twice a week. She is admitted to the hospital for dehydration. She is to receive fluid replacement for dehydration 4 times daily and total parenteral nutrition every 3 days for caloric needs. She is released from the hospital on day 6 and will be re-evaluated on an outpatient basis for nutritional needs.

Calculate the total daily calories needed for this patient. Assume amino acids = 0.75g/kg body weight and provides 4 kcal/g; lipids = 30% of total daily calories and provide 9 kcal/g; and dextrose = 3.4 kcal/g. Assume a stress factor adjustment of 1.2 due to hemodialysis. (Round the answer to the nearest **whole number**.)

Male = 66 + (13.7 × W) + (5 × H) - (6.8 × A)
Female = 655 + (9.6 × W) + (1.8 × H) - (4.7 × A)
A = age in years, W = weight in kg, H = height in cm

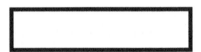

38. A pharmacist receives a prescription for Drug Y in a dose of 3 teaspoons every 8 hours for 14 days. How much Drug Y, in milliliters, will be dispensed?

a) 600 mL
b) 45 mL
c) 630 mL
d) 6.3 mL
e) 15 mL

39.

PATIENT PROFILE					
Patient Name: Caymen Atio			Address: 56 Longfellow, Sanctuary, PR		
Age: 37	Sex: M	Race: AA	Height: 5'7"	Weight: 153 lbs	
Allergies: Sulfa drugs			Diagnoses: 3rd degree burns on left arm, left leg		
MEDICATIONS					
Date	Rx#	Prescriber	Drug	Sig	Refills
1/23/21	555	Dr. Bug, MD	Gentamicin sulfate injection, 10 mg/mL	1.5 mg/kg IBW IM Q8-12hrs x 14 days	0

TEST	NORMAL VALUE	RESULTS
SCr	0.5- 1.1 mg/dL	0.8 mg/dL
01/29	Gentamicin dosing interval based on CrCl. Q8h for CrCl > 60 mL/min; Q12h for CrCl 40-60 mL/min; Q24h for CrCl 20-40 mL/min; <20 mL/min give loading dose and monitor levels	
01/28	Gentamicin sulfate comes in 10 mg/mL and 40 mg/mL sterile solution for injection	

What is an appropriate gentamicin dose and dosing interval for this patient?

a) 92 mg TID
b) 100 mg BID
c) 95 mg BID
d) 90 mg BID
e) 100 mg TID

40. How much water, in mL, must be added to a 0.12% solution to obtain 1 pint of a 0.07% solution? (1 fl oz = 29.57 mL)

a) 197
b) 192
c) 100
d) 97
e) 79

41. You receive the following order:

Amino Acids 8.5%	500 mL	Amino Acids 8.5%	
Dextrose 70%	500 mL	Dextrose 70%	
Sodium Chloride	20 mEq	NaCl 4 mEq/mL	
Potassium Chloride	15 mEq	KCl 2 mEq/mL	
Magnesium Sulfate	8 mEq	Magnesium Sulfate 4.08 mEq/mL	
Calcium Gluconate	12 mEq	Calcium Gluconate 0.465 mEq/mL	
Potassium Phosphate	23 mmol	Potassium Phosphate 3 mmol/mL	
Multi-Vitamins 12	10 mL	MVI-12 10 mL vial	

What is the total volume of the final hyperalimentation solution?

a) 1058 mL
b) 1061 mL
c) 1050 mL
d) 1060 mL
e) 1100 mL

42. You receive a compound for estrogen/progesterone sublingual drops.

Estrogen 0.8 g
Progesterone 0.8 g
Cherry Flavor 15 gtt
Almond Oil a.d. 20 mL

How many milliliters of cherry flavor is needed to prepare 50 mL of the Estrogen/Progesterone compound with a drop factor of 15 gtt/mL? (Round the answer to the nearest **tenths**.)

43.

PATIENT PROFILE					
Patient Name: Rose Blood			Address: 32 Resident Evil Way, Gambro, NC		
Age: 87	Sex: F	Race: W	Height: 6' 9"	Weight: 183 lbs	
Allergies: penicillins			Diagnoses: CKD, asthma, COPD		
MEDICATIONS					
Date	**Rx#**	**Prescriber**	**Drug**	**Sig**	**Refills**
8/29/21	655	Dr. Mo, MD	Proventil inhaler	1 puff q4-6h prn SOB	0

What is Mrs. Rose's estimated Ideal Body Weight (IBW)?

a) 95 kg
b) 94 kg
c) 96 kg
d) 92 kg
e) 93 kg

44. A 35-year-old, 5' 3", 166 lb man presented to the emergency department with severe dysphagia and has been receiving hemodialysis twice a week. He is admitted to the hospital for dehydration. He is to receive fluid replacement for dehydration 4 times daily and total parenteral nutrition every 3 days for caloric needs. He is released from the hospital on day 6 and will be re-evaluated on an outpatient basis for nutritional needs.

How many mL of a 7% amino acid solution are needed? Assume amino acids = 0.75 g/kg body weight and provides 4 kcal/g; lipids = 30% of total daily calories and provide 9 kcal/g; and dextrose = 3.4 kcal/g. Assume a stress factor adjustment of 1.2g/kg/day due to hemodialysis. (Round the answer to the nearest **whole number**.)

Male = 66 + (13.7 × W) + (5 × H) - (6.8 × A)
Female = 655 + (9.6 × W) + (1.8 × H) - (4.7 × A)
A = age in years, W = weight in kg, H = height in cm

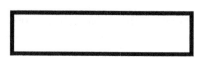

45.

PATIENT PROFILE					
Patient Name: Jin Lao			Address: 23 Forest View Way, Fresco, SC		
Age: 1	Sex: M	Race: W	Height: N/A	Weight: 13 lbs	
Allergies: penicillins			Diagnoses: asthma		
MEDICATIONS					
Date	Rx#	Prescriber	Drug	Sig	Refills
8/29/21	655	Dr. Ke, MD	Pantoprazole 15 mg/mL	1 mL BID	0

What is Jin's dose of pantoprazole in milligrams/kg/dose?

a) 5.91 mg/kg/dose
b) 2.54 mg/kg/dose
c) 5.1 mg/kg/dose
d) 7 mg/kg/dose
e) 4 mg/kg/dose

46. The pediatric dose of a drug is 375 mg/m^2. Determine the dose for an 8-year-old girl who is 3' 8" tall and weighs 70 lb. (Round the answer to the nearest **whole number**.)

47. You receive the following order:

Amino Acids 8.5%	500 mL	Amino Acids 8.5%
Dextrose 70%	500 mL	Dextrose 70%
Sodium Chloride	20 mEq	NaCl 4 mEq/mL
Potassium Chloride	15 mEq	KCl 2 mEq/mL
Magnesium Sulfate	8 mEq	Magnesium Sulfate 4.08 mEq/mL
Calcium Gluconate	12 mEq	Calcium Gluconate 0.465 mEq/mL
Potassium Phosphate	25 mmol	Potassium Phosphate 3 mmol/mL

What is the volume of potassium phosphate in the final solution? (Round the answer to the nearest **tenths**.)

48. How many moles of dietary sodium does a patient consume if he ingests 2 eggs (171 mg sodium/egg), 3 slices of bacon (192 mg sodium/slice), and 2 slices of toast (148 mg sodium/slice) with 4 tsp butter (27 mg sodium/tsp) for breakfast? (MW: Na = 23, Cl = 35.5)

a) 0.02
b) 23
c) 0.5
d) 0.06
e) 0.6

49. A pharmacist receives a prescription for lactulose 4 tablespoons every 8 hours for 48 hours. How much lactulose, in milliliters, will be dispensed?

    a) 150 mL
    b) 200 mL
    c) 180 mL
    d) 320 mL
    e) 360 mL

50. A 59-year-old, 227 lb man, presented to the emergency department with a pulse ox of 89, BP of 190/96, and HR of 136. He is administered O_2 via nasal cannula and 1 liter of normal saline over 4 hours. He has a history of diabetes and hypertension. He is admitted to the hospital on observational status to monitor. Once admitted, he is given Cipro®, 400 mg/200 mL, every 12 hours, infused at 500 mg/hr.

What is the flow rate (mL/hr) of the antibiotic?

    a) 280 mL/hr
    b) 230 mL/hr
    c) 250 mL/hr
    d) 300 mL/hr
    e) 200 mL/hr

Section 3: 50 questions, Time: 60 minutes

1.

PATIENT PROFILE						
Patient name: Melanie Pierce				Address: 123 Sesame Street, NY		
Age: 38	Sex: F		Race: AA	Height: 5' 3"	Weight: 130 lbs	
Allergies: sulfa drugs				Diagnoses: eye infection		
MEDICATIONS						
Date	Rx#	Prescriber	Drug	Quantity	Sig	Refills
12/19	765	Dr. Mo, MD	cefazolin sodium	0.35%	2 gtt OU BID	0
			thimerosal	0.002%		
			0.09% NaCl for Injection, USP	qs 15 mL		

The directions on a 500 mg vial of cefazolin for injection, USP indicates the addition of 2.0 mL of sterile water for injection, USP to the vial, 2.2 mL of cefazolin sodium solution is obtained. What volume of sterile cefazolin for injection, USP is required to provide the required amount of cefazolin in the prescription order? (Round the answer to the nearest **hundredths**.)

2. How many mL of a 25% w/v solution of calcium chloride must be mixed with a 10% solution to prepare 240 mL of a 15% solution?

    a) 80
    b) 60
    c) 40
    d) 20
    e) 100

3. A 34-year-old, 178 lb male hiker presents to urgent care with a rash covering his legs and feet. He is given 0.75 mg/kg dose of IM Depo-Medrol® (40 mg/mL) for immediate relief of urticaria and rash. He is also prescribed a topical calamine compound and a prednisone taper to be taken over 5 days.

Calamine	100 mg	Zinc Oxide	300 mg
Phenol	600 mg	Almond Oil	50 mg

    How much calamine is needed to make 30 grams of the topical calamine mixture?

    a) 2 g
    b) 4 g
    c) 3 g
    d) 5 g
    e) 1 g

4. How many mOsm are present when 950 mg of calcium chloride injection is dissolved in 1 liter of water? (MW: Ca = 40, Cl = 35.5) (Round the answer to the nearest **whole number**.)

5. 480 mL of a 15% w/v solution is mixed with 1 liter of water. What is the new strength, in % w/v, of this solution?

    a) 5.1%
    b) 4.0%
    c) 4.5%
    d) 4.9%
    e) 6%

6. A medication order is received for prednisolone 60 mg/m^2/day in 3 divided doses for 2 weeks followed by 45 mg/m^2/day in 2 divided doses for 2 weeks followed by 30 mg/m^2 once daily for 2 weeks followed by 20 mg/m^2 every other day for 2 weeks. Prednisolone is available as a 125 mg/5 mL solution. The patient is a 63-year-old man who is 346 lbs and 6' 11". What is this patient's body surface area? (Round the answer to the nearest **whole number**.)

7.

PATIENT PROFILE					
Patient name: Michael Jackson			Address: 46 TradePost Way, Wellpinit, WA		
Age: 38	Sex: M	Race: AA	Height: 5' 6"		Weight: 150 lbs
Allergies: sulfa drugs			Diagnoses: metabolic acidosis		
MEDICATIONS					
Date	**Rx#**	**Prescriber**	**Drug**	**Quantity**	**Sig**	**Refills**
01/19/21	7885	Dr. Qi, MD	sodium bicarbonate	180	Infuse IV	0
			potassium bicarbonate	150		
			sodium chloride	90		
			in sterile water for infusion, USP	2.5 L		

The molecular weights for the ingredients are as follows:
Sodium bicarbonate, 84 g/mole
Potassium chloride, 74.5 g/mole
Sodium chloride, 58.5 g/mole

The following sterile drug products are available:
Sodium Bicarbonate for Injection, USP, 8.4%
Potassium Chloride for Injections Concentrate, USP, 500 mEq/250 mL
Sodium Chloride for Injection Concentrate, USP, 14.6%

What volume of 8.4% Sodium Bicarbonate for Injection, USP should be added to the Sterile Water for Infusion, USP IV bag?

a) 400 mL
b) 450 mL
c) 500 mL
d) 600 mL
e) 300 mL

8. A pharmacist receives a prescription for lactulose 2 teaspoons every 8 hours for 48 hours. How much lactulose, in milliliters, will be dispensed? (Round the answer to the nearest **whole number**.)

9. A man is brought to the ED unresponsive and has a strong smell of alcohol on his breath. He begins to become slightly responsive and the staff is notified by the patient he is an alcoholic. The ED physician orders a "banana bag," to be administered over 6 hours.

> "Banana Bag"
> 1 L normal saline
> thiamine (100 mg/mL, 2 mL) 100 mg
> folic acid (5 mg/mL, 10 mL) 1 mg
> MVI (1 mL vial) 1 vial
> magnesium sulfate (0.5 g/mL, 2 mL) 3 g

The physician ordered 3 g of magnesium sulfate in the banana bag and it is to be infused at 0.5 g/hr. What is the flow rate of the banana bag if the drop factor is 18 gtt/mL?

a) 42 gtt/min
b) 45 gtt/min
c) 48 gtt/min
d) 50 gtt/min
e) 40 gtt/min

10. How many mL of a 17.5% w/v solution of calcium chloride must be mixed with a 5% solution to prepare 480 mL of a 15% solution?

a) 384 mL
b) 288 mL
c) 480 mL
d) 350 mL
e) 370 mL

11. How many mOsm are present when 550 mg of calcium chloride ($CaCl_2$) are dissolved in 1 liter of water? (MW: Ca = 40, Cl = 35.5)

a) 12 mOsm
b) 15 mOsm
c) 18 mOsm
d) 31 mOsm
e) 10 mOsm

12. An order is received for a new patient admitted to the hospital. The loading dose is 5 mg/kg ideal body weight. The maintenance dose is 2 mg/kg ideal body weight per hour. The patient is a 36-year-old female weighing 167 lbs. She is 5' 5" tall. What is the loading dose for this patient, in mg?

a) 280 mg
b) 300 mg
c) 285 mg
d) 330 mg
e) 250 mg

13. A 48-year-old, 142 lb man presented to the ED with a fever of 103.7°F for 3 days. He has an open ulceration on his right leg that is determined to be cellulitis. He is admitted to the hospital to receive IV antibiotics. A culture determines sensitivity to cephalosporins. Cefazolin at a dose of 1.5 g IV every 8 hours for 3 days is started. The physician orders the cefazolin (1 g/50 mL) to be infused at 2 g/hr. On the 4th day, the patient is released from the hospital and is prescribed cephalexin 500 mg 4 times daily for 7 days.

If cephalexin suspension contains 250 mg of cephalexin in each 5 mL dose, how many grams of cephalexin are contained in a 200 mL bottle of suspension? (Round the answer to the nearest **whole number**.)

14. You receive the following order:

Amino Acids 8.5%	500 mL	Amino Acids 8.5%	
Dextrose 70%	500 mL	Dextrose 70%	
Sodium Chloride	20 mEq	NaCl 4 mEq/mL	
Potassium Chloride	15 mEq	KCl 2 mEq/mL	
Magnesium Sulfate	8 mEq	Magnesium Sulfate 4.08 mEq/mL	
Calcium Gluconate	12 mEq	Calcium Gluconate 0.465 mEq/mL	
Potassium Phosphate	25 mmol	Potassium Phosphate 3 mmol/mL	

The physician orders this solution be infused at 200 mL/hr. At what flow rate (gtt/min) should it be infused if the drop factor is 15 gtt/mL? (Round the answer to the nearest **whole number**.)

15.

PATIENT PROFILE						
Patient name: Frazier Stevenson			Address: 46 TradePost Way, Wellpinit, WA			
Age: 33	Sex: M	Race: NA	Height: 5' 8"	Weight: 160 lbs		
Allergies: NKDA			Diagnoses: Burkitt's Lymphoma			
MEDICATIONS						
Date	Rx#	Prescriber	Drug	Quantity	Sig	Refills
03/19	8590	Dr. Sig, MD	vincristine sulfate	1.4 mg/m^2	IV in 50 mL NS over 15 minutes	0

What volume of a 2 mg/2 mL vincristine sulfate solution for injection should be injected into the 50 mL NS infusion bag? (Round the answer to the nearest **tenths**.)

16. A 31-year-old, 5' 3", 156 lb woman presented to the ED with severe dysphagia and has been receiving hemodialysis twice a week. She is admitted to the hospital for dehydration. She is to receive fluid replacement for dehydration 4 times daily and a total parenteral nutrition every 3 days for caloric needs. She is released from the hospital on day 6 and will be re-evaluated on an outpatient basis for nutritional needs.

How many kcal is provided from a 7% amino acid solution? Assume amino acids = 0.75 g/kg and provides 4 kcal/g; lipids = 30% of total daily calories and provide 9 kcal/g; and dextrose = 3.4 kcal/g. Assume a stress factor adjustment of 1.2 g/kg/day due to hemodialysis.

Male = 66 + (13.7 × W) + (5 × H) - (6.8 × A)
Female = 655 + (9.6 × W) + (1.8 × H) - (4.7 × A)
A = age in years, W = weight in kg, H = height in cm

  a) 210
  b) 230
  c) 200
  d) 213
  e) 221

17. A 59-year-old, 136 lb. female nurse presents to her family physician with hot flashes and fatigue. Her provider prescribes a compound for Estrogen/Progesterone sublingual drops. The directions for this compound are "Place 2 drops under the tongue once daily."

  Estrogen 0.5 g
  Progesterone 0.8 g
  Saccharin 100 mg
  Silica Gel 200 mg
  Fruity Tutti Flavor 8 gtt
  Sesame Seed Oil QS to 10 mL

How many grams of progesterone are needed to prepare 45 mL of the estrogen/progesterone compound?

  a) 3.6 g
  b) 4.5 g
  c) 5.1 g
  d) 3.0 g
  e) 2.6 g

18. A medication order is received for prednisolone 60 mg/m^2/day in 3 divided doses for 2 weeks followed by 45 mg/m^2/day in 2 divided doses for 2 weeks followed by 30 mg/m^2 once daily for 2 weeks followed by 20 mg/m^2 every other day for 2 weeks. Prednisolone is available as a 125 mg/5 mL solution. The patient is a 49-year-old woman weighing 246 lbs and standing 5' 11" tall. What is the total volume of prednisolone solution, in mL, needed to complete the course of therapy? (Round the answer to the nearest **tenths**.)

19. Drug X (826 mg) is dissolved in 500 mL of purified water. What is the resulting concentration, expressed as a ratio strength?

    a) 1:666
    b) 1:600
    c) 1:605
    d) 1:566
    e) 1:733

20. A 38-year-old, 5' 3", 156 lb woman presented to the emergency department with severe dysphagia and has been receiving hemodialysis twice a week. She is admitted to the hospital for dehydration. She is to receive fluid replacement for dehydration 4 times daily and total parenteral nutrition every 3 days for caloric needs. She is released from the hospital on day 6 and will be re-evaluated on an outpatient basis for nutritional needs.

    Calculate the resting metabolic energy according to the Harris-Benedict equation. Assume amino acids = 0.75 g/kg body weight and provides 4 kcal/g; lipids = 30% of total daily calories and provide 9 kcal/g; and dextrose = 3.4 kcal/g. Assume a stress factor adjustment of 1.2 g/kg/day due to hemodialysis. (Round the answer to the nearest **whole number**.)

    Male = 66 + (13.7 × W) + (5 × H) - (6.8 × A)
    Female = 655 + (9.6 × W) + (1.8 × H) - (4.7 × A)
    A = age in years, W = weight in kg, H = height in cm

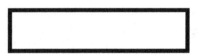

21.

PATIENT PROFILE						
Patient name: Fred Flintstone				Address: 4 Lane, Tacoma, Wyoming		
Age: 43		Sex: M	Race: W	Height: 6' 1"		Weight: 160 lbs
Allergies: NKDA				Diagnoses: knee replacement		
MEDICATIONS						
Date	Rx#	Prescriber	Drug	Quantity	Sig	Refills
04/19	8790	Dr. Kit, MD	fentanyl citrate	100 mcg	Slow IV pre-op	0

Fentanyl citrate (MW = 528.6 g/mole) is available as a sterile solution for injection containing fentanyl citrate, which the label indicates as equivalent to 50 mcg/mL fentanyl base (MW = 336.5 g/mole). What volume of the injectable solution should be administered to the patient to provide the indicated dose of fentanyl citrate?

    a) 1.20 mL
    b) 1.30 mL
    c) 63.7 mL
    d) 1.50 mL
    e) 1.27 mL

22. 300 mL of a 15% w/v solution is mixed with 200 mL of water. What is the new strength, in % w/v, of this solution?

    a) 8%
    b) 9%
    c) 10%
    d) 11%
    e) 5%

23. A pharmacist receives a prescription for Drug X in a dose of 4 tablespoons every 6 hours. How much Drug X, in liters, would be dispensed for a 30-day supply? (Round the answer to the nearest **tenths**.)

24. A hospital pharmacist receives an order for piperacillin/tazobactam sodium 3.375 g IV every 6 hours in 150 mL normal saline infused over 1 hour. If the administration set delivers 30 drops of solution per mL, how many drops per minute must be regulated to deliver the medication as prescribed? (Round the answer to the nearest **whole number**.)

25.

PATIENT PROFILE						
Patient name: Jack Sparrow				Address: 4 Pirate View Way, Smithson, Maine		
Age: 46	Sex: M		Race: W	Height: 5' 8"	Weight: 190 lbs	
Allergies: lisinopril				Diagnoses: asthma, allergies		
MEDICATIONS						
Date	Rx#	Prescriber	Drug	Quantity	Sig	Refills
06/19/21	8788	Dr. Bin, MD	Prednisone 60 mg	QS 30 days	Daily q3 days, then taper by 5 mg q3d to 10 mg daily	0

Prednisone 5 mg tablets are available to fill this patient's prescription. How many tablets should be dispensed to this patient to fill the order for the first 30 days? (Round the answer to the nearest **whole number**.)

26.

PATIENT PROFILE						
Patient name: Baja Blast			Address: 21 Baja Lane, Blast, Kansas			
Age: 6	Sex: M	Race: W	Height: 2' 8"		Weight: 30 lbs	
Allergies: penicillin			Diagnoses: allergies			
MEDICATIONS						
Date	Rx#	Prescriber	Drug	Quantity	Sig	Refills
02/19/21	8778	Dr. Fun, MD	Desloratadine 0.5 mg/mL	250 mL	5 mg PO QD PRN	0

If taken maximally every day as prescribed, how many days will Rx#8778 last this patient?

a) 20 days
b) 25 days
c) 30 days
d) 15 days
e) 10 days

27. What is the final concentration (as a ratio strength) of a solution if four 100 mg tablets are dissolved in 250 mL of water?

a) 1:625
b) 1:325
c) 1:525
d) 1:425
e) 1:250

28. A female patient is 5' 9" tall and weighs 190 pounds. She presents to the outpatient infusion center today to receive Herceptin® 6 mg/kg. Calculate, in grams, the dose of Herceptin® she will receive

a) 0.518 g
b) 518 g
c) 504 g
d) 0.504 g
e) 0.6 g

29.

PATIENT PROFILE						
Patient name: Clark Kent			Address: 24 Metropolis Lane, NY, NY			
Age: 29	Sex: M	Race: AA	Height: 5' 9"		Weight: 210 lbs	
Allergies: NKDA			Diagnoses: metabolic acidosis			
MEDICATIONS						
Date	Rx#	Prescriber	Drug	Quantity	Sig	Refills
05/19/21	8889	Dr. Doom, MD	Sodium Bicarbonate	180	Infuse IV	0
			Potassium Chloride	150		
			Sodium Chloride	90		
			In Sterile Water for infusion, USP	2.5 L		

The molecular weight of NaCl is 58.5 g/mole. What volume of 14.6% Sodium Chloride for Injection Concentrate, USP should be added to the Sterile Water for Infusion, USP IV bag? (Round the answer to the nearest **whole number**.)

30.

PATIENT PROFILE						
Patient name: Marcus Kent			Address: 453 Middle of, Nowhere, Kansas			
Age: 69	Sex: M	Race: W	Height: 5' 6"		Weight: 250 lbs	
Allergies: NKDA			Diagnoses: T2DM, HTN			
MEDICATIONS						
Date	Rx#	Prescriber	Drug	Quantity	Sig	Refills
06/19/21	889	Dr. Day, MD	Metformin 1000 mg	30	Take 1 tablet PO BID	2

What is the patient's BMI? (Round the answer to the nearest **whole number**.)

31. A 48-year-old, 193 lb. male retired teacher has undergone several rounds of chemotherapy for lung cancer. He was given this prescription for "Miracle Mouthwash" to help with mouth ulcerations he developed from chemotherapy. The directions for this compound are "Swish, gargle, and spit 1 teaspoonful every 6 hours as needed for sore throat."

1 part	viscous lidocaine 2%
2 parts	Maalox®
1 part	diphenhydramine (12.5 mg/5 mL)
1.8 parts	Nystatin 100,000 Units Suspension®

How many milliliters of Nystatin® should be used to prepare 240 mL?

a) 65.5 mL
b) 74.5 mL
c) 70 mL
d) 80 mL
e) 66 mL

32. A medication order is received for gentamicin 1.7 mg/kg IV every 8 hours in 50 mL NS. The patient is a 56-year-old woman with an ideal body weight of 75 kg. Gentamicin is available in a 2 mL single use vial (40 mg/mL).

How many vials of gentamicin solution are needed to prepare a 5-day course of therapy (assume all doses are prepared in the morning and the expiration is 24 hours)?

a) 28
b) 23
c) 25
d) 40
e) 20

33. Which of the following factors is the most appropriate for calculating the dose of a drug to achieve a specific plasma concentration?

a) Half-life
b) Volume of distribution
c) Bioavailability
d) Protein binding
e) Clearance

34.

PATIENT PROFILE						
Patient name: Thomas Smith			Address: 34 Road Circle, Blountstown, FL			
Age: 9	Sex: M	Race: AA	Height: 2' 9"		Weight: 56 lbs	
Allergies: NKDA			Diagnoses: allergies, hay fever			
MEDICATIONS						
Date	Rx#	Prescriber	Drug	Quantity	Sig	Refills
01/27	889	Dr. Slow, MD	Cefdinir 125 mg/5 mL	QS	7 mg/kg q12hrs x 7 days	0

What dose of cefdinir should the patient receive?

a) 6 mL every 12 hours for 7 days
b) 5 mL every 12 hours for 7 days
c) 3 mL every 12 hours for 7 days
d) 8 mL every 12 hours for 7 days
e) 7 mL every 12 hours for 7 days

35.

PATIENT PROFILE						
Patient name: Belinda Good			Address: 69 Road Circle, Oz, Kansas			
Age: 76	Sex: F	Race: W	Height: 162 cm		Weight: 79 kg	
Allergies: penicillin		SCr: 1.03	Diagnoses: hyperlipidemia			
MEDICATIONS						
Date	Rx#	Prescriber	Drug	Quantity	Sig	Refills
06/26/21	8764	Dr. Gel, MD	Crestor 10 mg	30	1 tablet PO daily HS	0

Using the Cockcroft-Gault equation, what is the best estimate of this patient's creatinine clearance? (Round the answer to the nearest **whole number**.)

36. You receive the following order for a 150 lb patient:

Amino Acids 8.5%	1.5 g/kg	Amino Acids 8.5%, 500 mL bottle
Dextrose 70%	5 g/kg	Dextrose 70%, 500 mL bottle
Sodium Chloride	20 mEq	NaCl 4 mEq/mL
Potassium Chloride	15 mEq	KCl 2 mEq/mL
Magnesium Sulfate	8 mEq	Magnesium Sulfate 4.08 mEq/mL
Calcium Gluconate	12 mEq	Calcium Gluconate 0.465 mEq/mL
Potassium Phosphate	25 mmol	Potassium Phosphate 3 mmol/mL

What volume of 8.5% amino acid solution is needed to prepare this hyperalimentation solution?

a) 1,200 mL
b) 1,250 mL
c) 1,203 mL
d) 1,215 mL
e) 1,220 mL

37. A 50-year-old, 153 lb female retired CIA agent has undergone several rounds of chemotherapy for breast cancer. She was given this prescription for "Miracle Mouthwash" to help with mouth ulcerations she developed from chemotherapy. The directions for this compound are "Swish, gargle, and spit 1 teaspoonful every 6 hours as needed for sore throat."

1 part	viscous lidocaine 2%
2 parts	Maalox®
1 part	diphenhydramine (12.5 mg/5 mL)
1.8 parts	Nystatin 100,000 Units Suspension®

How many milliliters of viscous lidocaine should be used to prepare 240 mL? (Round the answer to the nearest **hundredths**.)

38. Using the same case as #37, how many milliliters of Maalox® should be used to prepare 240 mL? (Round the answer to the nearest **tenths**.)

39. You receive the following order:

Amino Acids 8.5%	1.5 g/kg	Amino Acids 8.5%, 500 mL bottle
Dextrose 70%	5 g/kg	Dextrose 70%, 500 mL bottle
Sodium Chloride	45 mEq	NaCl 4 mEq/mL
Potassium Chloride	15 mEq	KCl 2 mEq/mL
Magnesium Sulfate	8 mEq	Magnesium Sulfate 4.08 mEq/mL
Calcium Gluconate	12 mEq	Calcium Gluconate 0.465 mEq/mL
Potassium Phosphate	25 mmol	Potassium Phosphate 3 mmol/mL

What is the volume of sodium chloride needed in the final solution? (Round the answer to the nearest **hundredths**.)

40. A 57-year-old, 156 lb. female nurse presents to her family physician with hot flashes and fatigue. Her provider prescribes a compound for estrogen/progesterone sublingual drops. The directions for this compound are "Place 1 drop under the tongue once daily."

Estrogen 0.5 g
Progesterone 0.8 g   Saccharin 100 mg
Silica Gel 200 mg   Fruity Tutti Flavor 8 gtt
Sesame Seed Oil QS to 10 mL

How many milligrams/days of estrogen is the patient receiving if the dropper delivers 15 gtt/mL? (Round the answer to the nearest **hundredths**.)

41. A 46-year-old male has been receiving vancomycin for 1 week for MRSA pneumonia. He is 5' 9" and weighs 160 lbs. His admission SCr was 1 mg/dL. His SCr is now 1.6 mg/dL.

> Vancomycin dosing: 750 mg IV Q24H at 2100 (stable regimen since 5/10/19)
> Last vancomycin dose given: 5/17/19 @ 2100
> Vancomycin level (random): 5/18/19 @ 1000 = 28 mg/L
> Vancomycin level (random): 5/18/19 @ 1300 = 24.7 mg/L

Calculate MK's vancomycin half-life. (Round the answer to the nearest **whole number**.)

42. Drug P03E6 has a volume of distribution of 80 L and a clearance of 9.37 L/hr. What is the half-life of this drug?

a) 4
b) 6
c) 3
d) 2
e) 5

43. A new antibiotic has the following properties listed in its monograph:

> Dosing (IV): 675 mg IV Q8H
> Dosing (PO): 675 mg PO TID
> Protein binding: 18%
> Metabolism: partially hepatic
> Half-life: 1.6 - 2.1 hours

What is this drug's bioavailability?

a) 1%
b) 90%
c) 100%
d) 40%
e) 50%

44. An oral drug is administered as a 225 mg dose. The resulting AUC is 52 mg x hr/mL. The bioavailability of the oral formulation is 50%. What is the clearance of this drug? (Round the answer to the nearest **hundredths**.)

45. Following a 400 mg dose of cefdinir, the terminal elimination rate constant was determined to be 0.38 hr^{-1}. Calculate the half-life of cefdinir. (Round the answer to the nearest **tenths**.)

2023-2024 NAPLEX® Practice Questions | RxPharmacist, LLC © 2023

46. Amoxicillin has a clearance of 4.5 L/hr and a volume of distribution of 65 L. Calculate the half-life of amoxicillin. (Round the answer to the nearest **whole number**.)

47. You gave a 400 mg dose of fluconazole IV, calculate the clearance if the area under the curve is measured at 38.0 mcg × hr/mL. (Round the answer to the nearest **whole number**.)

48. Following an oral dose of 400 mg of cefdinir, the terminal elimination rate constant was determined to be 0.38 hr^{-1}, and the AUC was determined to be 25.18 mg × hr/L. Calculate the volume of distribution of cefdinir. (Round the answer to the nearest **whole number**.)

49. What is the pH of a solution prepared to be 0.5 M sodium bicarbonate and 0.05 M ascorbic acid (pKa for ascorbic acid = 3.13)?

    a) 4.0
    b) 4.5
    c) 4.2
    d) 4.13
    e) 4.10

50. What is the conversion calculation from aminophylline to theophylline?

    a) Aminophylline × 0.3 = theophylline dose
    b) Aminophylline × 0.5 = theophylline dose
    c) Aminophylline × 0.6 = theophylline dose
    d) Aminophylline × 0.4 = theophylline dose
    e) Aminophylline × 0.8 = theophylline dose

Section 4: 20 questions, Time: 25 minutes

1. A pediatric regimen for drug A is 10 mcg/m^2 three times daily. A child has weight of 45 lb and height of 36 inches. How many micrograms is the total daily dose for this child? (Round the answer to the nearest **tenths.**)

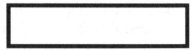

2. How many days will the following prescription last? (Round the answer to the nearest **whole number**.)

    Rx: Reglan® 5 mg tablets #70
    Sig: 1 tablet TID AC and 2 tablets HS

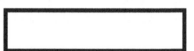

3. How many milliliters of 5% acetic acid solution is needed to make 1 liter of 1:400 (w/v) acetic acid solution? (Round the answer to the nearest **whole number**.)

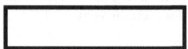

4. Consider the following prescription, how much lanolin cream is ordered?

    Rx:
    Zinc oxide powder (5 g)
    Talc powder (5 g)
    Starch powder aa 5 g
    Lanolin cream
    Petrolatum ointment aa qs a.d. 100 g

    a) 37.5 g
    b) 40 g
    c) 45 g
    d) 42.5 g
    e) 50.5 g

5. What is the final ratio strength of zinc oxide ointment prepared by combining 20 grams of 2.5% (w/w) zinc oxide ointment and 10 grams of 5% (w/w) zinc oxide ointment?

    a) 1:20
    b) 1:30
    c) 1:40
    d) 1:50
    e) 1:15

6. How many milligrams of sodium chloride is needed to make these eye drops isotonic with tears? (Round the answer to the nearest **whole number**.)

$E_{\text{ephedrine sulfate}} = 0.23$; $E_{\text{tetracycline HCl}} = 0.14$

Rx:
Ephedrine sulfate 0.2 g
Tetracycline HCl 0.5 g
Total volume: 30 mL

Questions 7-9 pertain to the following case:

A hospital pharmacy received the following parenteral nutrition order:

Patient A.A. (Room 101)
Female
Dr. Johns Hopeth
Height: 5' 6"
Weight: 140 lb

Central TPN:
        Amino acids 5%
        Dextrose 20%
        Sodium chloride 40 mEq/L
        Potassium acetate 20 mEq/L
        Potassium phosphate 20 mEq/L
        Magnesium sulfate 5 mEq/L
        Calcium gluconate 10 mEq/L
        Multivitamins 10 mL/day
        Trace elements 3 mL/day .

        Rate: 1500 mL/day at 62.5 mL/hour

        Plus 20% fat emulsion 500 mL per day

7. What is the total daily calorie (kcal)? (Round the answer to the nearest **whole number**.)

8. What is the non-protein calories to nitrogen ratio?

    a) 1:138
    b) 1:225
    c) 1:155
    d) 1:172
    e) 1:168

9. The pharmacy has a 70% dextrose solution stock bottle. How many milliliters of 70% dextrose are needed to prepare 1500 mL parenteral nutrition solution? (Round the answer to the nearest **whole number.**)

10. A patient is receiving 750 mL of 5% dextrose in water (E = 0.18). What is the tonicity of this solution?

    a) Isotonic
    b) Hypotonic
    c) Hypertonic
    d) Catatonic
    e) Not enough information to calculate

11. A pharmacist receives a prescription for a patient (female, 176 lb, 6'): 16 units/kg of heparin per hour as continuous infusion. The pharmacy has prepared heparin 25,000 units in 5% dextrose (in water) 500 mL. What is the infusion rate (mL/hour) this bag should be administered at?

    a) 20.2 mL/hour
    b) 25.6 mL/hour
    c) 36.2 mL/hour
    d) 90.56 mL/hour
    e) 67.2 mL/hour

12. How many milliliters of 25% dextrose solution and how many milliliters of 10% dextrose solution are required to prepare 500 mL of 12.5% dextrose solution?

    a) 70 mL of 25% dextrose, and 430 mL of 10% dextrose
    b) 103 mL of 25% dextrose, and 397 mL of 10% dextrose
    c) 120 mL of 25% dextrose, and 380 mL of 10% dextrose
    d) 233 mL of 25% dextrose, and 467 mL of 10% dextrose
    e) 83 mL of 25% dextrose, and 417 mL of 10% dextrose

13. Consider the following prescription. What is the percentage strength of the salicylic acid component? (Round the answer to the nearest **tenths.**)

    > Salicylic acid 1.7 g
    > Benzoic acid 4.3 g
    > Lanolin cream 45 g

14. If a source of drinking water contains 3.4 ppm of fluoride, how many micrograms (mcg) of fluoride are in one quart (950 mL) of water?

    a) 3230 mcg
    b) 3.23 mcg
    c) 6460 mcg
    d) 6.46 mcg
    e) 1.62 mcg

15. A 154 lb patient is to receive 1.5 mEq of NaCl per kilogram. How many milliliters of 0.9% sodium chloride solution should be administered? (MW: NaCl = 58.5) (Round the answer to the nearest **tenths**.)

16. The label of 1,000 mg dry powder for constitution into pediatric drops states that: when 16 mL of purified water are added to the powder, 20 mL of a pediatric suspension results, containing 50 mg/mL. How many milliliters of water should be added to have the dose in each 10 drops, if the dropper delivers 15 drops/mL, the infant weights 28 lb, and the dose of the drug is 2.5 mg/kg?

    a) 15.2 mL
    b) 5.7 mL
    c) 10.1 mL
    d) 11.7 mL
    e) 16.3 mL

17. The half-life of an isotope is 73 days. If 1 mCi of this substance is stored for 1 year (365 days), how many microCi will remain? (Round the answer to the nearest **tenths**.)

18. JL is a 52-year-old obese woman with a history of type 2 diabetes x 2 years.

    Her current diabetes regimen:
    Metformin XR 2000 mg PO daily
    Glyburide 5 mg PO daily

    Vital signs: BP 122/78 mmHg, HR 78 bpm, RR 20 rpm, Weight 65 kg, Height 5'2"
    Labs: SCr = 0.8 mg/mL; fasting BG: 228 mg/dL; most recent A1c: 10.6%

    Today, she admitted to the hospital due to sepsis. Her physician stopped her oral DM regimen and start insulin (basal-bolus) regimen while she is in the hospital with a total daily dose (TDD) of 0.4 units/kg. She is on 4 carb serving limit per meal. Only glargine and Lispro® are in the hospital formulary

    What is the **MOST APPROPRIATE** initial insulin regimen?

    a) 26 units of glargine QHS and 8 units of Lispro® AC
    b) 13 units of glargine QHS and 13 units of Lispro® AC
    c) 13 units of glargine QHS and 4 units of Lispro® AC
    d) 7 units of glargine QHS and 7 units of Lispro® AC
    e) 10 units of glargine QHS and 5 units of Lispro® AC

19. A pharmacist received a medication order to add 60,000 units of heparin sodium to 1 liter of D5W for a 180 lb patient. The rate of the infusion was prescribed as 2,000 units per hour. How long will the infusion run, in hours? (Round the answer to the nearest **whole number**.)

20. A pharmacist received a medication order to add 60,000 units of heparin sodium to 1 liter of D5W for a 200 lb patient. The rate of the infusion was prescribed as 2,000 units per hour. What is the dose of heparin sodium received by the patient, on a unit/kg/min basis?

    a) 0.11 units/kg/min
    b) 0.89 units/kg/min
    c) 33.3 units/kg/min
    d) 0.37 units/kg/min
    e) 21.98 units/kg/min

2023-2024 NAPLEX® Practice Questions | RxPharmacist, LLC © 2023

Pharmacotherapy and Case Questions

The following 5 sections each contain 50 general pharmacotherapy and case scenario questions to help you master your clinical knowledge. This section will be composed of brand/generic, compounding sterile/nonsterile products, reviewing/dispensing/administering drugs, and pharmacotherapy questions.

Practice Test 1: 50 questions, Time: 60 minutes

1. Another name for Enbrel® is:

   a) Efavirenz
   b) Etanercept
   c) Eptifibatide
   d) Enfuvirtide
   e) Etidronate

2. A patient asks the pharmacist about a severe hangover from drinking vodka last night. He awakened with heartburn, nausea, tremor, dizziness, fatigue, body aches, headache, and depression. What is the worst combination of ingredients for him?

   a) Caffeine, calcium carbonate
   b) Ibuprofen, calcium carbonate
   c) Naproxen, calcium carbonate
   d) Tums®
   e) Advil®, Maalox®

3. After you ask for her allergies, an elderly woman mentions that she is allergic to capsules. She says that capsules never seem to get into her throat correctly and she hates swallowing them. She says that even after a full glass of water she still feels the capsule right in her mouth. After looking at her profile, you find out that 4 out of 7 of her medications are capsules. Which of the following is likely to help her swallow?

   a) Do not use water
   b) Empty capsule contents into apple juice, then drink
   c) Extend head upward, when feeling capsule in back of throat swallow
   d) Take a sip of water with capsule, flex the head forward, and swallow
   e) Swallow with some food

4. Another name for Macrobid® is:

   a) Nitrofurantoin
   b) Gentamicin
   c) Bactrim DS
   d) Metronidazole
   e) Clarithromycin

5. Combivent® is also known as:

    a) Albuterol/Formoterol
    b) Albuterol/Fluticasone
    c) Albuterol/Salmeterol
    d) Albuterol/Budesonide
    e) Albuterol/Ipratropium

6. Another name for Bactrim® is:

    a) Bacitracin
    b) Baclofen
    c) Sulfamethoxazole/Trimethoprim
    d) Piperacillin/Tazobactam

7. Many dosage forms and medication delivery methods are considered suitable for nonprescription use. However, some are not available for nonprescription products. Which of the following is not available on a nonprescription basis?

    a) Inhalers
    b) Suppositories
    c) Enteric-Coated Tablets
    d) Injections
    e) Powders for Inhalation

8. Magnesium stearate is commonly used as what type of pharmaceutic ingredient in tablet preparation?

    a) Tablet lubricant
    b) Tablet disintegrant
    c) Tablet opaquant
    d) Tablet polishing agent
    e) Tablet glidant

9. A 17-year-old who is sexually active (gravida 0 para 0) presents with painful menstruation. This is accompanied by diarrhea, headache, nausea, and vomiting. She feels incapacitated for 48 to 72 hours during menstruation each period. She was tried on first-line medication with side effects which she claims she could not tolerate. Her doctor started her then on combination oral contraceptives. What is one of the effects of this medication?

    a) Osteoporosis
    b) Gallstone formation
    c) Vaginal dryness
    d) Increased cholesterol levels
    e) Blurry vision

10. A patient appearing to be aged in his 40s asks the pharmacist about a product to help his insomnia. He has only had it for 1 night and thinks it may be caused by worry over an upcoming CPA exam. It may also be caused by the fact that his enlarged prostate causes him to have to urinate several times a night. He takes glyburide for diabetes. What should the pharmacist tell him?

    a) Insomnia for 1 night requires a physician appointment
    b) Nonprescription insomnia products are contraindicated with prostate enlargement
    c) Nonprescription products are not indicated for short-term insomnia
    d) Nonprescription insomnia products are contraindicated in patients with diabetes
    e) Nonprescription insomnia products interact with glyburide

11. Which agent is available in a rectal formulation for relief of constipation?

    a) Bisacodyl
    b) Sorbitol
    c) Lubiprostone
    d) Methylcellulose
    e) Docusate sodium

12. A 24-year-old woman is studying for final exams and wants to know what she can do about several small vesicles that have formed a crust on the upper margin of her lip. The lesions are painful, and she would like to minimize discomfort in for an upcoming job interview. What is the most likely cause of infection?

    a) Fungal
    b) Viral
    c) Bacterial
    d) Candida
    e) Parasite

13. What is the appropriate needle gauge for a newly diagnosed diabetic patient requiring subcutaneous insulin?

    a) 25G, 1 inch
    b) 31G, 1 inch
    c) 33G, 5/16 inch
    d) 31G, 5/16 inch
    e) 25G, 5/16 inch

14. An 80-year-old patient comes to the pharmacy counter requesting assistance with choosing an appropriate medication to treat her cold symptoms. Her main symptom is nasal congestion. She is a routine customer in your pharmacy and is compliant with her blood pressure medications, glaucoma eye drops, and bisphosphonates for osteoporosis. What do you recommend to treat this patient's cold symptoms?

    a) Oral loratadine
    b) Nasal spray saline
    c) Oxymetazoline nasal spray
    d) Oral diphenhydramine
    e) Oral pseudoephedrine

15. A 17-year-old sexually active G1P1 female presents with white cheesy vaginal discharge. A speculum exam is performed, visualizing adherent white and erythematous vaginal membranes. Hyphae are seen on the KOH smear. The patient is diagnosed with vaginal candidiasis and is prescribed fluconazole for treatment. She has an allergy to penicillin, which causes anaphylaxis. Which of the following is a side effect this patient should be counseled about?

    a) Potential for anaphylaxis due to cross reactivity
    b) Injection site reaction
    c) Nausea and vomiting in conjunction with alcohol use
    d) Teeth discoloration
    e) Mild nausea and vomiting after a single pill use

16. A 20-year-old woman is studying for final exams and wants to know what she can do about several small vesicles that have formed a crust on the upper margin of her lip. The lesions are painful, and she would like to minimize discomfort in for an upcoming job interview. What OTC agent can be used to manage her condition?

    a) Carbamide peroxide 10%
    b) Benzocaine 20%
    c) Capsaicin
    d) Oxybenzone
    e) Camphor 20%

17. Which one of the following is a trigger for reactivation of fever blisters?

    a) Shingles
    b) Chicken Pox
    c) Avobenzone
    d) Ultraviolet Radiation
    e) Sulfonamides

18.

PATIENT PROFILE					
Patient name: Sleve McDichael			Address: 12 Bobson Road, Dugnutt, TX		
Age: 38	Sex: M		Race: NA	Height: 5' 6"	Weight: 150 lbs
Allergies: penicillin		SCr: 1.03		Diagnoses: metabolic acidosis	
MEDICATIONS					
Date	Rx#	Prescriber	Drug	Quantity	Sig	Refills
01/19	7885	Dr. Bonzalez, MD	Fentanyl Citrate	50 mcg	IM pre-op	0

Fentanyl Citrate Injection, USP is dispensed as a single dose in a syringe for use in surgery scheduled the same day the drug product is prepared. What would the appropriate storage conditions and beyond use date be for the dispensed product if it had been prepared under ISO Class 5 conditions?

    a) 14 days at cold temperature
    b) 30 hours at controlled room temperature
    c) 45 days in solid frozen state
    d) 48 hours at controlled room temperature
    e) 9 days at cold temperature

19. What dosage adjustment needs to be taken into consideration if a patient's phenytoin regimen needs to be changed from a capsule to a suspension?

    a) The dose needs to be decreased by 8%
    b) The dose needs to be increased by 8%
    c) The dose needs to be increased by 50%
    d) The dose needs to be decreased by 50%
    e) The dose needs to be increased by 10%

20. A patient purchasing Alli® (orlistat) asks the pharmacist whether there are any special instructions he should follow. What should the pharmacist tell him?

    a) Take with a fiber supplement to prevent Alli®-induced constipation
    b) Take 4-6 capsules daily to reach maximal weight-loss potential
    c) Take a multivitamin once daily at bedtime
    d) Take along with an herbal weight loss product
    e) Ingest 1 serving of fat with each meal to counteract fat malabsorption

21. A 56-year-old male presents to the urologist with complaints of urinary frequency, urgency, hesitancy and nocturia. Upon examination, it is determined that the prostate is enlarged and weighs approximately 50 grams. His current medications include atorvastatin 40 mg once daily, lisinopril 20 mg once daily, aspirin 325 mg once daily, HCTZ 25 mg once daily, Humalog® 7 units with meals, Lantus® 50 units at night. Pertinent data: PSA 4.6 ng/mL, BP 120-130/74-80, fasting glucose 106, HgbA1c 6.2%. The physician decides to initiate terazosin. Which of the following patient education points will you address first regarding this medication with this patient?

    a) Monitor your blood pressure for additional decreases
    b) It is important that you monitor your PSA levels annually for efficacy
    c) Common side effects of this medication include nausea, headache, and stomach upset
    d) If you notice that you are starting to feel depressed or have thoughts of hurting yourself, seek help immediately
    e) Women of childbearing age should not handle this medication

22. A mother is asking for assistance. Her 6-year-old son has white bumps on his fingers that appear to be warts. The warts do not seem to bother him, but he keeps injuring the warts. What concentration of salicylic acid do you recommend for her son?

    a) 10%
    b) 12%
    c) 17%
    d) 40%
    e) 35%

23.

Ingredient	Source
Cefazolin sodium	Cefazolin for Injection, USP Sterile Powder for Reconstitution, 500 mg vial
Thimerosal	Bulk thimerosal powder, non-sterile
0.9% Sodium chloride for injection, USP	0.9% Sodium Chloride for Injection, USP Sterile solution, 20 mL vial

The ingredients needed to prepare the formulation are listed in the table below. Based on this information, what USP <797> risk level and beyond-use-dating would you assign to this product?

    a) High risk, 9 days refrigerated
    b) High risk, 3 days refrigerated
    c) Medium risk, 14 days refrigerated
    d) Medium risk, 9 days refrigerated
    e) Medium risk, 3 days refrigerated

24. A 21-year-old male presents to his primary care physician with urethritis, proctitis, urethral discharge, dysuria, and itching. The microscopic findings of the urethral discharge include *C. trachomatis*. The patient admits to unprotected intercourse approximately 10 days ago. His medical record indicates he is allergic to clarithromycin and penicillin. Which of the following is the most appropriate treatment option?

    a) Acyclovir
    b) Penicillin G
    c) Doxycycline
    d) Azithromycin
    e) Cefdinir

25. This patient is prescribed the medication Latisse®. When she comes to the pharmacy to get the prescription filled, she asks how the medication should be stored. The package insert for Latisse® instructs the patient to store Latisse® at 2° to 25°C. Based on USP standards, how should the patient store their Latisse®?

    a) Cool
    b) Cold
    c) Frozen
    d) Warm
    e) Room temperature

26. Which of the following is an SSRI that is marketed as an isomer rather than a racemate?

    a) Citalopram
    b) Fluoxetine
    c) Escitalopram
    d) Paroxetine
    e) Sertraline

27. A mother is asking for assistance. Her 6-year-old son has white bumps on his fingers that appear to be warts. The warts do not seem to bother him, but he keeps injuring the warts. She is afraid someone else in the family will "get these things."

Salicylic acid for the nonprescription treatment of warts is contained in all of the following products except:

    a) Compound W Freeze Off®
    b) Occlusal-HP®
    c) Dr. Scholl's Clear Away®
    d) Wart-Off®
    e) Compound Wart Strips®

28. Omnipred® contains the following list of ingredients: prednisolone acetate 1%, benzalkonium chloride 0.01%, hypromellose, dibasic sodium phosphate, polysorbate 80, edetate disodium, glycerin, citric acid and/or sodium hydroxide, and purified water. What purpose does hypromellose serve in this formulation?

    a) Surfactant
    b) Viscous Vehicle
    c) pH adjuster
    d) Tonicity Adjuster
    e) Preservative

29. Which of the following is FDA-approved for treatment of infection *C. difficile*?

    a) Ciprofloxacin
    b) Metronidazole
    c) Vancomycin
    d) Streptomycin
    e) Clindamycin

30. Unless specified by a requirement in a USP monograph, in general the expiration date of a pharmaceutical product means that after that date, the product would lose what percentage of its original activity?

    a) 10%
    b) 20%
    c) 15%
    d) 5%
    e) 2%

31. Good oral hygiene is important to prevent a specific drug-related effect of which of the following drugs?

    a) Lamotrigine
    b) Phenytoin
    c) Phenobarbital
    d) Valproic acid
    e) Carbamazepine

32. A 46-year-old man inquiries about smoking cessation. He currently smokes 9 cigarettes per day. He admits that he is a chronic gum chewer and he is concerned about weight gain upon quitting. His past medical history is significant for hypertension, depression, epilepsy, and seasonal allergies. He has tried nicotine patches in the past with limited success. What is the most appropriate treatment option for this patient?

   a) Clonidine 0.1 mg patch daily
   b) Nicotine 21 mg patch daily
   c) Bupropion 150 mg twice daily
   d) Nicotine gum 4 mg every week
   e) Nortriptyline 25 mg twice daily

33. The formula for 33 grams of coal tar ointment is: 0.33 g of crude coal tar, 0.165 g of polysorbate 80, and 32.505 g of zinc oxide paste. What equipment should be used to measure the required amount of coal tar?

   a) Stirring rod
   b) 10 mL cylindrical graduate
   c) Oral or injectable syringe
   d) Spatula and electronic balance
   e) Spoon

34. Which of the following mathematical equations can be used to calculate the pH of an electrolyte solution?

   a) Henderson-Hasselbalch
   b) Arrhenius
   c) Cockcroft and Gault
   d) Michaelis-Menten
   e) Fundalis

35. Which of the following is an appropriate route for administration of heparin? (Select **ALL** that apply.)

   a) Heparin flush
   b) Subcutaneous
   c) IV infusion administered intermittently
   d) Intramuscular administration
   e) Continuous IV infusion

36. A 64-year-old male is brought to ER by his spouse after she found him wandering in the back yard. He was spraying grass when he experiences stomach pain with cramping. He had episodes of diarrhea and vomiting. He is currently somewhat confused, his eyes are watery, pupils constricted, and skin is flushed. His spouse tells you that he has several different pills at home which he takes for different conditions. They include the following: verapamil, hydrochlorothiazide, lisinopril, cetirizine, warfarin, codeine syrup, allopurinol, vitamin D, St. John's wort, lansoprazole, and ibuprofen. He does drink about a 6-pack of beer per day. Vital signs include: T 37°C (98.6°F), BP 120/68, P 58, RR 14. Which of the following is likely to be effective in the treatment of this patient?

   a) Naloxone
   b) Physostigmine
   c) 2PAM and atropine
   d) Activated charcoal
   e) N-acetylcysteine

37. A 23-year-old woman with plaque psoriasis on the scalp asks the pharmacist to recommend a product. Which of the following is effective?

   a) Head & Shoulders Intensive Treatment®
   b) DHS Tar Shampoo® (coal tar extract)
   c) Nizoral A-D® (ketoconazole)
   d) Zinc pyrithione
   e) Loma Lux® Psoriasis

38. What is the most appropriate storage temperature for biologicals?

   a) 85° C
   b) 20° C
   c) 2° to 10° C
   d) 15° to 20° C
   e) 2° to 8° C

39. Which of the following statements regarding the use of controlled-release analgesic formulations to provide longer-lasting analgesia is true?

   a) The formulations have higher C_{max} than immediate-release formulations
   b) The formulations have shorter T_{max} than immediate-release formulations
   c) The formulations have higher bioavailability than immediate-release formulations
   d) The formulations have same bioavailability as immediate-release formulations
   e) The formulations are designed to break down in the stomach for optimal absorption

40. A 54-year-old male patient complains of a rash between the eyes, in the eyebrows, down the sides of the nose, and in the ear canals. He says it burns and itches. The pharmacist notes reddened areas of skin in a symmetric pattern with indistinct borders, and greasy yellowish scaling flakes. What condition is most likely?

    a) Psoriasis
    b) Contact dermatitis
    c) Miliaria
    d) Tinea of the face
    e) Seborrheic dermatitis

41. You receive a prescription for crude coal tar ointment 33 grams. You have vials that contain triamcinolone acetonide suspension 40 mg/mL. What equipment would be most useful in compounding this preparation?

    a) Ointment tile
    b) Stirring rod
    c) Porcelain mortar and pestle
    d) Glass mortar and pestle
    e) Wood mortar and pestle

42. In an inpatient hospital pharmacy setting unit dose packaging refers to which of the following?

    a) Exact dose of the drug prescribed for the patient
    b) A specific route of administration for the drug
    c) The amount of the drug necessary for the patient's hospital course
    d) Half of the amount of the drug available in the pharmacy
    e) One dose of the drug to complete the entire patient regimen

43. The blood-brain barrier has which permeability characteristic?

    a) Impermeable to chloral hydrate
    b) Impermeable to dopamine receptor antagonists
    c) Semi-permeable barrier of the brain only
    d) Semi-permeable barrier of the spine only
    e) More easily penetrated by lipophilic molecules

44. It is essential that patients use a metered-dose inhaler properly as drug effectiveness may be reduced considerably by poor technique. The recommended techniques for using a metered-dose inhaler to achieve maximum benefit include which of the following?

    a) Exhale. Place inhaler in mouth. Begin inhaling slowly. Activate inhaler while continuing to inhale then hold breath for 10 seconds and exhale
    b) If a spacer device is used, breathe normally into spacer while activating inhaler
    c) Exhale. Place inhaler in mouth. Activate inhaler, then inhale and hold breath for a few seconds
    d) Exhale. Hold inhaler 4 inches from mouth and inhale as inhaler is activated. Repeat 2 to 3 times to insure sufficient inhalation of drug
    e) Rinse mouth with water and swallow after use of a steroidal inhaler

45. After which phase of the new drug development process is a New Drug Application (NDA) submitted to the FDA?

    a) Phase I
    b) Phase II
    c) Phase III
    d) Phase IV
    e) Preclinical testing phase

46. A 20-year-old female presents to her gynecologist with a greenish vaginal discharge with a strong odor and vaginal itching. She also mentioned that the last time she and her boyfriend had intercourse, it was very painful, and she bled afterward. Which of the following is this patient most likely experiencing?

    a) Trichomoniasis
    b) Gonorrhea
    c) Human Papilloma Virus
    d) Herpes Simplex Virus
    e) Syphilis

47. Which of these is a contraindication for Nicorette Gum®?

    a) Renal dysfunction
    b) Vivid dreams
    c) Hepatic dysfunction
    d) Skin eczema
    e) Stomach ulcers

48. A 45-year-old woman presents to the clinic with a complaint of a runny nose, coughing, and chest congestion. She made a New Year's resolution to lose weight and is looking to you for advice. The patient has a past medical history of hypertension (6 months), arthritis in the knees (2 years), and asthma (5 years). The patient is 5' 7", 165 lbs, and has a waist circumference of 36 inches. The patient states she eats a light breakfast and lunch. She eats skinless chicken and a salad for dinner. She has been on this diet for 2 weeks. She does not like to exercise but walks around the block twice a week. Which of the following is most appropriate to treat her weight concerns?

    a) Healthy eating habits
    b) Phentermine 37.5 mg daily
    c) Begin jogging 30-45 minutes at least 5 days/week
    d) Sibutramine 10 mg daily
    e) Orlistat 60 mg twice daily

49. A patient ingested a month's supply of amitriptyline 50 mg tablets in a suicide attempt. Her roommate found her approximately 2 hours after the ingestion and calls 911. When the patient arrives in the emergency room, the pharmacist is involved in the discussion of treatment options. Which of the following is most appropriate to treat this patient?

    a) Activated charcoal
    b) Syrup of ipecac
    c) Gastric lavage
    d) Hemodialysis
    e) Hydrating excessively

50. Compared to the typical antipsychotic agents, the newer atypical antipsychotic drugs are less likely to cause which of the following side effects?

    a) Orthostatic hypotension
    b) Sedation
    c) Akathisia
    d) Weight gain
    e) Agranulocytosis

Practice Test 2: 50 questions, Time: 60 minutes

1. Which of the following is true?

   a) Creams have a higher percentage of oil than lotions
   b) Lotions have a higher percentage of oil than ointments
   c) Lotions are water in oil preparations
   d) Ointments wash off the skin easily
   e) Creams provide a stronger skin barrier than ointments

2. An investigational drug in early development has a high therapeutic index. What does this mean?

   a) The drug is eliminated by the kidney
   b) The drug is unlikely to have any significant adverse effects
   c) The drug has minimal entry to the brain
   d) The drug has plasma concentrations monitored
   e) The drug has minimal interactions with other drugs

3. What clinical trial is designed to show that a treatment is no less effective than an existing treatment?

   a) Noninferiority
   b) Superiority
   c) Equivalence
   d) Cohort
   e) Randomized

4. A patient comes to the pharmacy to refill prescriptions; she brings a grocery bag full of prescription medications, dietary supplements, and over-the-counter medications. She pulls 2 medications out of the bag and tells you that she received them from a relative in Spain. She would like to receive a similar medication if it is available in the United States. What reference would you consult for information about the imported medications?

   a) Remington
   b) Martindale
   c) USP
   d) Facts & Comparisons®
   e) Micromedex®

5. Which of the following is an appropriate statistic to describe the most common value in data distribution?

   a) Mean
   b) Median
   c) Mode
   d) Standard Deviation
   e) Central Tendency

6. What statement is true regarding the primary objective of different clinical studies in drug development?

   a) Phase 4 study is performed for the determination of an appropriate dosage regimen to be used in a large number of patients
   b) Phase 3 study is performed for the purpose of post-marketing surveillance
   c) Phase 3 study is performed for evaluation of response in a large number of patients with the target disease
   d) Phase 2 study is performed for determination of the pharmacokinetic profile in a small number of healthy volunteers
   e) Phase 1 study is performed for determination of toxicity in a large number of patients

7. A multicenter randomized controlled phase III trial is designed to investigate whether a new drug, daclizumid, is better than placebo in the treatment of early breast cancer (stages I, II). Phase II trial has shown significant benefit over placebo in 42 women (open-label trial) in overall response rates and recurrence rates. Women ages 34 to 65 will be enrolled if they have unilateral breast cancer, have not had any prior chemotherapy, have normal serum creatinine and liver function tests, as well as MUGA tests. Patients who are HER2/neu positive, have other prior cancers, or have any comorbidity will be excluded. Following treatment, ER/PR + cancer patients will be offered tamoxifen therapy for 5 years. Interim analysis was performed in 2 years after opening of the study. What is the major limitation of this study?

   a) Interim analysis is performed too early
   b) Interim analysis needs to be completed before the first year
   c) Tamoxifen administration may skew results
   d) Exclusion of HER2/neu patients from study
   e) Study is unethical

8. A pharmacist receives a new prescription for an isotonic eye solution. He would like to consult a reference about isotonicity before compounding the prescription; what reference should he consult?

   a) Remington
   b) Martindale
   c) USP
   d) Facts & Comparisons®
   e) Micromedex®

9. A patient wants to attend a party tonight and drink alcohol. However, he will have to drive home alone. He wishes to purchase a product he saw advertised as minimizing alcohol absorption to allow him to drive safely and also to prevent hangover. What advice should he be given?

   a) He should ingest syrup of ipecac after drinking. The emesis will reduce the load of alcohol reaching his bloodstream
   b) No nonprescription product can minimize or prevent hangover
   c) He should simply stop drinking about 30 minutes before he needs to drive home
   d) A nonprescription product containing herbal ingredients
   e) Activated charcoal will reduce absorption of alcohol

10. Which of the terms is appropriate for measuring the variability of a data set?

    a) Mean
    b) Median
    c) Mode
    d) Standard Deviation
    e) Range

11. A patient's bone mineral density (BMD) test revealed a T score of -2.7. Based on this result, the patient was diagnosed with osteoporosis. The World Health Organization (WHO) criteria for osteoporosis compare an individual's BMD to that of which of the following?

    a) Age and gender-matched peers
    b) Postmenopausal women with previous fractures
    c) American woman at age 60
    d) Perimenopausal women with risk factors
    e) Young adult Caucasian women

12. During the counseling session with a patient, he is encouraged to make lifestyle recommendations to reduce the likelihood of future gouty attacks. Which of the following dietary recommendations must be reviewed with this patient?

    a) Add more protein in the form of seafood
    b) Reduce purine-rich foods
    c) Decrease sodium intake
    d) Increase fructose intake
    e) Reduce fruit intake

13. What is the therapeutic target range for hemoglobin in patients receiving erythropoiesis-stimulating agent?

    a) 10 to 11 g/dL
    b) 10 to 13 g/dL
    c) 11 to 12 g/dL
    d) 12 to 13 g/dL
    e) 9 to 12 g/dL

14. Which of the following is an appropriate therapeutic target for erythropoietic therapy?

    a) Improved quality of life
    b) Improved cognitive function
    c) Increase in hemoglobin concentration from baseline
    d) Reduction in hemoglobin concentration from baseline
    e) Increased platelet count

15. A patient receiving warfarin 5 mg Mon/Wed/Fri and 3 mg all other days presents with an INR result of 3.7. His readings usually fall between 2.4 and 2.7. The patient was diagnosed with atrial fibrillation 6 months ago. When should the patient return for the next INR?

    a) 2 weeks
    b) 1 week
    c) 5 days
    d) 3 months
    e) 6 months

16. What laboratory test should be monitored in a patient taking allopurinol?

    a) Serum amylase
    b) Serum potassium
    c) Serum uric acid
    d) Blood glucose
    e) Serum Sodium

17. A patient comes for counseling and to initiate warfarin therapy. The patient is post-myocardial infarction with high risk for left ventricular thromboembolism requiring oral vitamin K antagonism. What is the most appropriate INR therapeutic range for this patient's therapy?

    a) 1.0 – 2.0
    b) 2.0 – 3.0
    c) 1.5 – 4.0
    d) 2.5 – 3.0
    e) 2.5 – 4.5

18. Which of the following antibacterial agents is judged to be "probably safe" and can be recommended for administration to a pregnant patient?

    a) Azithromycin
    b) Metronidazole
    c) Tetracycline
    d) Doxycycline
    e) Erythromycin estolate

19. What would be the desirable gastric pH that should be achieved with antacid administration?

    a) 4.5
    b) 3.5
    c) 2.5
    d) 6.5
    e) 5.5

2023-2024 NAPLEX® Practice Questions | RxPharmacist, LLC © 2023

20. Antimicrobial resistance is usually associated with which of the following factors?

    a) Increased use of broad-spectrum antibiotics
    b) Restriction of use imposed by formulary
    c) Decreased treatment failure
    d) Decreased use of antibiotics
    e) Increased costs of antibiotics

21. What lipid class combination/risk factor(s) most closely identifies the need to institute pharmacotherapy?

    a) An LDL cholesterol of >110; no history of coronary heart disease (CHD)
    b) An HDL cholesterol of >60; cigarette smoking
    c) An HDL of <40; age (men >45 yrs, women >55 yrs)
    d) VLDL of <100; diabetes
    e) A total cholesterol of <200; hypertension (BP >140/90)

22. The patient presents with a 36-hour history of excruciating pain in his right great toe. The patient admits to nonadherence to medications because he "just forgets to refill them". The patient received prescriptions for Zyloprim® and Naprosyn EC® the last time he had a similar episode, but he claims the medications did not seem to work. What is the most likely explanation?

    a) Naprosyn EC® is not indicated for treatment of an acute gouty attack
    b) There is a drug-drug interaction between Zyloprim® and another medication this patient is taking which results in decreased efficacy of Zyloprim®
    c) The patient has a history of nonadherence, so it is unlikely that he administered them correctly
    d) Uricosurics such as Zyloprim® are not effective in an acute gouty attack
    e) Nonsteroidal anti-inflammatory drugs are not effective more than 24 hours after the start of an acute gouty attack

23. A 46-year-old male receives a prescription for fluoxetine 10 mg daily for his first episode of generalized anxiety disorder. He is reluctant to take medications but agrees to adhere to therapy if it will make him feel better. 3 months later, he returns and is in remission. How soon can he stop this medication?

    a) Discontinue the medication today
    b) Treatment is usually lifelong
    c) Discontinue the medication in 2 years
    d) Discontinue the medication in 1 year
    e) Discontinue the medication in 3 months

24. A new patient presents to the pharmacist-run clinic for counseling and to initiate warfarin therapy. The patient recently underwent surgery for placement of a bileaflet mechanical valve in the mitral position. What is the most appropriate INR therapeutic range for this patient's therapy?

    a) 3.0 – 4.0
    b) 2.0 – 3.0
    c) 2.5 – 3.5
    d) 1.5 – 2.5
    e) 1.0 – 2.0

25. A 54-year-old male presents for non-productive cough, headache, runny nose, and chest pain. He was previously seen 2 weeks ago with the same symptoms. Physical exam at that time demonstrated coarse breath sounds. Chest x-ray demonstrated left lower lobe consolidation. CT scan showed ground-glass pattern with centrilobular nodules. EKG was unremarkable. His final diagnosis upon discharge was pneumonia due to *Mycoplasma pneumonia,* for which he was given a prescription for erythromycin 250 mg 4 times/day for 2 weeks. Which of the following is the most likely explanation for persistence of patient symptoms?

   a) Inadequate duration of treatment
   b) Wrong drug
   c) Antibiotic resistance
   d) Wrong diagnosis
   e) Non-compliance

26. A patient comes with c/o congestion, thick yellow nasal discharge, pain in sinus areas, and sore throat. She had a cold about 2 weeks ago, with symptoms persisting. She is allergic to penicillin and she is currently taking ketoconazole. She is diagnosed with acute sinusitis. Which antibiotic of the following would be the best treatment option for this patient?

   a) Amoxicillin
   b) Ciprofloxacin
   c) Bactrim
   d) Telithromycin
   e) Gentamicin

27.

PATIENT PROFILE	
Patient Name: Bojack Horseman	Address: 67 Famous Way, Hollywoo, CA
Age: 46 Sex: M Race: W	Height: 5' 6" Weight: 70 kg
Allergies: NKDA	FH: none
ADMITTING DIAGNOSIS: Seizure, admitted to emergency department overdosed with phenytoin	**PAST MEDICAL HISTORY:** T2DM, atrial fibrillation, peptic ulcer, gout
CURRENT MEDICATION LIST: Phenytoin 300 mg qHS Quinidine 300 mg four times daily (increased 1 week ago) Cimetidine 200 mg qHS (increased 1 week ago) Insulin NPH/Reg 20U/20U qAM and 10U/15U qPM Probenecid 500 mg bid	**PE:** VS: 120/86, 92 (regular), 39° C, 18 HEENT: Nystagmus on lateral gaze COR: WNL Chest: WNL ABD: WNL Neuro: Alert and oriented x 3, slight gait ataxia All WNL except the 2 levels of phenytoin (45 and 34 mcg/L).

What would be an appropriate target HbA1C level in patients with diabetes, per ADA guidelines?

   a) 7.5%
   b) 6%
   c) 6.5%
   d) 7%
   e) 8%

28. What drug has been shown to have a **positive effect** on mortality in patients with heart failure?

    a) Furosemide
    b) Hydrochlorothiazide
    c) Diltiazem
    d) Digoxin
    e) Captopril

29. A 27-year-old female recently received prescriptions for lorazepam and paroxetine for treatment of generalized anxiety disorder. When counseling the patient, it is important to tell her that the full therapeutic effects of lorazepam will occur within how many days?

    a) 60 days
    b) 43 days
    c) 28 days
    d) 7 days
    e) 3 days

30. Which anti-Parkinson's medications could be used for once-daily dosing?

    a) Rasagiline
    b) Pramipexole
    c) Amantadine
    d) Carbidopa/levodopa
    e) Ropinirole

31. Before counseling a pregnant woman about the use of a medication that she has been prescribed, you should first check which of the following?

    a) The metabolism induced by CYP2E1 because she enjoys alcoholic drinks
    b) The metabolism induced by CYP1A2 because she is a smoker
    c) Whether it passes into breast milk
    d) Its teratogenic classification
    e) How the drug works

32. A patient comes in and asks you what his blood pressure goal should be. His past medical history includes hypertension, type II diabetes, angina, GERD, and hypercholesterolemia. What should you respond to this patient?

    a) <130/$\leq$80 mm Hg
    b) <130/$\leq$90 mm Hg
    c) <120/$\leq$80 mm Hg
    d) <150/$\leq$90 mm Hg
    e) <120/$\leq$90 mm Hg

33. Which of the following drugs cannot be prescribed by a general practitioner in any state?

    a) Schedule III
    b) Schedule I
    c) Schedule II
    d) Schedule IV
    e) Schedule V

34. A 55-year-old male patient with a past medical history of Type II diabetes, hyperlipidemia, and hypertension comes into your pharmacy. His past blood pressure reading is 142/93 mmHg. According to ACC/AHA guidelines, what is the recommended blood pressure goal for this patient based on the information given?

    a) <150/90 mmHg
    b) <120/80 mmHg
    c) <130/80 mmHg
    d) <135/90 mmHg
    e) <130/90 mmHg

35. Sara is a 54-year-old female patient with a past medical history of rheumatoid arthritis x 10 years, hypertension, and dyslipidemia. She currently takes methotrexate 5 mg and folic acid 1 mg. During a recent visit with the rheumatologist, Sara reported a gradual increase in morning stiffness, joint pain, and swelling over the last 2 months. The rheumatologist would like to initiate combination therapy to help control her symptoms and prevent disease progression. Her current disease activity level is considered moderate. Which of the following is the most appropriate option to add to her current regimen?

    a) Rituximab
    b) Abatacept + etanercept
    c) Sulfasalazine
    d) Sulfasalazine + leflunomide
    e) Infliximab

36. A patient comes for counseling and to initiate warfarin therapy. The patient recently experienced a DVT secondary to oral contraceptive therapy. What is the most appropriate INR therapeutic range for this patient's therapy?

    a) 2.0 – 3.0
    b) 2.5 – 3.5
    c) 3.0 – 3.5
    d) 2.5 – 3.0
    e) 1.5 – 2.5

37. A father wishes to purchase NoDoz Maximum Strength® (caffeine) for his 10-year-old daughter, who has perennial allergic rhinitis. The physician believes she has chronic fatigue due to a sleep disorder and requested further evaluation before prescribing any type of medication. The father only wants to use NoDoz® until she can be seen by a sleep laboratory. What should the pharmacist advise him to do?

    a) Recommend against its use, as caffeine is contraindicated with allergic rhinitis
    b) Recommend against its use, as it is only for patients aged 12 and above
    c) Ask the child to drink large quantities of caffeine-containing beverages
    d) Use Vivarin® (caffeine) instead, as it is labeled for her condition
    e) Use NoDoz®, but purchase the regular strength product instead

38. Which of the following defines pharmacokinetics?

    a) What the kidney does to the drug
    b) What the drug does to the body
    c) What the body does to the drug
    d) What the liver does to the drug
    e) What the drug does to the microorganism

39. What is the definition of a Type II error?

    a) The clinical trial was not large enough to detect a meaningful difference between treatment groups
    b) The null hypothesis is true, but is rejected in error
    c) The null hypothesis is false, but it is rejected in error
    d) The null hypothesis is false, but is accepted in error
    e) The null hypothesis is true, but it is accepted in error

40. In biostatistics, what is meant by the median of a group of values?

    a) The relative risk reduction
    b) The value in the middle of the list
    c) The average
    d) The variance squared
    e) The value that occurs most frequently

41. Marital status (married, single, divorced) can be described as what type of data?

    a) Ordinal
    b) Nominal
    c) Continuous
    d) Random
    e) Interval

42. Blood pressure, hemoglobin A1C and LDL cholesterol can each be described as what type of data?

    a) Ordinal
    b) Nominal
    c) Continuous
    d) Random
    e) Discrete

43. Which of the following statements regarding specificity are true? (Select **ALL** that apply.)

    a) The percentage of time a test is negative when disease is not present
    b) The percentage of time a test is positive when disease is not present
    c) The percentage of time a test is negative when disease is present
    d) The percentage of time a test is positive when disease is present
    e) It is equal to 1 – type I error

44. A patient has tested positive for the HLA-B*5701 allele. Which of the following statements is correct?

    a) The patient can receive Epzicom®
    b) The patient cannot be dispensed abacavir
    c) The patient can receive Trizivir®
    d) The patient would be expected to launch an aggressive immune response against HIV
    e) The patient is not at risk for hypersensitivity reactions with any of the HIV medications

45. Jamie developed hives and got a swollen face from using sulfamethoxazole. Which of the following drugs should be avoided? (Select **ALL** that apply.)

    a) Sulfasalazine
    b) Sulfisoxazole
    c) Zonisamide
    d) Celecoxib
    e) Morphine sulfate

46. Jason has a peanut allergy. His aunt will need to be instructed about an anaphylactic reaction. Which of the following instructions are true? (Select **ALL** that apply.)

    a) If Jason has an anaphylactic reaction, he will need to receive epinephrine
    b) If Jason has an anaphylactic reaction, he should wait 1 hour before going to the ED
    c) If he is just wheezing slightly, you can give him some loratadine
    d) Swollen airways can be quickly fatal
    e) Jason should receive the EpiPen if he has difficulty breathing

47. What is the name of the FDA's adverse event reporting system program?

    a) ISMP
    b) MedCoAlert
    c) MedWatch
    d) MedAware
    e) MedAction

48. What is the name of the accreditation body for more than 21,000 health care organizations and programs in the U.S. including hospitals, health care networks, long term care facilities, home care organizations, office-based surgery centers and independent laboratories?

    a) Institute of Medicine
    b) The Joint Commission
    c) Institute for Safe Medication Practices
    d) National Institutes of Health
    e) Food and Drug Administration

49. Dr. Davis wrote this prescription: *1.0 teaspoonful of oral suspension. UAD*

    The pharmacist wanted to verify the dose, but neither the child's age nor weight was provided. What are possible sources of medication errors found in this prescription? (Select **ALL** that apply.)

    a) Using "as directed" for patient instructions
    b) Not providing the route of administration
    c) Using a "teaspoonful" to indicate the dose
    d) Not providing the patient's weight to verify the dose, or the indication
    e) Use of a trailing zero

50. Which of the following practices should be followed to ensure sterility in a laminar flow hood? (Select **ALL** that apply.)

    a) Do not interrupt the flow of air by placing items in the hood all lined up across the front of the hood; items should be placed in a straight line behind one another
    b) Use of a mask that covers the nose and mouth is required for regular hoods, but not for laminar flow hoods
    c) Preparation should be at least six inches into the hood
    d) Items such as pens and calculators should remain outside the hood
    e) Laminar flow hoods should be cleaned at least at the start of each shift, but more frequently depending on use

Practice Test 3: 50 questions, Time: 60 minutes

1. A hospital pharmacist dispensed the wrong vaccine for an infant, who then had to be re-inoculated. The same pharmacist pulled the wrong type of insulin from the refrigerator to send to the floor. Which of the following represents the most reasonable method to help the pharmacist avoid this type of error in the future?

   a) Indications for use on the prescription
   b) Placing the medications in high-risk bins, with notations on the front of the bins regarding name mix-ups and other relevant alerts
   c) Having the pharmaceutical companies present more information on their drugs at grand rounds
   d) The use of standardized protocols
   e) Patient discharge education

2. A pharmacist works in a small city hospital that has a medical doctor who is an orthopedist. He does several hip replacements and several knee replacements at this hospital per month. The pharmacist hopes to implement patient-controlled analgesic (PCA) devices for the orthopedic patients. However, the medical staff at the hospital is overburdened and the head of the nursing team is not interested in changing to a new system. What is the primary reason why PCA devices may not be appropriate in this setting?

   a) PCAs cannot be used in small hospitals
   b) PCAs require an educated, coordinated health care team
   c) PCAs are not used in orthopedic surgeries due to higher-than-normal DVT risk
   d) PCAs are only used in outpatient clinics
   e) The use of a PCA would increase costs too much for a small hospital to manage

3. Which of the following represents a common cause of hospital-acquired (nosocomial) infections?

   a) UTIs, due to the use of broad-spectrum antibiotics
   b) UTIs, due to enlarged prostates
   c) UTIs, due to the use of parenteral nutrition and "PICC" lines
   d) UTIs, due to uterine prolapse
   e) UTIs, due to indwelling catheters

4. One of the largest causes of needlestick infections is due to the use of glucose meters in healthcare settings that are used to test many patients. Another cause of needlestick infections is due to vials of medicine, such as insulin, that are used in more than one patient. Which of the following statements are correct? (Select **ALL** that apply.)

   a) If a glucose meter travels from room-to-room, the nursing staff must replace the lancet tip prior to testing each patient
   b) If the same injection vial will be used for multiple patients, it is imperative never to re-insert a needle that has already been used on a patient into the vial
   c) It is preferable to avoid the use of multi-use vials in different patients; it is preferable to label the multi-use vial with one patient's name only
   d) The ISMP recommends using insulin pens to avoid contamination from using insulin in multiple patients
   e) Glucose meters should not be used in the hospital; blood sugar can be tested with the daily labs

5. Which of the following are High-Alert drugs per ISMP?

    a) Hypertonic saline and fosphenytoin
    b) Vancomycin and potassium chloride injection
    c) Potassium chloride injection and hypertonic saline
    d) Vancomycin and gentamicin
    e) Insulin and 0.45% sodium chloride

6. What is the purpose of the FDA REMS program?

    a) To ensure that the benefits of dangerous drugs outweigh the risks
    b) To help control drug costs
    c) To get unsafe OTC drugs off the market
    d) To educate patients about herbals and other natural products
    e) To employ more government workers

7. What is the primary purpose of Phase III studies?

    a) To determine safety, efficacy, and dose-response relationships in the population
    b) To put the drug manufacturing system in place and ready for FDA approval
    c) To determine the profit potential of the drug
    d) To evaluate safety after the drug has been approved and released for sale
    e) To rate the drug against a panel of known drug inducers and inhibitors

8. Which of the following designations describes equivalence between two products?

    a) BC
    b) BX
    c) AX
    d) AB
    e) ABC

9. What is the primary purpose of Phase II studies?

    a) To find the treatment dose
    b) To evaluate side effects
    c) To determine efficacy
    d) To determine the drug's profit potential
    e) To review the marketing approach

10. Which of the following agents can be used for anxiety? (Select **ALL** that apply.)

    a) Garlic
    b) Chamomile tea
    c) Lemon balm
    d) Ginseng
    e) Valerian root

11. A patient with recently diagnosed active tuberculosis was prescribed isoniazid, rifampin, pyrazinamide and ethambutol. Which vitamin is recommended?

    a) Vitamin B1
    b) Vitamin B12
    c) Vitamin B2
    d) Vitamin B3
    e) Vitamin B6

12. Select the correct vitamin name and abbreviation match. (Select **ALL** that apply.)

    a) Vitamin B6 – Pyridoxine
    b) Vitamin B1 – Riboflavin
    c) Vitamin B12 – Cobalamin
    d) Vitamin B3 – Thiamine
    e) Vitamin A – Retinol

13. It is a priority to increase folic acid intake among women of child-bearing age. Why is this important?

    a) To reduce the risk of low bone density in young women
    b) To reduce the risk of serious birth defects in children born to women with low folic acid intake
    c) To reduce the risk of ovarian cancer in young women
    d) To reduce the risk of endometrial cancer in young women
    e) To make money for the manufacturer of folic acid

14. Mary developed a UTI and received a 3-day course of an antibiotic. She tells the pharmacist that she used to get diarrhea when she took antibiotics but does not expect this to happen now because she uses a probiotic. What should you say?

    a) Do not use the probiotic during the 3 days you are using antibiotic; wait until the therapy is complete
    b) If you take the antibiotic in the morning and at night, take the probiotic in the middle of the day
    c) It would be best to replace the probiotic with lycopene
    d) It would be best to replace the probiotic with saw palmetto
    e) It would be best to replace the probiotic with comfrey

15. A patient brings in a prescription for orlistat. Which of the following vitamins should the pharmacist recommend the patient also take? (Select **ALL** that apply.)

    a) Vitamin A
    b) Vitamin B6
    c) Vitamin D
    d) Vitamin E
    e) Vitamin K

16. Which natural products can be useful for migraine headache prophylaxis? (Select **ALL** that apply.)

    a) Feverfew
    b) Saw palmetto
    c) Ginger
    d) Magnesium
    e) Riboflavin

17. Which calcium supplement is absorbed better in an acidic environment and is taken with meals?

    a) Calcium citrate
    b) Citracal®
    c) Os-Cal®
    d) Citrucel®
    e) None of these should be taken with food

18. Which of the following agents is required for calcium absorption?

    a) Folic acid
    b) Vitamin C
    c) Vitamin D
    d) Vitamin E
    e) Vitamin K

19. Which agent is a precursor to androgens (male sex hormones)?

    a) GABA
    b) Lysine
    c) Chondroitin
    d) SAMe
    e) DHEA

20. Which of the following statements are true regarding vitamin D supplements?

    a) 50,000 units of vitamin D (the large green capsules), taken daily, is acceptable for most patients
    b) Vitamin D intake is acceptable in most patients in the United States
    c) Vitamin D2 should not be recommended
    d) Vitamin D3 should not be recommended
    e) Cholecalciferol is vitamin D3 and is the preferred source

21. Which calcium supplement is absorbed well on either an empty stomach or with food?

    a) Tums®
    b) Citracal®
    c) Os-Cal®
    d) Rolaids®
    e) Caltrate®

22. Jamie recently became involved in a sexual relationship. She went to the clinic and was prescribed *Loestrin® Fe* 1/20. She believes in natural healing and takes a handful of supplements daily: a fish oil capsule, a B vitamin complex, a multivitamin, a vitamin E 400 IU capsule, St. John's wort, kava and a probiotic supplement. She uses melatonin when she has trouble sleeping. Despite strict adherence with her birth control pill regimen, Jamie became pregnant. What was the most likely cause of the pregnancy?

    a) Concurrent use of birth control pills and fish oils
    b) Concurrent use of birth control pills and St. John's wort
    c) Concurrent use of birth control pills and lactobacillus
    d) Concurrent use of birth control pills and melatonin
    e) Concurrent use of birth control pills and high-dose vitamin E

23. Mary uses *Imitrex®* for migraines 2-4 times each month. Recently she began to use *Sarafem®* 10 mg daily for premenstrual dysphoric disorder. In addition, she uses meperidine once or twice daily for headache relief. Which of the following symptoms is Mary is at risk for? (Select **ALL** that apply.)

    a) Tremor, agitation, confusion, hallucinations
    b) Tachycardia, sweating
    c) Diarrhea
    d) Muscle rigidity, shivering
    e) Acute bradycardia

24. Drug A is a substrate of 2C9 and a potent 3A4 inhibitor. Drug B is a substrate of 2D6 and 1A2 as well as a potent inhibitor of 2C19. Drug C is a substrate of 3A4 and a potent inhibitor of 2D6. If all three drugs were given together, what would the expected levels of each drug to do?

    a) Drug A levels would stay the same, Drug B levels increase, Drug C levels increase
    b) Drug A levels would increase, Drug B levels decrease, Drug C levels increase
    c) Drug A levels would decrease, Drug B levels decrease, Drug C levels increase
    d) Drug A levels would increase, Drug B levels stay the same, and Drug C levels decrease
    e) Drug A, B, and C levels would all increase

25. Mart uses ibuprofen for pain. Mart has hypertension. He takes two over-the-counter ibuprofen tablets twice daily on workdays. Lately, he has noticed his blood pressure is elevated more than usual. Which of the following would be safe options that would not elevate his blood pressure? (Select **ALL** that apply.)

    a) Advil® or Aleve®
    b) ThermaCare Activated Heat Wraps®
    c) Acetaminophen
    d) A topical menthol analgesic patch, such as Bengay®
    e) Aspirin

26. Which of the following statements concerning drug interactions are correct? (Select **ALL** that apply.)

    a) If a compound is a P-gp pump inhibitor, it can cause the levels of P-gp substrates to decrease if given concurrently
    b) If a compound is a P-gp pump inducer, it can cause the levels of P-gp substrates to decrease if given concurrently
    c) Inducers cause more metabolism of drugs that are substrates of the enzymes
    d) Inhibitors reduce or knock out the ability of the enzyme to work; this increases metabolism of the substrates
    e) Tacrolimus is a substrate of the P-gp efflux pump

27. A patient is at risk for atrial fibrillation; she has had this atrial fibrillation in the past. The medical team has asked the pharmacist to check for drugs on her profile which can increase her risk of arrhythmia. Which of the following medications should the pharmacist include?

    a) Xolair®
    b) Lamictal®
    c) Ziprasidone
    d) Proscar®
    e) Xalatan®

28. Sandra is about to get on the waiting list for a kidney transplant. She has a creatinine clearance of 16 mL/min and experiences frequent bouts of hyperkalemia. She cannot use any medicines that elevate potassium because in this patient even small increases in potassium trigger an arrhythmia. Which medications elevate potassium and would put Sandra at risk for arrhythmia? (Select **ALL** that apply.)

    a) Altoprev®
    b) Dyazide®
    c) Inspra®
    d) Aldactone®
    e) Yasmin®

29. Ann lives in Florida and occasionally eats grapefruit. Whichi of the following statements is true regarding grapefruit-drug interactions? (Select **ALL** that apply.)

    a) Do not use grapefruit with cyclosporine
    b) Do not use grapefruit with buspirone
    c) If a drug interacts with grapefruit, use a long gut separation period, such as taking the grapefruit two hours before or four hours after the interacting drug
    d) Do not use grapefruit with rivaroxaban
    e) Do not use grapefruit with valproate

30. A patient is using digoxin. Which of the following drugs will need to have its dose decreased if prescribed?

    a) Diazepam
    b) Phenytoin
    c) Cyclosporine
    d) Carbamazepine
    e) Cancidas®

31. A 76-year-old woman had been taking metoprolol extended-release 100 mg daily and warfarin 4 mg daily (both for atrial fibrillation) and amitriptyline 50 mg QHS (for migraine prophylaxis) for several years. Shortly after the death of her spouse, she experienced very sad mood swings. Initially she was prescribed citalopram 40 mg daily. When this was not very effective, the physician added on paroxetine 10 mg daily (as he did not wish to increase the citalopram dose). What is this patient at risk for due to the drug combinations?

    a) Increased bleeding risk but decreased risk of arrhythmia
    b) Increased risk of clotting but decreased risk of bleeding
    c) Increased risk of bleeding and increased risk of arrhythmia
    d) Increased risk of worsening depression
    e) Worsening depression and increased clotting risk

32. Which of the following statins has the lowest risk of drug interactions?

    a) Atorvastatin
    b) Pravastatin
    c) Lovastatin
    d) Simvastatin
    e) Fluvastatin

33. Sara has been using a monoamine oxidase inhibitor. Which of the following drugs can be dispensed to Sara and will not cause concern? (Select **ALL** that apply.)

    a) Prempro®
    b) Boniva®
    c) Zolmitriptan
    d) Xalatan®
    e) Sumatriptan

34. Jess worries that she will have a hip fracture. What agents increase the risk of Jess having a fall? (Select **ALL** that apply.)

    a) Flexeril®
    b) Remeron®
    c) Nuvigil®
    d) Bactrim®
    e) Restoril®

35. RM is a 48-year-old female patient who is hospitalized with chest pain. She uses many drugs, including Cozaar®, Coumadin®, Coreg®, Lasix® and Micro-K®. An INR is taken and is reported as a critical lab value. At this hospital, the critical value for warfarin is an INR ≥ 4. Which of the following best describes a critical value?

    a) A value that can be life-threatening if corrective action is not taken quickly
    b) A value that can cause the patient to suffer physical or psychological harm
    c) A value that has to be acted on within 6 hours
    d) A value that has to be acted on within 8 hours
    e) A value that has to be acted on within 2 hours

36. A patient has G6PD-deficiency. What will occur if the patient receives primaquine for malaria prophylaxis?

    a) The patient will be at higher risk of catching malaria
    b) The patient will be at higher risk of developing primaquine-induced neurotoxicity
    c) The patient will be at risk for serious internal bleeding
    d) The patient will have increased renal excretion of electrolytes
    e) The patient will develop leukopenia

37. A male is hospitalized with a pulmonary embolism. He is receiving unfractionated heparin for VTE treatment. Which of the following lab values would indicate heparin-induced thrombocytopenia?

    WBC: 13.5 (3.5-12)   HGB: 16.1(13.4-17.7)
    HCT: 48.2 (40-53)   MCV: 93 (80-97)
    PLT: 73 (150-420)   BUN: 22 (6-23 mg/dL)
    Creatinine: 1.9 (0.7-1.6 mg/dL)

    a) The hemoglobin
    b) The hematocrit
    c) The glucose
    d) The platelets
    e) The CBC

38. What lab values will be present in a patient with a metabolic acidosis?

    a) Low pH, low serum bicarbonate
    b) Low pH, high serum bicarbonate
    c) High pH, low serum bicarbonate
    d) High pH, high serum bicarbonate
    e) Low pH, low alkaline phosphatase

39. A patient presents with a butterfly-shaped rash on her face and achy joints. The patient's chronic medications include Klor-Con®, Lasix®, Toprol XL®, BiDil®, Atacand® and Inspra®. Which of the daily medication is most likely contributing to this presentation?

    a) Lasix®
    b) Toprol®
    c) BiDil®
    d) Atacand®
    e) Inspra®

40. Select the name of the lab test used to distinguish between a microcytic and a macrocytic anemia:

    a) RDW
    b) MCH
    c) MCV
    d) MCHC
    e) TIBC

41. An 82-year-old male with COPD, has difficulty breathing and finds little relief from daily Advair Diskus® and Spiriva®. Which condition is most likely in this patient?

    a) Respiratory acidosis
    b) Respiratory alkalosis
    c) Anion gap acidosis
    d) Lactic acidosis
    e) Diabetic ketoacidosis

42. Sam has a creatinine clearance of 38 mL/min. Which of the following statements are accurate concerning this degree of renal impairment? (Select **ALL** that apply.)

    a) This is classified as severe renal insufficiency
    b) This is defined as Stage 3 CKD
    c) The patient may need to have the erythropoietin level checked if anemic
    d) ACE inhibitors or Angiotensin Receptor Blockers should be initiated if there are no contraindications to use
    e) The blood pressure should be controlled to less than 110/70 mmHg with this degree of impairment

43. A patient who was receiving enalapril and spironolactone develops renal insufficiency. An ECG is obtained in the emergency department which demonstrates electrolyte changes consistent with hyperkalemia. What should be administered to this patient to reverse the effects of hyperkalemia on the heart?

    a) Albuterol
    b) Sodium bicarbonate
    c) Dextrose
    d) Calcium chloride
    e) Kayexalate

44. Tom has end stage renal disease and uses many medications, including Renagel®. Previously he was using PhosLo®. What is a possible reason that Tom needed to stop using PhosLo®?

    a) Cost; Renagel® is less expensive than PhosLo®
    b) Higher calcium levels
    c) Lower calcium levels
    d) Hyperphosphatemia
    e) Lower efficacy

45. Which of the following statements concerning bone metabolism abnormalities in chronic kidney disease (CKD) is correct?

    a) Initially, bone metabolism abnormalities are caused by a rise in calcium
    b) Hyperphosphatemia causes an increase in the release of parathyroid hormone
    c) A benefit of hyperphosphatemia is improved bone health
    d) To counteract the increase in phosphate levels, it is necessary to give injectable phosphate binders
    e) Treatment of secondary hyperparathyroidism is restricting dietary calcium

46. Sam has lupus-related renal disease. Her serum creatinine today is 2.7 g/dL and potassium is 6.2 mEq/L. The physician has prescribed sodium polystyrene sulfonate (SPS). Which of the following statements regarding sodium polystyrene sulfonate is true?

    a) The brand name is Gabitril®
    b) This drug is a cation exchange resin that binds potassium in the gut
    c) This drug may stabilize cardiac tissue to reduce arrhythmia risk
    d) The potassium should be lowered to 3.2 mEq/L
    e) SPS increases appetite

47. A patient who has a history of hypothyroidism has become pregnant. You want to provide their prescriber with information about hypothyroidism treatment during pregnancy. Which of the following statements are true? (Select **ALL** that apply.)

    a) Propylthiouracil is Pregnancy Category D and is used during the first trimester
    b) Methimazole is Pregnancy Category D and is used during the first trimester
    c) Methimazole is Pregnancy Category D and is used after the first trimester
    d) Methimazole has a higher risk of hepatotoxicity than propylthiouracil
    e) Both agents can cause serious liver damage

48. Which of the following medication(s) can increase the level of theophylline?

    a) Smoking
    b) Lithium
    c) Erythromycin
    d) Estrogen-containing contraceptive
    e) Verapamil

49. A pharmacist is counseling a 45-year-old man with new prescription for Spiriva Handihaler®. Which of the following information is/are the correct counseling points? (Select **ALL** that apply.)

    a) Do not swallow the capsule
    b) Advise patient to clean the inhaler device weekly
    c) Do not rinse the inhaler with water
    d) After you close your lips around the mouthpiece, breathe in deeply and fully. Hold your breath for a few second
    e) You must inhale twice for each capsule

50. A patient with severe COPD experiences exacerbation. She is currently on Arcapta Neohaler® and azithromycin. The doctor decides to start her on Daliresp®. Which of the following medication(s) will be contraindicated to this patient? (Select **ALL** that apply.)

    a) Lovastatin
    b) St. John's Wort
    c) Rifampin
    d) Amiodarone
    e) Phenytoin

Practice Test 4: 50 questions, Time: 60 minutes

1. Your patient is taking digoxin, with a current level is 0.25 ng/mL. You know that the normal levels of digoxin are 0.5 to 0.8 ng/mL. You take another digoxin level 2 hours after giving the medication to the patient and notice that the levels are now 1.5 ng/mL. What should you do?

    a) This is a toxic level, reduce the patient's digoxin dose
    b) Check the patient's level in 2 hours
    c) Check the patient's level in 4 hours
    d) Increase the dose, digoxin displays a 2-hour compartment model
    e) Check the patient's level in 6 hours

2. SJ is a patient coming into your clinical to be evaluated for statin therapy. He is 60 years old and has an LDL-C level of 170 mg/dL. His only comorbid condition is peripheral artery disease. What statin therapy should you start SJ on?

    a) Simvastatin 10 mg
    b) Atorvastatin 20 mg
    c) Atorvastatin 40 mg
    d) None, his LDL-C levels are not greater than 190 mg/dL
    e) Lovastatin 10 mg

3. SM is a 14-year-old male who has attention deficit hyperactivity disorder (ADHD). He also has a history of substance abuse. What drug should be recommended for him?

    a) Guanfacine
    b) Clonidine
    c) Atomoxetine
    d) Lovastatin
    e) Methylphenidate

4. Guy Simpton is a 74-year-old male with atherosclerotic cardiovascular disease (ASCVD) and hyperlipidemia. He is on atorvastatin 40 mg once daily. Labs were drawn and his LDL-C was 285 mg/dL. One year later, he comes back into clinic after intensive diet and exercise regimens. His LDL-C comes back at 205 mg/dL. His provider asks you what he should do. What do you recommend?

    a) Increase to atorvastatin 80 mg once daily
    b) Switch to rosuvastatin 40 mg once daily
    c) Switch to rosuvastatin 20 mg once daily
    d) Lower his dosage as he is 74 years old and should be on a moderate-intensity statin
    e) Decrease to atorvastatin 20 mg once daily

5. Francisca comes into your clinic with a T score of -2.5 with recent vertebral fracture. She is currently only taking calcium and vitamin D supplements. She reports debilitating pain and is taking the maximum 4,000 mg acetaminophen daily dose for pain. What do you recommend for Francisca's osteoporosis management?

   a) Calcitonin
   b) Raloxifene
   c) Alendronate
   d) Zoledronic acid
   e) Calcitriol

6. CJ is an African-American male with bacterium for 14 days and is being treated for a urinary tract infection (UTI). He has black urine and is symptomatic. What does CJ have?

   a) Sickle cell crisis
   b) Hepatic necrosis
   c) Hemorrhagic cystitis
   d) Benign prostatic hyperplasia
   e) Sickle cell disease

7. CJ is a 37-year-old female who comes into your clinic with a past medical history of breast cancer. She recently got a CT scan with IV radiographic contrast media. Her current medications are metformin 1000 mg once daily. Two days after her CT scan, she comes back in and her SCr is 4.6 mg/dL. What caused her SCr level to increase?

   a) Acute tubular necrosis due to her metformin
   b) Acute tubular necrosis due to her CT contrast dye
   c) Acute tubular necrosis due to the lactic acidosis
   d) Acute tubular necrosis due to her breast cancer
   e) Acute tubular necrosis due to her age

8. What statistical test would you use in a cohort study?

   a) Relative risk
   b) Odds ratio
   c) Correlation
   d) Regression
   e) Analysis

9. What statistical test would you use in a case-control study?

   a) Relative risk
   b) Odds ratio
   c) Correlation
   d) Regression
   e) Analysis

10. The CDC releases official guidelines related to vaccines. Where are these located?

   a) FDA
   b) Pink Sheet
   c) Weekly publication
   d) MMWR
   e) CMS

11. CJ is a 46-year-old female who has a history of a transient ischemic attack (TIA), intracranial hemorrhage, and is notated to have an ST-elevation on her leads. She is taking omeprazole and lives in a rural area so is being medically managed instead of receiving a percutaneous coronary intervention (PCI). Her provider knows that she needs antiplatelet therapy. What do you recommend?

   a) Clopidogrel
   b) Prasugrel
   c) Ticagrelor
   d) Ticlopidine
   e) Atorvastatin

12. Trejon is a 64-year-old man who has a foley catheter in place and was treated for a urinary tract infection (UTI). His past medical history includes type 2 diabetes. The nurse staff suspected he had an infection and took a culture of his foley catheter. His culture came back positive for *E. coli,* so he was diagnosed with bacteriuria and started on board-spectrum antibiotics. A urinalysis came back positive for *C. albicans*. Trejon currently does not state he has any symptoms. What do you recommend treating for his *C. albicans*?

   a) Fluconazole
   b) Vancomycin
   c) Erythromycin
   d) No treatment is needed for now
   e) Voriconazole

13. FooFoo is a 59-year-old male patient who comes into your clinic to be pharmacologically cardioverted after 7 days of consistent atrial fibrillation symptoms. He has a past medical history of atrial fibrillation and a heart failure exacerbation with reduced left ventricular ejection fraction of 25%. What do you recommend to cardiovert FooFoo?

   a) Dofetilide
   b) Propafenone
   c) Diltiazem
   d) Adenosine
   e) Ticagrelor

14. Which of the following adverse drug reaction should be reported to the prescriber about montelukast?

    a) Increased serum creatinine
    b) Increased risk of respiratory tract infection
    c) Decreased serum albumin
    d) Dizziness
    e) Palpitation

15. Which of the following medications should the pharmacist counsel to "not swallow the capsule"? (Select **ALL** that apply.)

    a) Tudorza Pressair®
    b) Breo Ellipta®
    c) Utibron Neohaler®
    d) Spiriva Handihaler®
    e) Arcapta Neohaler®

16. AB (34-year-old female) presents to the clinic. She is concerned that she may have HIV because her husband had a confirmed HIV positive result last week. Which of the following should a pharmacist do? (Select **ALL** that apply.)

    a) Confirm HIV negative status using HIV antibody test
    b) Screen AB for hepatitis B and sexually transmitted infections
    c) Tell the patient to get an OTC HIV test and come back later to determine if she should be on antiretroviral therapy
    d) Immediately recommend Biktarvy® to treat HIV
    e) When the patient has negative HIV result, start her on Truvada® once daily and counsel on safe sex reduction practices

17. JM is a 32-years old woman with a history of hypertension (3 years) and type 2 diabetes and has been compliant with her regimen. Two weeks ago, she came to the clinic with a chief complaint of vaginal pain. At that time, she also shared that one of her sexual partners was HIV positive, so she got blood drawn for a comprehensive test of HIV, sexually transmitted infections, pregnancy, and renal function test. Today, she presents to the clinic to follow up on an HIV-positive result. Which of the following regimens should you recommend to her?

Allergies: sulfa – hives

PMH:
DM II - 2 years
HTN - 3 years

Medications:
Zestril® 20 mg PO daily
Metformin 1000 mg ER PO daily
Ibuprofen 200 mg PO every 6 hours as needed for headache
MVI

Labs:
Na (mEq/L) = 140 (135 – 145)
K (mEq/L) = 3.8 (3.5 – 5)
Cl (mEq/L) = 100 (95 – 103)
HCO_3 (mEq/L) = 27 (24 – 30)
BUN (mg/dL) = 20 (7 – 20)
SCr (mg/dL) = 1.11, eGFR 67
Fast BG (mg/dL) = 190 (100 – 125)
Ca (mg/dL) = 9.4 (8.5 – 10.5)
PO_4 (mg/dL) = 4 (2.3 – 4.7)
Mg (mg/dL) = 2.1 (1.3 – 2.1)

A1C (%) = 8.0
AST (IU/L) = 33 (10 – 40)
ALT (IU/L) = 35 (10 – 40)
LDL (mg/dL) = 65
HDL (mg/dL) = 67
TG (mg/dL) = 125
TC (mg/dL) = 157
hCG: (-)
HIV: (+)

a) Truvada®
b) Complera®
c) Symtuza®
d) Biktarvy®
e) Atripla®

18. KN comes to the pharmacy to pick up his new HIV regimen that his primary care provider just changed today. The new prescription reads: Complera® 1 tablet PO, take with food. While waiting for his prescription to get filled, he brings a bottle of Prevacid® and a bottle of Tums®. Which of the following actions should you take?

a) Tell him to take Tums and Prevacid® 2 hours after Complera®
b) Tell him to not take Prevacid® more than 2 tablets per day while he is on Complera®
c) Tell him that he should not take Tums if he takes Prevacid®
d) Tell him to not take Prevacid® while he is on Complera® because Prevacid® is contraindicated with Complera®. He can take Tums® two hours before Complera®
e) Tell him to not take Tums because it will interfere the absorption of Complera®

19. AM (13-year-old male) presents to the clinic for his annual checkup with his mom. Per his mom, besides annual influenza, he has not been vaccinated for two years. His pediatrician wants to administer the HPV vaccine. Which of the following vaccines would you recommend for AM?

>   **PMH:** Type 1 diabetes and COPD
>   **Immunization:** TDaP (completed), HepB (completed), and influenza (13 months ago).

   a) Gardasil®, Fluzone®, Prevnar®, Tdap
   b) Gardasil®, Fluzone®, Prevnar®
   c) Gardasil®, Fluzone®, Pneumovax®
   d) Gardasil®, Fluzone®, Pneumovax®, Tdap, and Menveo®
   e) Fluzone®, Pneumovax®, Tdap, Menveo®

20. A 40-year-old male comes to your pharmacy to pick up his medications. He has a history of hypertension and is two years post kidney transplant. He excitedly tells you his plans to travel out of the country, but he concerned about catching an infection while on vacation. He asks you for a recommendation on travel vaccines. His current medications include lisinopril, Prograf®, Cellcept®, and prednisone. Which of the following vaccines could be safely received, if needed?

   a) Vivotif®
   b) Typhim Vi®
   c) YF-VAX®
   d) DenguVax®
   e) Vaxchora®

21. A 70-year-old woman with a history of type 2 diabetes, COPD (an acute exacerbation that occurred 2 months ago), heart failure, and uncomplicated UTI (a month ago and was on Keflex®) presents to the clinic. After assessment, the patient was diagnosed with CAP but does not require admission to the hospital.

>   **Vital:** T°C = 38.4°C; RR: 22 BPM; HR: 98 BPM.
>   **Culture:** pending
>   **Allergies:** Lasix®, Celebrex®, and Glucotrol®

Which of the following regimens should be recommended to the patient empirically?

   a) Zithromax®
   b) Amoxil®
   c) Cipro®
   d) Doxycycline and Avelox®
   e) Cefuroxime and Zithromax®

22. TM (55-year-old man) presents to the clinic with recurrent *C. difficile* diarrhea for the 3rd time. As reviewing his profile, you noticed that he took oral vancomycin and metronidazole for his past episodes.

> **Vital:** TC = 36.8°C; RR: 18 BPM; HR: 78 BPM.
> **Labs:**
> Na (mEq/L) = 140 (135 – 145)
> K (mEq/L) = 3.8 (3.5 – 5)
> Cl (mEq/L) = 100 (95 – 103)
> HCO3 (mEq/L) = 27 (24 – 30)
> BUN (mg/dL) = 20 (7 – 20)
> SCr (mg/dL) = 1.11, eGFR 67
> Ca (mg/dL) = 9.4 (8.5 – 10.5)
> PO4 (mg/dL) = 4 (2.3 – 4.7)
> Mg (mg/dL) = 2.1 (1.3 – 2.1)
> WBC (cells/mm3) = 16 (4-10)

Which of the following would be the **APPROPRIATE** regimen(s) for him?

   a) Oral Vancomycin
   b) Rifaximin
   c) Fidaxomicin
   d) Clindamycin
   e) Metronidazole

23. A 34-year-old male was brought to the emergency department by his wife due to his altered mental status (confusion and lethargy). A lumbar puncture was taken for CFS culture. The ED physician wants to initiate an empiric regimen for the patient while waiting for susceptibility to return.

> **Labs (from CSF sample):**
> **Culture:** Pending
> **Gram-stain:** many Gram-negative diplococci
> WBC (cells/µL) = 500 (0-5) (neutrophils are predominant)
> Glucose (mg/dL) = 25 (> 60% of serum glucose)
> Protein (mg/dL) = 450 (< 45 mg/dL)
> **Opening pressure:** elevated
> **Allergy:** NDKA

Which of the following is the **APPROPRIATE** regimen that the ED pharmacist should recommend?

   a) Moxifloxacin + gentamicin
   b) Gentamicin + ampicillin
   c) Ampicillin + ceftriaxone + vancomycin
   d) Ceftriaxone + vancomycin
   e) Cefotaxime + gentamicin

24. NY (38-year-old male) was brought to the ED after a car accident and sustained close head trauma and pulmonary injury with underlying rib fracture on lower left side of his chest on 6/22. He was immediately intubated and admitted in the ICU. NY remains intubated since admission (today is day 8; 6/30).

Medical history: Asthma and type 2 of diabetes
Allergies: NKDA
Social history: IVDU and drink 2 wine per night

Vitals:
Height: 5'7"; weight: 180 pounds
BP: 105/58 mmHg; HR: 102 bpm; RR: 29 bpm;
Temp = 102.3°F; Pain: 7/10

Labs (6/30):
Na (mEq/L) = 140 (135 – 145)
K (mEq/L) = 3.8 (3.5 – 5)
Cl (mEq/L) = 100 (95 – 103)
HCO3 (mEq/L) = 27 (24 – 30)
BUN (mg/dL) = 18 (7 – 20)
SCr (mg/dL) = 1.11, eGFR 67
Ca (mg/dL) = 9.4 (8.5 – 10.5)
PO4 (mg/dL) = 4 (2.3 – 4.7)
Mg (mg/dL) = 2.1 (1.3 – 2.1)
Glucose (mg/dL) = 136 (100 – 125)
A1C = 7.2%

CBC:
WBC (cells/mm^3) = 17 (4-11 x10^3)
Hgb (g/dL) = 12
Hct (%) = 42
Plt (cells/mm^3) = 220 (150 – 450 x10^3)
AST (IU/L) = 36 (10 – 40)
ALT (IU/L) = 27 (10 – 40)
Albumin (g/dL) = 4 (3.5 – 5)

Tests:
Chest X-ray: Patchy consolidation and infiltrate
Culture (endotracheal aspirate sample): Gram-positive cocci (cluster)

Based on the lab results, he was diagnosed with ventilator acquired pneumonia (VAP). The medicine team wants to start him on an empiric regimen until the susceptibility is available. Which of the following regimen(s) are **APPROPRIATE** to treat VAP empirically?

a) Ceftriaxone + azithromycin
b) Vancomycin + tobramycin + Zosyn®
c) Vancomycin + Zosyn®
d) Linezolid + ceftriaxone + Zosyn®
e) Daptomycin + tobramycin + Zosyn®

25. A patient was admitted to the hospital with ascites secondary to alcoholic cirrhosis. After the assessment, the patient was diagnosed with primary peritonitis. The patient has no known drug allergies. Which of the following would be the **MOST APPROPRIATE** regimen to this patient?

a) Ceftriaxone 1 gram IV QD for 5-7 days
b) Vancomycin 750 mg IV Q8H for 7 days
c) Ciprofloxacin 750 mg PO QD for 14 days
d) Nafcillin 6 g IV QD for 5-7 days
e) Gentamicin 1 mg/kg IV Q12H for 7-10 days

26. A patient has a hip fracture repair. Which of the following antibiotic are used as the first-line agent for antibiotic prophylaxis?

    a) Ceftriaxone
    b) Vancomycin
    c) Cefazolin
    d) Clindamycin
    e) Doxycycline

27. A patient shows up to an urgent care with a chief complaint of "I think I get flu". Her symptoms include fever, chills, muscle aches and a severe headache. As talking to her, a physician noticed that she had a 5-day camping trip in South Carolina with her friends. After examination, the patient appears to have a tick bite. The physician orders a *Rickettsia ricketsii* serology as he suspects that the patient might get Rocky Mountain spotted fever. Which is the drug of choice to treat the patient for now while waiting for the lab result?

    a) Rifampin
    b) Clotrimazole
    c) Valacyclovir
    d) Gentamicin
    e) Doxycycline

28. A 47-year-old woman is diagnosed with gonorrhea today in the clinic. She does not have drug allergy. Which of the following regimen is appropriate to treat her?

    a) Amoxicillin + doxycycline
    b) Doxycycline + azithromycin
    c) Azithromycin + ceftriaxone
    d) Penicillin G
    e) Metronidazole

29. A patient brings a box of AZO® to the counseling window and asks the pharmacist how to take it and what to expect. Which of the following points should the pharmacist tell the patient? (Select **ALL** that apply.)

    a) AZO® is an OTC that can help to relieve urinary pain
    b) AZO® is not a urinary antibiotic, so if you suspect that a UTI is causing your pain, you should contact your PCP
    c) AZO® can only be used up to 2 days (no more than 2 days)
    d) AZO® can turn your body fluids into red-orange coloring (including your urine, tears); it may also stain your clothes and contact lenses
    e) You should take it with 8 oz of water and with meal right after to minimize stomach upset

30. A patient is admitted to the hospital for her fourth cycle of chemotherapy (5 days of treatment course). She is receiving posaconazole suspension as a prophylaxis due to prolonged neutropenia and mucositis, which has occurred after each cycle of her chemotherapy. Her mucositis is improved on day 5, and she requests to take posaconazole as pills rather than liquid upon discharge. Which of the following statement(s) is/are correct about posaconazole dosage form (dose conversion)? (Select **ALL** that apply.)

   a) PO (tablet) : PO (suspension) = 1:1
   b) PO (suspension) : IV injection = 1:1
   c) PO (tablet) : IV injection = 1:1
   d) PO (tablet) : PO (suspension) is not 1:1
   e) PO (tablet) : IV injection = 1.25 :1

31. JM presents to the clinic for a follow-up appointment for his asthma since his regimen was changed a month ago (add on Dulera®). While doing examination, his physician notices a white film on his tongue and throat. The patient states that he does not rinse his mouth after each dose because he often takes it at work. Which of the following drugs that can be used to treat his oral thrush?

   a) Doxycycline
   b) Amoxil® (high dose)
   c) Keflex®
   d) Bio-statin®
   e) Bactrim®

32. A 26-year-old man comes to the pharmacy to pick up influenza medication for him (positive with influenza B) and his wife (not infected, but for prophylaxis).

   His Rx (Rx1): Tamiflu® 75 mg BID for 5 days #10
   His wife's Rx (Rx2): Tamiflu® 75 mg QD for 10 days #10

   Which of the following is the APPROPRIATE action that the pharmacist should take?

   a) Contact the physician to change the frequency and quantity
   b) Dispense as written
   c) Contact the physician to change the strength for Rx2
   d) Contact the physician to change the strength of Rx1
   e) Contact the physician to change the regimen because Tamiflu® only covers influenza A

33. GA presents to the clinic for the first time after being discharged from the hospital post-kidney transplant. She requires a medication to prevent *Pneumocystis* pneumonia (PCP) for 6 months post-transplant. However, she reports that she has recently developed allergy with Bactrim® (hives) and wants to try something else. Her current med list is as follows:

> Prograf® 3mg BID
> Cellcept® 750 mg BID
> Prednisone 30 mg QD
> Valcyte® 900 mg QD (due to CMV donor +/recipient+)
> Bactrim® DS 3x/week (Mon/Wed/Fri) for 6 months
> Zestril® 5 mg QD
> Lasix® 20 mg QD PRN for edema
> Tylenol 350 mg q4-6H PRN for mild pain
> Oxycodone 5 mg q4-6H PRN for mod-severe pain
> Prevacid® 30 mg BID for GERD
> Miralax® one-half to 1 packet QD + Senna 17.6 mg QD for constipation

Which of the following drugs should be recommended to the patient if she cannot take Bactrim®?

   a) Ganciclovir
   b) Dapsone
   c) Valcyte®
   d) Ethambutol
   e) Foscarnet

34. A pharmacy technician is sanitizing the class II biological safety cabinet (BSC) (for preparing sterile hazardous drugs). What is the correct order of cleaning the class II BSC?

   1. Disinfect with 70% isopropyl alcohol (IPA)
   2. Neutralize bleach or peroxide-containing agents with sterile water to minimize corrosion on the stainless-steel surfaces
   3. Deactivate and decontaminate with 2% bleach or peroxide-containing agents
   4. Allow the surface dry before starting compounding

   a) 2, 3, 1, 4
   b) 3, 1, 2, 4
   c) 1, 2, 3, 4
   d) 3, 2, 1, 4
   e) 4, 3, 2, 1

35. A pharmacy technician has prepared IV doxorubicin and spilled the solution on his personal protective equipment (PPE) including his gloves and gown. He also feels that the drug may get in his eyes as they start to burn and irritate. What should the technician do? (Select **ALL** that apply.)

   a) Immediately remove the garb (gloves and gown)
   b) Obtain medical attention
   c) Immediately cleanse any affected skin with soap and water
   d) Since his eyes may get exposure to the drug, flush the affected eyes at an eyewash fountain and wash with isotonic water for at least 5 minutes
   e) Document the incident in the employee's record

36. After compounding IV vincristine, a half of the solution remains in the vial. Which of the following color waste bin should be used to dispose the vial?

    a) Red
    b) Blue
    c) Green
    d) Black
    e) Yellow

37. A pharmacist is preparing a water-in-oil emulsion and would like to choose the most lipophilic emulsifier that is available in the pharmacy. Which of the following is the **MOST APPROPRIATE** option? HLB is hydrophilic-lipophilic balance.

    a) Span 60 (HLB = 4.7)
    b) Tween 81 (HLB = 10)
    c) Tween 85 (HLB = 11)
    d) PEG 400 monostearate (HLB = 3.8)
    e) Sorbitan tristearate (HLB = 2.1)

38. AK (38-year-old female) is brought to the ED for further evaluation because she has had symptoms of fatigue, chest pain, lower extremity edema (but cold and discoloration).

Allergies: NKDA

Past Medical history:
HIV (on Symtuza®)
Current pregnancy (2nd trimester)

Vitals:
Height: 5'7"; **weight**: 180 pounds
BP: 115/62 mmHg; **HR:** 102 BPM; **RR:** 29 BPM;
SatO2: 86%; **Temp** = 98.3°F; **Pain:** 2/10

ROS:
General appearance: appears to be in mild distress
CV: Regular rate and rhythm
Lungs: Faint crackles
Abdomen: normal bowel sounds
Extremities: 2+ pitting edema (bilaterally), cold and discolor

Tests:
ECG: regular rhythm, no ST or T-wave abnormalities
Chest X-Ray: No infiltrates or fibrosis
Right heart catheterization: not respond to vasodilatory testing; PAP = 47 mmHg
Echocardiogram: LVEF: 34%

Labs:
Na (mEq/L) = 138 (135 – 145)
K (mEq/L) = 4 (3.5 – 5)
Cl (mEq/L) = 100 (95 – 103)
HCO3 (mEq/L) = 29 (24 – 30)
BUN (mg/dL) = 13 (7 – 20)
SCr (mg/dL) = 1.11, eGFR 67
Ca (mg/dL) = 9 (8.5 – 10.5)
PO4 (mg/dL) = 4.1 (2.3 – 4.7)
Mg (mg/dL) = 1.8 (1.3 – 2.1)
Glucose (mg/dL) = 116 (100 – 125)

CBC:
WBC (cells/mm^3) = 8.8 (4-11 x10^3)
Hgb (g/dL) = 13.4
Hct (%) = 42.6
Plt (cells/mm^3) = 320 (150 – 450 x10^3)
AST (IU/L) = 29 (10 – 40)
ALT (IU/L) = 30 (10 – 40)
Albumin (g/dL) = 4 (3.5 – 5)

AK is diagnosed with pulmonary hypertension (non-responsive to vasodilatory testing). The ED resident asks a pharmacist for a recommendation for her. Which of the following is the **MOST APPROPRIATE** regimen for AK?

a) Diltiazem
b) Flolan®
c) Bosentan®
d) Riociguat®
e) Macitentan®

39. TN (20-year-old female) comes to the pharmacy to refill her asthma prescriptions including Flovent HFA® 2 inhalations daily and Ventolin HFA® 1-2 inhalations every 4-6H PRN for symptoms. While waiting for her prescriptions, she asks if she should see her PCP because she has had breathing problems when she practices aerobic exercise that she signed up two weeks ago. What would be the **MOST APPROPRIATE** recommendation that a pharmacist should provide?

a) Yes, she should see her PCP because she has a risk of respiratory exacerbation without a treatment
b) She can take 4 inhalations of Ventolin HFA® one hour before exercise
c) She can take 2 inhalations of Flovent HFA® 5-15 minutes before exercise
d) She should see her PCP to get prednisone 10 mg PO and take it one hour before exercise
e) She can take 2 inhalations of Ventolin HFA® 5-15 minutes before exercise

40. A patient comes to the pharmacy for counseling on her new inhaler prescription, Ventolin HFA®. Which of the following instructions for proper Ventolin HFA® technique below in the correct order?

    1. Press the top of the canister while breathing in deeply and slowly
    2. Breath out fully to expel as much air from the lungs as possible
    3. Hold breath as long as possible (up to 10 seconds)
    4. Shake for 5 seconds
    5. Place the mouthpiece into the mouth and close lips around it

    a) 4, 2, 5, 1, 3
    b) 4, 5, 2, 1, 3
    c) 4, 2, 1, 5, 3
    d) 2, 4, 5, 1, 3
    e) 2, 3, 4, 5, 1

41. Which of the following adverse effects is most likely to occur when using Spiriva Respimat®?

    a) QT prolongation
    b) Depression
    c) Muscle pain
    d) Dry mouth
    e) Oral thrush

42. Which one of the following medications does NOT have a Boxed Warning for increasing risk of asthma-related death?

    a) Serevent Diskus®
    b) Dulera®
    c) Advair Diskus®
    d) Symbicort®
    e) Xopenex HFA®

43. In the ED, a mother reported that her 3-year-old child might have ingested unknown amount of iron tablets (only 4 or 5 tablets left in the bottle) approximately one hour ago. Iron overdose can be fatally toxic in children. What is the antidote for iron overdose?

    a) Methylene blue
    b) Narcan®
    c) Sodium bicarbonate
    d) Pralidoxime
    e) Desferal®

44. A patient is admitted to the hospital with intracranial hemorrhage due to a car accident. A pharmacist receives an order of IV Kcentra® and IV Phytonadione. Which of the following medication(s) would the pharmacist expect to see in his home medication list?

    a) Aspirin 81 mg QD
    b) Coumadin® 5 mg QD
    c) Clopidogrel 75 mg QD
    d) Eliquis® 5 mg BID
    e) Pradaxa® 150 mg BID

45. AJ comes to a pharmacy to pick up Pulmozyme® (with nebulizer and compressor system) for her 3-year-old son who was diagnosed with cystic fibrosis. What counseling points would you tell AJ? (Select **ALL** that apply.)

    a) Store the ampules in the room temperature
    b) Protect from light
    c) Mix it with other inhaled drug(s) in the nebulizer
    d) This drug will decrease mucus viscosity in the lungs
    e) Do not mix it with other drug(s) in the nebulizer

46. A 28-year-old man comes to a pharmacy for a recommendation on which strength of nicotine patch he should start on as he is ready to quit smoking. What is the **MOST APPROPRIATE** question you should ask him?

    a) Ask if he has any pulmonary conditions such as COPD and asthma
    b) How long have you been smoking?
    c) When do you take his first cigarette in a day?
    d) How many cigarette(s) do you smoke per day?
    e) Refer him to his PCP

47. NY (38-year-old male) was brought to the ED due to a car accident with a close head trauma and pulmonary injury with underlying rib fracture on lower left side of his chest on 6/22. NY was immediately intubated and admitted in the ICU. He remains intubated since admission (today is day 8; 6/30).

Medical history: Asthma and type 2 diabetes
Allergies: NKDA
Social history: IVDU and drink 2 glasses of wine per night

Vitals:
Height: 5' 7"; weight: 180 pounds
BP: 105/58 mmHg; HR: 102 BPM; RR: 29 BPM; Temp = 102.3°F; Pain: 7/10

Labs (6/30):
Na (mEq/L) = 140 (135 – 145)
K (mEq/L) = 3.2 (3.5 – 5)
Cl (mEq/L) = 100 (95 – 103)
HCO3 (mEq/L) = 27 (24 – 30)
BUN (mg/dL) = 18 (7 – 20)
SCr (mg/dL) = 1.11, eGFR 67
Ca (mg/dL) = 9.4 (8.5 – 10.5)
PO4 (mg/dL) = 4 (2.3 – 4.7)
Mg (mg/dL) = 2.1 (1.3 – 2.1)
Glucose (mg/dL) = 136 (100 – 125)
A1C = 7.2%

CBC:
WBC (cells/mm^3) = 17 (4-11 x 10^3)
Hgb (g/dL) = 12
Hct (%) = 42
Plt (cells/mm^3) = 220 (150 – 450 x 10^3)
AST (IU/L) = 36 (10 – 40)
ALT (IU/L) = 27 (10 – 40)
Albumin (g/dL) = 4 (3.5 – 5)

Tests:
Chest X-ray: Patchy consolidation and infiltrate
Culture (endotracheal aspirate sample): Gram-positive cocci (cluster)

Based on the lab results, a medical resident ordered 40 mEq KCl infusion in 500 mL NS. How long (in hours) will the bag of KCl last (if we infuse with the allowed maximum infusion rate as possible)?

a) 4 hours
b) 6 hours
c) 2 hours
d) 5 hours
e) As quick as 30 minutes

48. A 57-year-old man was found on the street and brought to the emergency department with symptoms of altered mental status, headache, and neck stiffness. He has a history of IVDU, alcohol withdrawal, HIV, and hypertension. After examination, an ED doctor suspects him to have meningitis and want to start empiric regimen while waiting for the CSF culture.

PATIENT PROFILE				
Patient Name: AJ				
Age: 57	**Sex:** Male	**Race:** AA	**Height:** 5'8"	**Weight:** 140 lbs
Allergies: Lisinopril (angioedema)				
DIAGNOSES: Meningitis (CSF culture: pending)	**HOME MEDICATIONS:** (last refilled: 4 months ago) Multivitamin 1 tab PO daily Biktarvy® 1 tab PO daily Hydrochlorothiazide 25 mg daily Thiamine 1 tab PO daily			

Which of the following is the **MOST APPROPRIATE** regimen to AJ?

a) Vancomycin + Zosyn®
b) Vancomycin + ceftriaxone + gentamycin
c) Ceftriaxone + ampicillin + Zosyn®
d) Cefotaxime + ampicillin + gentamicin
e) Vancomycin + ceftriaxone + ampicillin

49. A 57-year-old man was found on the street and brought to the emergency department with symptoms of altered mental status, headache, and neck stiffness. He has a history of IVDU, alcohol withdrawal, HIV, and hypertension. After examination, an ED doctor suspects him to have meningitis and want to start empiric regimen while waiting for the CSF culture.

PATIENT PROFILE					
Patient Name: AJ					
Age: 57	Sex: Male	Race: AA		Height: 5'8"	Weight: 140 lbs
Allergies: Lisinopril (angioedema)					
DIAGNOSES: Meningitis		HOME MEDICATIONS: (Last refilled: 4 months ago) Multivitamin 1 tab PO daily Biktarvy® 1 tab PO daily Hydrochlorothiazide 25 mg daily Thiamine 1 tab PO daily			

LAB/DIAGNOTIC TESTS				
Test	**Normal Value**	**Results**		
		Date: 1/7	**Date: 1/8**	**Date: 2/8**
Na	135 – 146 mEq/L	138	139	140
K	3.5 – 5.3 mEq/L	4.2	4.0	4.4
Cl	98 – 110 mEq/L	105	101	103
CO2	21 – 33 mEq/L	28	26	24
BUN	7 – 25 mg/dL	22	22	22
SCr	0.6 – 1.2 mg/dL	1.4	1.2	1.0
Glucose	70 – 100 mg/dL	148	138	143
Albumin	3.5 – 5 g/dL	4	4.0	4
TG	< 150 mg/dL	178	-	-
HDL	>65 mg/dL	76	-	-
TC	<200 mg/dL	180	-	-
AST	0 - 40 U/L	32	-	-
ALT	0 – 40 U/L	24	-	-
WBC	4-11 x10^3/mm^3	13	11	10
Hgb	13-17 g/dL	14	14.1	14.2
Hct	40-52%	46	45.2	46
MCV	80-100 fL	88	87	88
HIV viral load	undetectable	pending		143,240
CSF culture	negative	pending		*S. pneumonia*

PROGRESS NOTES	
Date	Notes
3/17	Vitals: BP 156/96, HR 89 BPM, T: 37.8C; patient admitted to the ED with suspected meningitis. CSF culture: pending. Plan: Start empiric regimen and reassess when CSF is available. Continue on all home medications.
3/18	Vitals: BP 154/93, HR 82 BPM, T: 37.2C; patient remains stable on current medications. HIV viral load: 143, 240 copies/mL. CSF culture: *S. pneumonia*, d/c Vancomycin and ampicillin.

As noticing AJ's BP is elevated since admission, a medical resident suggests starting patient on Diovan HTC® 160 mg/12.5 mg 1 tab PO daily on rounds. What would be the **MOST appropriate** action a pharmacist should take?

a) Put in this verbal order and schedule every morning
b) Add Norvasc® 5 mg PO daily to his current HTN regimen
c) Suggest changing the frequency: daily to twice a day
d) Increase dose to 320 mg/25 mg 1 tab PO daily
e) Change to Lopressor HCT® (100 mg/25 mg) 1 tab PO daily

50. A pharmacy technician prepared ampicillin in NS and placed it in an amber IV bag. She is bringing it to a pharmacist for a final check before dispending it to the unit. What would the pharmacist do?

    a) Remake the IV ampicillin in D5W
    b) Remake the IV ampicillin in a non-PVC bag or glass
    c) Discard the amber IV bag and verify the order
    d) Place an auxiliary label "Shake well before using" on the bag and verify the order
    e) Place an auxiliary label "Chemotherapy: Dispose of Properly"

Practice Test 5: 50 questions, Time: 60 minutes

1. A new pharmacy technician is preparing IV Sulfatrim® bag. She knows that there is a specific instruction to prepare Sulfatrim®, but she cannot recall what they are and asks a floor pharmacist. What would a pharmacist tell to do to prepare this order? (Select **ALL** that apply.)

    a) In-line filter (0.22 micron) is required
    b) Place an auxiliary label "Do not refrigerate" on the bag
    c) Dilute Sulfatrim® in D5W
    d) Protect it from light by using an amber bag
    e) Place an auxiliary label "Check for peanut or soy allergy"

2. A woman drops off a new prescription: Tylenol® #3, 1 table every 4-6 hours as needed for severe pain, quantity #30, for her 17-year-old daughter who just got her root canal done this morning. As reviewing patient's profile, a pharmacist notices that she had tonsillectomy surgery 2 years ago and has a history of COPD. She has allergy with sulfa (anaphylaxis). She currently takes ProAir® PRN, EpiPen® and amoxicillin (prophylaxis for her dental procedure). Which of the following would the pharmacist do?

    a) Dispense the prescription
    b) Contact the dentist to change frequency
    c) Contact the dentist to change drug
    d) Contact the dentist to change quantity
    e) None of the above

3. A resident is planning to discharge a 36-year-old postpartum woman (2 days after delivery). She has a social history of smoking (10 cigarettes per day); otherwise, she is healthy and no known allergy. The resident calls a pharmacist for a recommendation on a birth control pill for her. Which of the following contraceptive is the **MOST APPROPRIATE** to this patient?

    a) Nora-BE
    b) Yaz®
    c) Yasmin®
    d) NuvaRing®
    e) Junel Fe®

4. NM (32-year-old female) with major depression disorder is currently being treated with Paxil® 20 mg daily for 4 months. She has noticed that she often feels sleepy and low energy throughout the day, which makes her not involved in any activities and low libido. She also concerns about weight gain, "I have gained 6 pounds since I started taking this drug." She wonders if she has any other option to help her depression, but it does not cause issues that she has had. Which is the **MOST APPROPRIATE** recommendation would you make?

    a) Switch Paxil® to Remeron®
    b) Switch Paxil® to Wellbutrin®
    c) Switch Paxil® to fluvoxamine
    d) Tell her to take Paxil® at bedtime; this drug causes weight gain for only the first three months of the treatment. Therefore, she should continue it.
    e) Switch Paxil® to Elavil®

5. RP (50-year-old female) comes to clinic with a chief complaint of fatigue and headache. She has a history of type 2 diabetes and GERD.

Allergies: NKDA
PMH: Type 2 of diabetes - 10 years, GERD, Post menopause

Vitals:
Height: 5'5"; **weight**: 140 pounds
BP: 125/85 mmHg; **HR:** 89 BPM; **RR:** 18 BPM;
SatO2: 99%; **Temp** = 37.3°C

Current Medication List:
Metformin 1000 mg PO BID
Invokana® 100 mg PO QD
Multivitamin 1 tab PO QD
Biotin for hair
Prilosec® 20 mg QAM

Labs:
Na (mEq/L) = 140 (135 – 145)
K (mEq/L) = 3.8 (3.5 – 5)
Cl (mEq/L) = 100 (95 – 103)
HCO3 (mEq/L) = 27 (24 – 30)
BUN (mg/dL) = 20 (7 – 20)
SCr (mg/dL) = 1.11, eGFR 62
Fast BG (mg/dL) = 140 (100 – 125)
A1C (%) = 8.0
Ca (mg/dL) = 9.4 (8.5 – 10.5)
PO4 (mg/dL) = 4 (2.3 – 4.7)
Mg (mg/dL) = 2.1 (1.3 – 2.1)
AST (IU/L) = 33 (10 – 40)
ALT (IU/L) = 35 (10 – 40)
LDL (mg/dL) = 65
HDL (mg/dL) = 67
TG (mg/dL) = 125
TC (mg/dL) = 157
Folate (ng/mL) = 2 (3.1 – 17.5)
VitB12 (mg/dL) = 160 (211 – 946)

CBC:
WBC (1000 cells/mm^3) = 8 (4-11)
RBC (million cells/mm^3) = 3.4 (4-5)
Hgb (g/dL) = 10.6 (12 – 16)
Hct (%) = 32 (36 – 46)
MCH (pgm) = 28 (27-31)
MCV (μm^3) = 122 (80-100)
Plt (1000/mm^3) = 252 (150 – 400)
ANC (1000 cells/mm^3) = 3.2 (1.5 – 6)

Iron (mcg/dL) = 54 (37 – 145)
Ferritin (ng/mL) = 65 (13 – 150)
TIBC (mcg/dL) = 320 (250 – 450)
Free T4 (ng/dL) = 1.2 (0.93 – 1.7)
TSH (μIU/mL) = 2.5 (0.27 – 4.2)

Which of the following are correct diagnosis and regimen for RP?

a) Macrocytic anemia, folate 1 mg QD and Vitamin B12 1 tab PO QD
b) Macrocytic anemia, ferrous sulfate 325 mg PO BID
c) Microcytic anemia, ferrous sulfate 325 mg PO BID
d) Normocytic anemia, Epogen®
e) Hypothyroidism, Synthroid® 25 mg QD

6. Mary was recently prescribed Imitrex® 50 mg tablets for her severe migraines. What is the maximum number of tablets that Mary can take per day?

a) 4
b) 5
c) 2
d) 1
e) 3

7. Michael comes into the emergency room with complaints of unexpected weight loss, rapid heart rate, fatigue, diarrhea, and sweating. A series of labs are conducted to determine the cause of Michael's symptoms. Which lab value do you expect to be decreased in this patient?

    a) HCG
    b) Na
    c) TSH
    d) Troponin
    e) INR

8. Jenny is being discharged from the hospital after complaints of green vaginal discharge, burning during urination, fever, and pain during sexual intercourse. Jenny has normal renal function and has an allergy to penicillin. Which of the following is an acceptable treatment regimen for her symptoms? (Select **ALL** that apply.)

    a) IM ceftriaxone 250 mg x 7 days
    b) SC azithromycin 1000 mg x 5 days
    c) PO azithromycin 1000 mg x 1 day
    d) PO doxycycline 100 mg TID x 7 days
    e) IM ceftriaxone 250 mg x 1 day

9. A pregnant woman presents to the emergency room with a blood pressure of 189/110. Which of the following is the most appropriate regimen for this patient?

    a) Coreg® 6.25 mg PO BID
    b) Zestril® 5 mg PO QD
    c) Lopressor® 15 mg IV
    d) Methyldopa® 250 mg PO BID up to 1000 mg PO every 8 hours
    e) Catapres® 0.1 mg PO QD

10. A patient with a sulfa allergy requires treatment for their hyperglycemia. Which of the following regimens should be used with caution in this patient? (Select **ALL** that apply.)

    a) Metformin 500 mg BID
    b) Repaglinide 2 mg TID
    c) Glipizide 5 mg daily
    d) Canagliflozin 100 mg daily
    e) Glimepiride 2 mg daily

11. George is receiving treatment for his pulmonary arterial hypertension in the ER. Which of the following immunizations should nurses make sure are up to date and received annually? (Select **ALL** that apply.)

    a) Influenza
    b) Hepatitis B
    c) Varicella
    d) Yellow Fever
    e) Pneumococcal

12. A 4-year-old is being prescribed montelukast tablets for his asthma management. What would be the appropriate dosing regimen for this patient based on his age?

    a) 10 mg daily in the evening
    b) 5 mg daily in the evening
    c) 5 mg BID in the morning and evening
    d) 4 mg BID in the morning and evening
    e) 4 mg daily in the evening

13. Casey is looking for a medication to help her quit smoking. She has tried nicotine gum and patches that they have not worked, and she is looking for a prescription option. The pharmacist recommends varenicline. Casey should be counselled on all the potential sides effects of varenicline EXCEPT which of the following?

    a) Nausea
    b) Insomnia
    c) Abnormal dreams
    d) Diarrhea
    e) Constipation

14. In addition to being a long-time smoker, Casey also takes metformin 500 mg twice daily, lisinopril 40 mg once daily, and has a 10-year ASCVD risk of 13%. What is the target blood pressure goal for a patient with these comorbidities according to ADA guidelines?

    a) 140/90 mmHg
    b) 130/80 mmHg
    c) 120/80 mmHg
    d) 140/80 mmHg
    e) 130/90 mmHg

15. A dialysis patient with a CrCl of 15 mL/min requires treatment for their diabetes. Which of the following medication should be avoided in this patient?

    a) Glimepiride
    b) Metformin
    c) Saxagliptin
    d) Pioglitazone
    e) Glipizide

16. A 26-year-old female is admitted to the emergency room with a myxedema coma. Which of the following is the best therapeutic option for this patient?

    a) IV levothyroxine
    b) PO levothyroxine
    c) IV liothyronine
    d) PO liothyronine
    e) PO Armour Thyroid®

17. AC weighs 76 kg. What is the full replacement dose of levothyroxine that she should be receiving per day?

    a) 88 mcg per day
    b) 122 mg per day
    c) 121 mg per day
    d) 122 mcg per day
    e) 121 mcg per day

18. A patient in the emergency room is experiencing a thyroid storm. What is the preferred hyperthyroidism treatment?

    a) Levothyroxine
    b) Potassium iodide
    c) Methimazole
    d) Propylthiouracil (PTU)
    e) Liothyronine

19. June is a 35-year-old pregnant woman that just found out that she is 6 weeks pregnant. June has been diagnosed with hyperthyroidism. Which of the following medications should be avoided during the first trimester due to its risk for fetal toxicity?

    a) Levothyroxine
    b) Potassium iodide
    c) Methimazole
    d) Propylthiouracil (PTU)
    e) Liothyronine

20. A patient presents to the pharmacy looking for a cream for her son's rash. She is asking for the most potent medication that she can purchase without a prescription. Which of the following medications would be the best option for her son?

    a) Cortisone
    b) Hydrocortisone
    c) Betamethasone
    d) Methylprednisolone
    e) Triamcinolone

21. AJ is a 62-year-old who has been discharged from the hospital after being treated for a diabetic foot. AJ should be instructed to avoid which of the following activities.

    a) Wearing clean, dry socks
    b) Cutting nails straight across
    c) Wearing socks to bed
    d) Walking barefoot
    e) Using an antiperspirant on the soles of his feet

22. George is working in a hospital pharmacy and is about to take a vial of insulin up to a patient. He notices frosted lumps in the vial. What should George do with this vial of insulin?

    a) Heat the vial to dissolve the crystals
    b) Discard the vial
    c) Place the vial back in the fridge
    d) Gently roll the vial
    e) Disregard the lumps. The insulin can still be used

23. A patient was recently prescribed Tamsulosin 0.4 mg for this enlarged prostate. What is the mechanism of action of this medication?

    a) Selective alpha-1 receptor agonist
    b) Selective alpha-1 receptor antagonist
    c) Nonselective alpha-1 receptor antagonist
    d) Selective beta-blocker
    e) Nonselective beta-blocker

24. Sulfamethoxazole and trimethoprim 200 mg/40 mg per 5 mL should be dispensed in which of the following:

    a) Clear glass container
    b) Clear plastic container
    c) Air protective container
    d) Original manufacturer packaging
    e) Light protective container

25. Patients should be counseling on limiting grapefruit juice when taking all of the following medications except:

    a) Amiodarone
    b) Buspirone
    c) Carbamazepine
    d) Tacrolimus
    e) Fluvastatin

26. Which of the following if a CYP inhibitor?

    a) Ketoconazole
    b) St. John's Wort
    c) Phenytoin
    d) Carbamazepine
    e) Rifampin

27. MJ was recently admitted to the hospital where he was given antibiotics for salmonella poisoning. His doctor recommends that he receive the Vivotif® vaccine to avoid further infections. How long should his nurse wait before administering this vaccine?

   a) At least 36 hours
   b) At least 24 hours
   c) At least 48 hours
   d) At least 72 hours
   e) Vivotif® can be administered immediately regardless of antibiotic administration

28. Which of the following vaccines is administered subcutaneously?

   a) Flumist®
   b) Varicella
   c) Vivotif®
   d) Vaxchora®
   e) BCG

29. Clozapine as a black box warning for all of the following conditions except which of the following?

   a) Fecal impaction
   b) Agranulocytosis
   c) Myocarditis
   d) Increased mortality in elderly
   e) Other cardiovascular and respiratory effects

30. A patient requires immediate reversal of heparin. What is the only approved antidote for unfractionated heparin?

   a) Protamine
   b) Activated charcoal
   c) Praxbind®
   d) Vitamin K
   e) Andexanet alfa

31. Which of the following medications may increase triglycerides and should be used with caution in patients with a triglyceride level greater than 250 mg/dL?

   a) Fenofibrate
   b) Colesevelam
   c) Ezetimibe
   d) Omega-3 ethyl esters
   e) Simvastatin

32. Jerry is a 57-year-old male that has been on atorvastatin 10 mg daily for 5 years. His LDL level is still not at goal. His cholesterol levels are TC 270 mg/dL, LDL-C 200 mg/dL, HDL 35, and TG 176. Which of the following changes should be made at his next doctor's appointment to lower his lipid levels?

    a) Switch from atorvastatin 10 mg to simvastatin 20 mg daily
    b) Add ezetimibe 10 mg daily
    c) Add omega-3 ethyl esters
    d) Increase atorvastatin 10 mg to 80 mg
    e) Discontinue his statin and recommend lifestyle modifications

33. Simvastatin should be limited to only 20 mg a day due to an increased risk of myopathy with which of the following medications?

    a) Metformin
    b) Hydroxyzine
    c) Verapamil
    d) Amlodipine
    e) Hydrochlorothiazide

34. Which of the following is true regarding amlodipine?

    a) Dosed at 5-10 mg three times daily for hypertension
    b) Approved for off label treatment for peripheral edema
    c) Peripheral edema is a common adverse drug reaction
    d) Classified as a beta-blocker
    e) FDA approved for diabetic nephropathy

35. Which of the following medications may mask the symptoms of hypoglycemia?

    a) Verapamil
    b) Lisinopril
    c) Propranolol
    d) Imitrex®
    e) Olmesartan

36. Jordan was just prescribed isosorbide dinitrate to treat his recurrent chest pain. This medication is dosed twice daily. When should Jordan be advised to take this medication?

    a) 8am and 8pm
    b) 8am and 6pm
    c) 8am and 3pm
    d) 8am and 10 pm
    e) 8am and 12 pm

37. Which of the following is a non-pharmacological treatment method for patients with cystic fibrosis?

    a) Fluid restriction
    b) Low-carb diet
    c) Chest percussion
    d) Avoidance of caffeine
    e) Low-fiber diet

38. Which of the following medications need to be heated to dissolve crystals prior to IV infusion?

    a) Heparin
    b) Insulin
    c) Amphotericin B
    d) Mannitol
    e) Fosphenytoin

39. Enoxaparin is available as a prefilled syringe in all of the following dosage strengths **except** which of the following?

    a) 160 mg
    b) 40 mg
    c) 80 mg
    d) 120 mg
    e) 60 mg

40. Which of the following medications requires a renal dose adjustment?

    a) Warfarin
    b) Ciprofloxacin
    c) Clindamycin
    d) Ceftriaxone
    e) Metronidazole

41. Kendra reports to the ER with complaints of fever, flank pain, and sudden onset of labor following IV drug use. The doctor orders 1 unit per 1 mL of heparin in D10W to be administered intravenously at 1 mL per hour. This heparin is most likely being used for which of the following reasons?

    a) Maintain renal function
    b) Prevent thromboembolism
    c) Treatment of DVT
    d) Treatment of hyperbilirubinemia
    e) Maintain catheter patency

42. Sarah is in the hospital and is currently receiving Lovenox® 40 mg subcutaneously daily following an abdominal procedure. Her creatinine clearance is 15 mL/min. Doctors are concerned about her bleeding risk. Which of the following lab tests should be assessed to determine the level of anticoagulation in this patient?

    a) INR
    b) Liver enzymes
    c) Bleeding time
    d) Anti Xa activity
    e) aPTT

43. Amara receives a prescription for Atripla® 30 mg by mouth daily. Which of the following medications is included in Amara's antiretroviral regimen?

    a) Acyclovir
    b) Zidovudine
    c) Ritonavir
    d) Efavirenz
    e) Isoniazid

44. Stacy was recently prescribed Seroquel XR® for her bipolar depression. Which of the following should be monitored while she is on this medication? (Select **ALL** that apply.)

    a) INR
    b) aPTT
    c) Lipid panel
    d) Blood pressure
    e) Fasting glucose

45. Tracy comes to the pharmacy requesting a tetanus booster immunization booster. She states that she last received a booster shot 4 years ago. When can Tracy receive her next tetanus booster?

    a) In 2-6 weeks
    b) In 6 years
    c) Annually
    d) In 9 years
    e) The same day

46. RJ, a 70-kg male, comes into your emergency department with diabetic ketoacidosis (DKA). His blood glucose is down to 250 mL/dL with an anion gap of 32 mEq/L. Which of the following do you suggest treating your patient initially?

    a) Stop insulin infusion 0.1 units/kg/hour drip when the glucose normalizes, and the anion gap is 12 mEq/L
    b) Continue insulin drip and add dextrose
    c) Continue insulin drip and add fluids while monitoring potassium levels
    d) Monitor potassium and serum ketones
    e) None of the above

47. Your outpatient clinic wants to improve safety with vitamin K. What would you recommend to your safety officer to prevent vitamin K overdose and ensure safe use?

   a) Ensure vitamin K is not available inpatient care areas and restrict to guideline recommendation
   b) Place vitamin K in kits in all patient care areas
   c) Place vitamin K only in crash carts in the ER
   d) Educate the staff on appropriate vitamin K use
   e) None of the above

48. RJ is an-HIV positive male patient who comes into your clinic for follow-up. His current medication regimen is the following: abacavir, lamivudine, and ritonavir & lopinavir combination. He is also taking simvastatin. Which of the following would you recommend?

   a) Change abacavir and lamivudine to tenofovir DF and emtricitabine
   b) Change ritonavir and lopinavir to raltegravir and efavirenz
   c) Change ritonavir and lopinavir to darunavir and cobicistat
   d) Change abacavir and lamivudine to tenofovir disoproxil fumarate
   e) None of the above

49. MJ is a 30-year-old female who is pregnant, HIV-positive, and in her second trimester. Her HIV is well controlled, and her current medication regimen includes: raltegravir 400 mg BID, emtricitabine and tenofovir disoproxil fumarate. She has GERD and wants to take an OTC antacid to treat. What do you recommend?

   a) Advise her to take pantoprazole
   b) Advise her to take an H2 antagonist blocker such as famotidine and use standard twice daily
   c) Advise she may use H2 antagonist or calcium carbonate antacids
   d) Recommend aluminum/magnesium antacid for quick relief
   e) None of the above

50. RJ is a 46-year-old man taking carbidopa and levodopa. He was recently started on ephedrine OTC and metoclopramide. He complains of experiencing Parkinson's-like symptoms. Which drug likely caused the symptoms, and by what mechanism?

   a) The symptoms are likely due to ephedrine and its dopamine receptor antagonism
   b) The symptoms are likely due to metoclopramide and its dopamine receptor antagonism
   c) The symptoms are likely due to metoclopramide and its dopamine receptor agonism
   d) The symptoms are likely due to ephedrine and its dopamine receptor agonism
   e) None of the above

Practice Test 6: 50 questions, Time: 60 minutes

1. The bugs that can induce AmpC production are often referred to as "SPACE" bugs. Which of the following are included in "SPACE"? Select all that apply.

   a) *Serratia spp.*
   b) *Pseudomonas spp.*
   c) *Acinetobacter spp.*
   d) *Citrobacter spp.*
   e) *Enterococcus spp.*

2. Which of the following antibiotic classes can cause QT prolongation? Select all that apply.

   a) Fluoroquinolones
   b) Penicillins
   c) Cephalosporins
   d) Macrolides
   e) Aminoglycosides

3. KPC-producing bacteria would be resistant to which antibiotic/antibiotic class?

   a) Ciprofloxacin
   b) Cephalosporins
   c) Carbapenems
   d) Clindamycin
   e) Chloramphenicol

4. Which of the following antibiotics are concentration-dependent?

   a) Ciprofloxacin
   b) Vancomycin
   c) Amikacin
   d) Moxifloxacin
   e) Aztreonam

5. Which of the following antibiotics needs to be renally adjusted?

   a) Ceftriaxone
   b) Clindamycin
   c) Rifampin
   d) Erythromycin
   e) Cefepime

6. Which of the following insulins can be stored at room temperature for up to 28 days? Select all that apply.

   a) Insulin detemir (Levemir®) vial
   b) Insulin aspart (Novolog®) vial
   c) Insulin glargine (Lantus®) pen
   d) Insulin lispro (Humalog®) vial
   e) NPH Novolin® pen

7. A 70/30 Humulin® pen can be stored at room temperature up to how many days?

   a) 10 days
   b) 14 days
   c) 28 days
   d) 42 days
   e) 56 days

8. A patient is prescribed unfractionated heparin for a VTE. What is the prophylactic dose of unfractionated heparin?

   a) 1000 units SQ q8-12h
   b) 5000 units SQ q8-12h
   c) 30 mg SQ q12h
   d) 1 mg/kg SQ q12h
   e) 1.5 mg/kg SQ q12h

9. A patient is prescribed enoxaparin for a VTE. What is the prophylactic dose of enoxaparin?

   a) 1000 units SQ q8-12h
   b) 5000 units SQ q8-12h
   c) 30 mg SQ q12h
   d) 1 mg/kg SQ q12h
   e) 1.5 mg/kg SQ q12h

10. A patient is prescribed rivaroxaban to treat their VTE. What is the appropriate dose?

   a) 30 mg PO BID for 21 days, then 20 mg PO daily
   b) 20 mg PO BID for 21 days, then 15 mg PO daily
   c) 10 mg PO BID for 21 days, then 15 mg PO daily
   d) 15 mg PO BID for 21 days, then 20 mg PO daily
   e) 15 mg PO BID for 21 days, then 10 mg PO daily

11. Which of the following anticoagulants is NOT correctly matched with its reversal agent/antidote?

   a) Warfarin and vitamin K
   b) Rivaroxaban and andexanet alfa
   c) Unfractionated heparin and protamine
   d) Dabigatran and idarucizumab
   e) Enoxaparin and andexanet alfa

12. Which of the following people should NOT receive one dose of PPSV23?

   a) 30-year-old woman who smokes
   b) 29-year-old man with alcoholism
   c) 48-year-old person with type 2 diabetes
   d) 23-year-old person with asplenia
   e) 52-year-old woman with congestive heart failure

13. Truvada® is composed of which medications?

   a) Tenofovir disoproxil fumarate + emtricitabine
   b) Tenofovir alafenamide + emtricitabine
   c) Tenofovir disoproxil fumarate + emtricitabine + efavirenz
   d) Tenofovir alafenamide + emtricitabine + bictegravir
   e) Tenofovir alafenamide + emtricitabine + rilpivirine

14. A patient with HIV has a CD4+ cell count of 100 cells/mm^3. Which of the following therapies can they use? Select all that apply.

   a) Juluca®
   b) Odefsey®
   c) Complera®
   d) Truvada®
   e) Triumeq®

15. Which of the following HIV medications contains a protease inhibitor? Select all that apply.

   a) Evotaz®
   b) Combivir®
   c) Kaletra®
   d) Prezcobix®
   e) Symtuza®

16. "Triple DMARD" therapy is often used to treat rheumatoid arthritis. What three medications are included in a Triple DMARD?

    a) Leflunomide + hydroxychloroquine + sulfasalazine
    b) Methotrexate + hydroxychloroquine + sulfasalazine
    c) Methotrexate + abatacept + sulfasalazine
    d) Methotrexate + leflunomide + abatacept
    e) Methotrexate + hydroxychloroquine + sarilumab

17. Which of the following treatments can be used for drug-induced lupus? Select all that apply.

    a) Hydroxychloroquine
    b) Cyclophosphamide
    c) NSAIDs
    d) Azathioprine
    e) Procainamide

18. Which of the following should not be used to treat gout?

    a) Allopurinol
    b) Febuxostat
    c) Aspirin
    d) Colchicine
    e) Prednisone

19. A pregnant woman comes up to your pharmacy and complains of constipation. What do you recommend she take?

    a) Dulcolax®
    b) Fleet enema®
    c) Metamucil®
    d) Mineral oil
    e) Miralax®

20. A pregnant woman comes up to your pharmacy and complains of diarrhea. What do you recommend she take?

    a) Loperamide
    b) Kaopectate
    c) Lomotil®
    d) Pepto Bismol®
    e) Castor oil

21. Which of the following medications would increase the bleeding risk but not change the INR if used together with warfarin?

a) Naproxen
b) Fluconazole
c) Metronidazole
d) Amiodarone
e) Bactrim

22. Which of the following drugs should be initially selected as hypertension treatment for JP, an African American 34-year-old with a blood pressure of 142/94?

a) Lisinopril
b) Valsartan
c) Microzide®
d) Vasotec®
e) Benicar®

23. KP is a patient who presented with weakness and fatigue. Lab results showed that KP is hypokalemic and ECG analysis revealed a QT interval of 510ms. Which of the following drugs should be avoided? (Select all that apply)

a) Ciprofloxacin
b) Scopolamine
c) Procainamide
d) Amitriptyline
e) Repaglinide

24. LM is a patient who has chronic systolic heart failure. Which of the following class of medications have a mortality benefit for heart failure? (Select all that apply)

a) ACE inhibitors
b) Angiotensin receptor blockers (ARBs)
c) Beta blockers
d) Alpha 1 agonist
e) Aldosterone receptor antagonists

25. FP presents to the hospital with loose stools, fever, vomiting, and bloody diarrhea. FP reports that he has recently traveled overseas and ingested the local food or water where he believes he was contaminated. Physicians were able to identify it as traveler's diarrhea. What is the preferred treatment for FP?

a) Ceftriaxone
b) Clindamycin
c) Doripenem
d) Azithromycin
e) Metronidazole

26. GH is a 26-year-old female who presents with urgency and frequency including nocturia. What is the preferred empiric treatment for acute uncomplicated cystitis in GH?

a) Ciprofloxacin 500mg BID
b) Levofloxacin 750mg QD
c) Azithromycin 250mg QD
d) Rifaximin 200mg TID
e) Nitrofurantoin 100mg BID

27. How many days of ceftriaxone treatment is needed for spontaneous bacterial peritonitis (SBP)?
    a) 1-3 days
    b) 3-5 days
    c) 5-7 days
    d) 7-10 days
    e) 10-14 days

28. AJ is 35-year-old male who presents with shortness of breath and edema. An ultrasound of the heart confirmed the presence of systolic heart failure for AJ. Which of the following drugs should be avoided for AJ that may worsen his condition? (Select all that apply)

    a) Saxagliptin
    b) Amlodipine
    c) Diltiazem
    d) Naproxen
    e) Ramipril

29. PJ was undergoing heparin treatment at the hospital when on the 5th day of treatment, his platelet count was observed to be decreasing to around 80,000/microL. What is the drug of choice for PJ considering his treatment setting?

    a) Argatroban
    b) Fondaparinux
    c) Pradaxa$^{®}$
    d) Lovenox$^{®}$
    e) Eliquis$^{®}$

30. A patient on warfarin wants to switch to another anticoagulant. His INR is <2. Which of the following should the patient be switched to after stopping warfarin? (Select all that apply)

    a) Edoxaban
    b) Rivoraxaban
    c) Apixaban
    d) Dabigatran
    e) Fondaparinux

31. What is the appropriate regimen for treating Mycobacterium avium complex (MAC) infection if ART is not started immediately?

a) SMX/TMP DS daily
b) Azithromycin 1,200mg weekly
c) Fluconazole 200mg daily
d) Valganciclovir 450mg daily
e) Atovaquone 1,500mg weekly

32. Which of the following conditions increases the risk for digoxin toxicity? (Select all that apply)

a) Hyperkalemia
b) Hypomagnesemia
c) Hypercalcemia
d) Hypernatremia
e) Hyperthyroidism

33. TP is a patient with a known hypersensitivity to sulfonamide derived drugs. Which of the following medications should TP avoid? (Select all that apply)

a) Chlorthalidone
b) Amlodipine
c) Amoxicillin
d) Sulfasalazine
e) Dapsone

34. AM is a 65-year-old male with a FEV1/FVC < 0.7, CAT score of 8 and three exacerbations in the past year, one of which led to a hospital admission. AM reports getting short of breath when hurrying on ground level and when walking up a hill. Which of the following is an appropriate initial pharmacologic therapy for AM?

a) Atrovent®
b) Spiriva Handihaler®
c) Advair Diskus®
d) Symbicort®
e) Stiolto Respimat®

35. What is the appropriate dose of methotrexate in treating rheumatoid arthritis for initial therapy?

a) 1mg once daily
b) 2-7.5mg once daily
c) 2-7.5 mg once weekly
d) 7.5-20mg once daily
e) 7.5-20mg once weekly

36. TM is a 72-year-old patient presenting with frequent urination and incomplete emptying of the bladder including leaking as well as dribbling. Testing and exams revealed that TM suffered from benign prostatic hyperplasia. Which of the following drugs should TM avoid? (Select all that apply)

a) Caffeine

b) Benztropine
c) Escitalopram
d) Pseudoephedrine
e) Naproxen

37. Which of the following side effects is listed as a boxed warning for all anthracyclines?

a) Hepatoxicity
b) Neurotoxicity
c) Anemia
d) QT prolongation
e) Myocardial toxicity

38. What is the primary treatment for restless leg syndrome? (Select all that apply)

a) Mirapex®
b) Requip®
c) Neupogen®
d) Neurontin®
e) Anaprox®

39. A family comes to the pharmacy and requests a ODT formulation for GERD treatment in their infant who is unable to swallow tablets/capsules. Which of the following medications is available as an oral disintegrating tablet? (Select all that apply)

a) Omeprazole
b) Esomeprazole
c) Lansoprazole
d) Pantoprazole
e) Ranitidine

40. TM is a 42-year-old patient presenting for the first time with multiple loose stools after being on an intensive antibiotic therapy. TM's WBC count is less than 15,000 cells/mm^3 and SCr is less than 1.5 mg/dL. What is the most appropriate regimen for TM?

a) PO vancomycin 125mg QID as tapered regimen
b) PO vancomycin 125mg QID for 10 days
c) IV fidaxomicin 100mg BID for 10 days
d) PO fidaxomicin 100mg BID for 10 days
e) PO metronidazole 50mg BID for 10 days

41. Triumeq® is made up of which of the following combination drugs?

a) Bictegravir/ Emtracitibine / Tenofovir alafenamide
b) Dolutegravir / Abacavir / Lamivudine
c) Dolutegravir/ Emtracitibine/ Tenofovir alafenamide
d) Dolutegravir/ Lamivudine
e) Dolutegravir/Abacavir/ Tenofovir alafenamide

42. PJ is a 45-year-old patient urgently admitted to the hospital for severe hyperkalemia caused by taking potassium supplements with his ramipril. Which of the following interventions should be prioritized for PJ?

    a) Administer Sodium polystyrene sulfonate
    b) Administer furosemide
    c) Administer sodium bicarbonate
    d) Administer calcium gluconate
    e) Begin hemodialysis

43. Which of the following interventions removes potassium from the body as opposed to shifting potassium intracellularly? (Select all that apply)

    a) Furosemide
    b) Regular Insulin
    c) Dextrose
    d) Sodium polystyrene sulfonate
    e) Patiromer

44. Which of the following drugs does NOT require dose adjustment in renal impairment?

    a) Allopurinol
    b) Lithium
    c) Ranitidine
    d) Ciprofloxacin
    e) Doxycycline

45. What is the appropriate regimen of Bactrim DS for Pneumocystis Pneumonia (PCP) prophylaxis?

    a) 1 DS tablet daily
    b) 1 DS tablet BID
    c) 1 DS tablet TID
    d) 1 DS tablet QID
    e) 1 SS tablet BID

46. AG is a 52-year-old patient who presents to an outpatient clinic with shortness of breath and a fever of 102°F along with a productive cough. A chest X-ray revealed a right lower lobe infiltrate. What is the most appropriate empiric regimen in this outpatient with community acquired pneumonia?

    a) Rifampin
    b) Amoxicillin
    c) Cefazolin
    d) Ampicillin
    e) Moxifloxacin

47. TG is a 56-year-old patient who is taking simvastatin to control his cholesterol levels. Which of the following should TG avoid to prevent any interactions? (Select all that apply)

   a) Grapefruit
   b) Ritonavir
   c) Erythromycin
   d) Amlodipine
   e) Fluconazole

48. Which of the following side effects is listed as a boxed warning of ACE inhibitors?

   a) Hepatoxicity
   b) Neurotoxicity
   c) Nephrotoxicity
   d) Fetal toxicity
   e) QT prolongation

49. Which of the following are contraindications for the use of alteplase in acute ischemic stroke management? (Select all that apply)

   a) Active internal bleeding
   b) History of autoimmune disease
   c) History of recent stroke
   d) Sinus bradycardia
   e) Severe uncontrolled hypertension

50. What is the appropriate dose of enoxaparin for the prophylaxis of VTE?

   a) 10mg SC Q12H
   b) 40mg SC daily
   c) 20mg SC Q12H
   d) 20mg SC daily
   e) 30mg SC daily

Practice Test 7: 50 questions, Time: 60 minutes

1. A patient is currently taking warfarin for mitral valve replacement. The addition of which medication would cause a pharmacist to recommend a 50% decrease in the warfarin dose?
   a) Keppra
   b) Trazodone
   c) Nardil
   d) Pacerone
   e) Famotidine

2. Which of the following medications are CYP3A4 inhibitors? Select all that apply
   a) Lanoxin
   b) Neoral
   c) Cartia XT
   d) Modafanil
   e) Amiodarone

3. Which medications should not be taken concurrently with Nardil. Select all that apply.
   a) Flexeril
   b) Wellbutrin
   c) Dextromethorphan
   d) Elavil
   e) Prozac

4. A female patient at your pharmacy has been using an oral contraceptive for the past 2 years. She recently became pregnant despite using her oral contraceptive correctly after the addition of a new herbal supplement. Which of the following herbal supplements could have decreased the effectiveness of her contraceptive?
   a) St. John's Wort
   b) N-acetylcysteine
   c) Omega-3 fatty acids
   d) Black cohosh
   e) Calcium

5. Which of the following medications would require HLA-B*1501 testing before initiating? Select all that apply.
   a) Imuran
   b) Triumeq
   c) Carbamazepine
   d) Epzicom
   e) Trizivir

6. Which of the following antifungals inhibits P-glycoprotein?
   a) Micafungin
   b) Diflucan
   c) Vfend
   d) Noxafil
   e) Sporanox

7. Which of the following antifungals have pH dependent absorption? Select all that apply.
   a) Nizoral
   b) Diflucan
   c) Vfend
   d) Noxafil
   e) Sporanox

8. Which of the following medications would *not* be an appropriate first-line medication for a patient newly diagnosed with hypertension with no comorbidities?
   a) Norvasc
   b) Zestril
   c) Tenormin
   d) Avapro
   e) Altace

9. A patient is switching from warfarin to Eliquis. What INR must the patient be at or below to begin taking Eliquis?
   a) 3
   b) 2.5
   c) 2
   d) 1.5
   e) Baseline

10. Which of the following cardiac medications cannot be taken with Viagra?
    a) Bidil
    b) Toprol XL
    c) Aldactone
    d) Vasotec
    e) Entresto

11. Which cardiac arrythmia can be treated with adenosine?
    a) Atrial fibrillation
    b) Ventricular fibrillation
    c) Torsades de Pointes
    d) Paroxysmal supraventricular tachyarrhythmias
    e) Bradycardia

12. What is the dose of Activase for ischemic stroke?
    a) 0.75 mg/kg
    b) 0.9 mg/kg
    c) 0.9 mg/kg up to 90 mg
    d) 0.9 mg/kg up to 100 mg
    e) 1 mg/kg

13. Which of the following medications can cause drug induced hemolytic anemia? Select all that apply.
    a) Isoniazid
    b) Levodopa
    c) Carboplatin

d) Epogen
e) Rifampin

14. How long should a female patient avoid becoming pregnant after discontinuing therapy with Droxia?
    a) 30 days
    b) 60 days
    c) 90 days
    d) 180 days
    e) 1 year

15. Which of the following medications can cause a patient to experience visual color distortions?
    a) Humira
    b) Amiodarone
    c) Vfend
    d) Hydroxychloroquine
    e) Cialis

16. What is the INR goal of a patient that requires anticoagulation with warfarin for pulmonary arterial hypertension?
    a) 1.5 to 2.5
    b) 2 to 3
    c) 2.5 to 3.5
    d) 3 to 4
    e) Warfarin is never indicated for pulmonary arterial hypertension.

17. Which CYP enzyme does smoking tobacco induce?
    a) CYP3A4
    b) CYP2D6
    c) CYP2C9
    d) CYP1A2
    e) CYP2C19

18. Which injectable GLP-1 agonists are injected once weekly? Select all that apply.
    a) Trulicity
    b) Byetta
    c) Victoza
    d) Bydureon
    e) Ozempic

19. Which vaccines should not be given to a pregnant patient? Select all that apply.
    a) MMR
    b) Zostavax
    c) Vivotif
    d) YF-VAX
    e) Intranasal influenza vaccine

20. Which of the following vaccinations can only be given subcutaneously? Select all that apply.
    a) TdAP
    b) MMR

    c) YF-VAX
    d) Varivax
    e) Ixiaro

21. Which antibiotic is contraindicated if used concurrently with unfractionated heparin?
    a) Ceftriaxone
    b) Firvanq
    c) Orbactiv
    d) Bactrim
    e) Cubicin

22. Which of the following are indications for Flagyl? Select all that apply.
    a) Clostridium difficile infections
    b) Endocarditis
    c) Bacterial Vaginosis
    d) Trichomoniasis
    e) MRSA

23. At what weight is Plan-B (levonorgestrel) less effective?
    a) >150 lbs
    b) >165 lbs
    c) >175 lbs
    d) >200 lbs
    e) >250 lbs

24. Which of the following classes of medications can increase the risk of osteoporosis? Select all that apply.
    a) Depo-Provera
    b) Anticonvulsants
    c) Loop diuretics
    d) Calcium channel blockers
    e) Aromatase inhibitors
    f)

25. Which of the following medications are indicated for the treatment and prevention of osteoporosis?
    a) Fosamax
    b) Forteo
    c) Evista
    d) Prolia
    e) Duavee

26. Which of the following medications can worsen erectile dysfunction? Select all that apply.
    a) Venlafaxine
    b) Coreg
    c) Vancomycin
    d) Catapres
    e) Prozac

27. What equation is used to calculate carboplatin dosing?
    a) DuBois BSA Equation

b) Cockgroft Gault Equation
c) CKD-EPI Equation
d) Calvert Formula
e) Mosteller BSA Equation

28. What pharmacogenomic test must a chronic myelogenous leukemia patient have to begin treatment with Gleevec?
    a) BRAF V600E positive
    b) KRAS wildtype
    c) Philadelphia chromosome positive
    d) EGFR mutation positive
    e) ALK mutation positive

29. How far apart must stimulants be started after stopping an MAO inhibitor?
    a) 3 days
    b) 7 days
    c) 14 days
    d) 30 days
    e) Stimulants and MAO inhibitors may be taken together

30. Which of the following are MAO inhibitors?
    a) Marplan
    b) Zyban
    c) Nardil
    d) Emsam
    e) Anafranil

31. A pharmacist performing a double check on a prescription accidentally permits a high dose to a patient. Following the event, the Medication Safety Team reviews the incident and its cause. Which of the following describes a safety and evaluation process that the Medication Safety Team can perform to analyze the current pharmacy workflow for medication checks and identify areas of improvement to prevent similar incidents in the future?

    a) FMEA
    b) RCA
    c) CQI
    d) MERP
    e) REMS

32. If a filter is used for a CSP, which of the following is a test that must be done to determine the integrity of the filter used?

    a) Visual inspection
    b) UV light inspection
    c) Pyrogen test
    d) Bubble-point test
    e) None of the above

33. According to best safety practices recommended by ISMP, which of the following medications cannot be placed in an automated dispensing cabinet?

   a) A patient's home medication in an adult medicine unit
   b) Hydromorphone 10 mg/mL vials in a cardiac telemetry unit
   c) Amiodarone 600mg tablets in an adult medicine unit
   d) Pitocin 25 mcg unit doses (split from 100 mcg tablets) in a mother/baby unit
   e) Rocuronium 10mg/mL vials in a surgery unit

34. A 1-year-old patient is preparing for their heart transplant by ensuring all immunizations are up to date. Which of the following routine childhood immunizations is the **most important** for preventing infection in solid organ transplant patients?

   a) Hepatitis A
   b) Rotavirus
   c) DTap
   d) Hepatitis B
   e) Varicella

35. Which of the following spots can a Climera® patch be placed? Select **ALL** that apply.

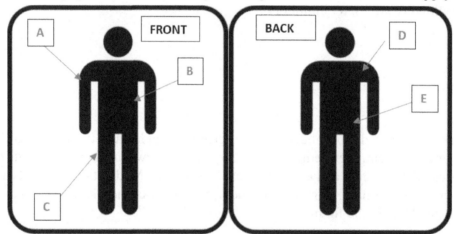

   a) A (upper arm)
   b) B (lower abdomen)
   c) C (thigh)
   d) D (shoulder)
   e) E (upper buttocks)

36. Which of the following spots can a Xulane® patch be placed? Select **ALL** that apply.

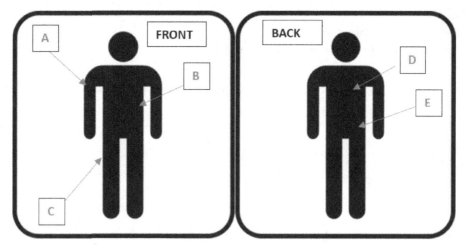

a) A (upper arm)
b) B (lower abdomen)
c) C (thigh)
d) D (back)
e) E (upper buttocks)

37. A 38-year-old patient is planning a climbing trip and expresses concerns about acute mountain sickness (AMS). Which of the following is recommended as primary prophylaxis for AMS?

a) Diamox®
b) Transderm Scop®
c) Dramamine®
d) Reglan®
e) Phenergen®

38. Which one of the following vaccines should be stored in a freezer? Select **ALL** that apply.

a) Zostavax®
b) Prevnar13®
c) Boostrix®
d) Gardisil-9®
e) Vaxchora®

39. Which of the following is not an early cancer warning sign based on recommendations from the ACS? Select **ALL** that apply.

a) Unusual bleeding
b) A sore with delayed healing
c) Nagging cough or hoarseness
d) Change in bowel habits
e) Unusually out of breath

40. Which of the following are high risk indicators for HIV infection? Select **ALL** that apply.

a) History of tuberculosis
b) History of hepatitis

c) History of SUD
d) Sexual history with multiple partners
e) Sexual history of possible exposure through bodily fluids

41. Which of the following is an example of a buffered temperature probe used for vaccine storage?

a) Glycol-encased probe
b) Glass thermometer
c) Electronic probc
d) Aluminum-encased probe
e) Sand-encased probe

42. A 38-year-old patient comes in with a recent diagnosis of heart failure with reduced ejection fraction (HFrEF). Patients should call their PCP in which of the following scenarios? Select **ALL** that apply.

a) Weight gain of 5 lbs in 1 week
b) Increased shortness of breath
c) Patient has just fainted
d) Patient is feeling confused
e) Increased coughing

43. An IV preparation of mitoxantrone would be which of the following colors?

a) Red
b) Yellow
c) Orange
d) Blue
e) Black

44. A neonate (29-week gestational age) is born with an initial APGAR score of 3, and a 5-minute APGAR score of 5. Per ACOG, what APGAR score range does not require additional medical intervention?

a) 5-10
b) 8-12
c) 7-10
d) 6-10
e) 9-12

45. Which type of hypersensitivity is being assessed with a penicillin test?

a) Type I
b) Type II
c) Type III
d) Type IV
e) None of the above

46. Which of the following drugs and genetic test pairings do not match? Select **ALL** that apply.

a) Plavix®-CYP2C9
b) Cerebyx®-HLA-B*1502
c) Tegretol®-HLA-B*1502
d) Trimumeg®-HLA-B*5701
e) Fluorouracil-DPD

47. Which of the following antipsychotic and boxed warning label pairings do not match? Select **ALL** that apply.

a) Thioridazine-QT prolongation
b) Clorazil®-QT prolongation
c) Clorazil®-Seizures
d) Haldol®-Increased risk of death in elderly patients
e) Zyprexa Relprev®-Delirium

48. Which of the following accurately describes the mechanism of action of Abilify®? Select **ALL** that apply.

f) D2 antagonist
g) D2 partial agonist
h) 5-HT1A partial agonist
i) 5-HT2A partial agonist
a) 5-HT2A antagonist

49. Which of the following will cause an increase in lithium levels?

a) Increased salt intake
b) Increased caffeine intake
c) NSAID use
d) Taking Prozac® concurrently with lithium
e) Taking carbamazepine concurrently with lithium

50. A 52-year-old patient is starting on a new drug regimen for weight loss. If they start their treatment weighing 230 lbs, which of the following should be their **minimum** weight loss goal before they should consider switching to a different medication?

a) 15 lbs in 4 weeks
b) 15 lbs in 8 weeks
c) 10 lbs in 10 weeks
d) 12 lbs in 12 weeks
e) 20 lbs in 12 weeks

Practice Test 8: 45 questions, Time: 55 minutes

1. A 34-year-old patient is picking up her son's prescription for Diastat Acudial®. Which of the following does not accurately describe a procedure for dispensing and administering the Diastat Acudial®?

a) Diastat Acudial® is a seizure-preventing medication for patients at risk of long-lasting seizures
b) Diastat Acudial® is packaged with two prefilled syringes
c) The pharmacist must dial the dose and lock the syringes before dispensing
d) Once a syringe is locked, it cannot be unlocked
e) The Diastat Acudial® syringe should be disposed of immediately after use in a garbage away from children

2. At which part of the nephron does Osmitrol® work?

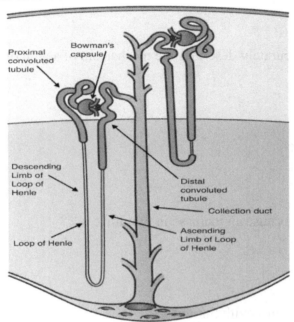

Image Credit: Kidney Nephron by Holly Fischer is licensed with CC BY 3.0 https://creativecommons.org /licenses/by/3.0

a) Descending Loop of Henle
b) Ascending Loop of Henle
c) Distal convoluted tubule
d) Proximal convoluted tubule
e) Bowman's capsule

3. A 34-year-old patient comes into the pharmacy to ask for an OTC product recommendation. The patient has a history of frequent headaches and occasional migraines. Initially, she started using Excedrin® to manage symptoms. However, over the past six weeks, she has used Excedrin® 4-5 times a week and continues to have daily headaches. She wonders if the pharmacy carries another alternative she can try. What advice should the pharmacist convey to the patient?

a) Continue to try Excedrin® for another three weeks to see if there is an improvement in the frequency of her headaches
b) Call PCP
c) Suggest a trial of CoQ10 supplements with the current Excedrin® regimen and see if the frequency of her headaches decreases
d) Reduce Excedrin® use to 2-3 times per week at the most

e) Suggest looking into Botox® injections for migraine prophylaxis

4. Which of the following references is used to help practitioners apply best vaccine practices?

a) CDC Yellow Book
b) CDC Pink Book
c) CDC Green Book
d) CDC Blue Book
e) CDC Purple Book

5. List the following 1st generation antipsychotics from the lowest to the highest level of potency.

a) Chlorpromazine
b) Loxapine
c) Perphenazine
d) Thioridazine
e) Haloperidol

6. A 92-year-old female patient walks up to the pharmacy counter and asks for an OTC recommendation to help alleviate her seasonal allergies. She identifies nasal congestion as the most bothersome symptom she seeks relief from. Which of the following drugs should be avoided?

a) Diphenhydramine
b) Claritin
c) Allegra
d) Saline nasal spray
e) Fluticasone nasal spray

7. A 50-year-old male patient is currently taking doxazosin. After a recent visit to his doctor, he receives a prescription for tadalafil. Which adverse event is most likely to become exacerbated as a result of this new addition?

a) Flatulence
b) Burping
c) Snoring
d) Dizziness
e) Increased blood pressure

8. A 33-year-old female who suffers from osteoporosis, diabetes, and hypothyroidism would like a recommendation regarding suitable birth control options. She is currently taking metformin, levothyroxine, and alendronate. She also mentions that she would like a fast return to fertility once she gets off of birth control, as she doesn't have much time left to bear children at her age. Which contraceptive method would NOT be appropriate for her?

a) Seasonique
b) Nexplanon
c) Yaz
d) Depo-Provera injection
e) Yasmin

9. A patient's medication profile contains aspirin, hydrochlorothiazide, metformin, furosemide, valproic acid, levothyroxine, and docusate. Which medications can increase his uric acid level? Select all that apply.

a) Aspirin
b) Furosemide
c) Hydrochlorothiazide
d) Docusate
e) Metformin

10. A patient's medication profile contains metformin, rosuvastatin, spironolactone, lisinopril, BiDil, and metoprolol succinate. He walks up to the pharmacy counter and hands you a prescription for Viagra. What is your main concern?

a) No concerns, fill the prescription
b) The patient is on BiDil, which is contraindicated with Viagra
c) The patient is on spironolactone, which is contraindicated with Viagra
d) You should recommend that he only take half a tablet of Viagra per day
e) There is a boxed warning for an increased risk of death

11. Which of the following criteria warrant a dose reduction of Eliquis for stroke prevention in the setting of atrial fibrillation? Select all that apply.

a) Age ≥ 80 years
b) Age ≥ 70 years
c) CrCl < 60 mL/min
d) SCr ≥ 1.5 mg/dL
e) A body weight < 65kg

12. You are a clinical pharmacist at a hospital. A 25-year-old female is admitted after suffering a fall at her house. She complains of some nausea and dizziness. While reviewing the patient's profile, you note that she is HCG-positive. What is your recommendation for anticoagulation therapy?

a) Warfarin
b) Lovenox
c) Heparin
d) Pradaxa
e) Bivalirudin

13. A 20-year-old female was recently diagnosed with epilepsy. Her medication profile includes Jolessa, carbamazepine, and metformin. Which of the following are important counseling points that the patient should be made aware of? Select all that apply.

a) Carbamazepine causes hyponatremia; monitor sodium electrolytes
b) Carbamazepine decreases the effectiveness of Jolessa
c) Carbamazepine is a CYP 3A4 inducer
d) Carbamazepine increases the effectiveness of Jolessa
e) Carbamazepine is a CYP 3A4 inhibitor

14. A patient wishes to receive the Zoster vaccine. He informs you that he has undergone IVIG treatment about a week ago. What should you do next? Select all that apply.

   a) One week has passed; he can receive the vaccine
   b) Refuse to administer the vaccine
   c) Inform him that he must wait for at least 3 months to receive this vaccine
   d) Inform him that he must wait for at least 2 weeks to receive this vaccine
   e) Inform him that he must wait for at least 4 weeks to receive this vaccine

15. A patient with type II diabetes is complaining of severe diarrhea that is interfering with his quality of life. His current medication profile includes lisinopril, metformin, and simvastatin. What can be done to help this patient?

   a) Change simvastatin to pravastatin
   b) Titrate the metformin dose down, then go up as tolerated
   c) Titrate the metformin dose up, then go down as needed
   d) Change simvastatin to atorvastatin
   e) Change lisinopril to irbesartan

16. You are a clinical pharmacist rounding with the internal medicine team at St. Mary's hospital. The team is discussing a particular heart failure patient that does not appear to be improving despite multiple treatment attempts. His current medications include carvedilol, bumetanide, Vasotec, heparin, and Bactrim. The attending physician asks you for your opinion on initiating spironolactone. What are your thoughts? (Current Labs: K=6 mmol/L, Na=140 meq/L, Ca=9 mg/dl)

   a) The patient is not a candidate given his increased potassium levels
   b) The patient is a candidate given his uncontrolled symptoms of fluid overload
   c) Recommend he switches the patient to Entresto (36-hour washout period)
   d) Recommend he discontinues carvedilol, as it is not appropriate for heart failure
   e) Recommend he initiates atenolol

17. A 45-year old male with hypertension, diabetes, hyperlipidemia, and hypothyroidism was just admitted to the hospital for a hypertensive crisis. He is allergic to sulfa (anaphylaxis) and eggs (rash). His medication profile includes lisinopril, levothyroxine, rosuvastatin, and Lantus. Once he is stabilized, the doctor would like to optimize the patient's drug regimen by adding a second anti-hypertensive agent. Which of the following choices would not be appropriate? Select all that apply.

   a) Amlodipine
   b) Hydrochlorothiazide
   c) Valsartan
   d) Diltiazem
   e) Zestoretic

18. Despite your best efforts to persuade the doctor, a patient was placed on theophylline for asthma. As a pharmacist, you are aware that theophylline is a drug that can lower seizure thresholds. Which other medication would put the patient at a heightened risk of experiencing a seizure?

   a) Doxycycline

b) Lisinopril
c) Valsartan
d) Buprenorphine
e) Minoxidil

19. You are in charge of monitoring an epileptic patient who is currently on IV phenytoin while inpatient. What is the therapeutic range of phenytoin?

a) 5-10 mcg/mL
b) 10-20 mcg/mL
c) 20-25 mcg/mL
d) 25-35 mcg/mL
e) 35-40 mcg/mL

20. You are in charge of monitoring the serum theophylline levels of a newly admitted patient at the hospital. What is the therapeutic range of theophylline?

a) 5-15 mcg/mL
b) 6-16 mcg/mL
c) 7-17 mcg/mL
d) 8-18 mcg/mL
e) 15-20 mcg/mL

21. You are asked about the dose of Lovenox to treat a DVT in a patient with a CrCl=22. Which one of the following doses is appropriate for this patient?

a) 40 mg SQ qd
b) 30 mg SQ q12h
c) 30 mg SQ qd
d) 1 mg/kg q12h
e) 1 mg/kg q24h

22. You are asked about heparin prophylaxis for a patient with a CrCl=80. Which one of the following doses is appropriate for this patient?

a) 1000 U q8-12h
b) 2000 U q8-12h
c) 3000 U q8-12h
d) 4000 U q8-12h
e) 5000 U q8-12h

23. A pregnant patient asks for your recommendation for a painkiller. She states that her head is throbbing from a headache that started earlier this morning. What is the most appropriate OTC choice for pain relief in this case?

a) Imitrex
b) Codeine
c) Aspirin
d) Acetaminophen

e) Advil

24. A patient's medication profile includes digoxin, metformin, metoprolol, theophylline, Yasmin, and levothyroxine. She begins to experience blurry vision, yellow halos, nausea, vomiting, and confusion. Which medication is most likely the cause of this toxicity?

a) Metformin
b) Levothyroxine
c) Theophylline
d) Digoxin
e) Metoprolol

25. A patient's medication profile includes metformin, metoprolol, theophylline, Jolessa, clopidogrel, and levothyroxine. He is complaining of some acid reflux. His doctor gave him a prescription for Prilosec. What should you do? Select all that apply.

a) Fill it, there are no drug interactions
b) Do not fill, there is an interaction between Prilosec and clopidogrel
c) Recommend famotidine instead of Prilosec
d) Recommend Nexium instead of Prilosec
e) Tell the patient to just deal with it

26. Which of the following medications do not require shaking prior to use? Select all that apply.

a) Flovent HFA
b) Serevent Diskus
c) QVAR RediHaler
d) Breo Ellipta
e) Dulera

27. This medication is contraindicated in moderate to severe liver impairment.

a) Atrovent HFA
b) Anoro Ellipta
c) Brovana
d) Daliresp
e) Spiriva HandiHaler

28. Which of the following medications is administered by turning the clear base until it clicks, opening the cap and closing your lips around the mouthpiece, and then pressing the dose-release button and inhaling?

a) Striverdi Respimat
b) Trelegy Ellipta
c) Spiriva HandiHaler
d) Incruse Ellipta
e) Atrovent HFA

29. Which of the following are MDIs? Select all that apply.

a) Arcapta Neohaler

b) Incruse Ellipta
c) Stiolto Respimat
d) Turdoza Pressair
e) Alvesco

30. Which of the following is not a side effect of Perforomist?

a) Nervousness
b) Tremor
c) Oral candidiasis
d) Decreased potassium level
e) Coughing

31. How often should the Combivent Respimat mouthpiece be cleaned?

a) Daily
b) Every three days
c) Weekly
d) Every two weeks
e) Monthly

32. Which of the following medications has a lower risk for GI complications, but an increased risk for MI/stroke?

a) Voltaren
b) Aleve
c) Toradol
d) Ecotrin
e) Yosprala

33. Which of the following medications have a black box warning to not consume alcohol while taking the drug, as it can result in fatal drug plasma levels? Select all that apply.

a) Duragesic
b) Kadian
c) Oxymorphone ER
d) Norco
e) Zohydro ER

34. A patient with a documented drug allergy to Norco is being treated for pain. Which of the following is an acceptable treatment option?

a) Oxycontin
b) Kadian
c) Vicodin
d) Dolophine
e) Dilaudid

35. Which of the following analgesics have a risk of causing seizures? Select all that apply.

a) Ultram
b) Movantik

c) Dolophine
d) Demerol
e) Sublimaze

36. Which of the following is a permitted adhesive film dressing for Duragesic?

a) Tape
b) Tegaderm
c) Bioclear
d) Alfenta
e) Dsuvia

37. What is the brand name for dolutegravir/abacavir/lamivudine?

a) Dovato
b) Biktarvy
c) Genvoya
d) Juluca
e) Triumeq

38. Which of the following is a single tablet HIV regimen?

a) Symfi
b) Norvir
c) Prezista
d) Isentress
e) Retrovir

39. Which of the following is an NRTI?

a) Isentress
b) Tivicay
c) Reyataz
d) Viread
e) Sustiva

40. Which medication is often capped at 2 mg/dose?

a) Vincristine
b) Vinblastine
c) Xeloda
d) Trexall
e) Bleomycin

41. All the following are considered crystalloids except which solution?

a) D5W
b) Normal saline
c) Dextran
d) Plasma-Lyte
e) Lactated Ringer's

42. What is a suitable alternative for Alzheimer's patients experiencing GI side effects from Aricept? Select all that apply.

   a) Exelon patch
   b) Namenda
   c) Aricept ODT
   d) Sinemet CR
   e) Mirapex ER

43. Which of the following drugs can lower the seizure threshold? Select all that apply.

   a) Plavix
   b) Wellbutrin
   c) Ultram
   d) AndroGel
   e) Levaquin

44. SP reported anaphylaxis after taking Zosyn. Which of the following medications should be avoided? Select all that apply.

   a) Vancocin
   b) Primaxin
   c) Invanz
   d) Zyvox
   e) Flagyl

45. Which of the following is an antidote used to reverse the effects of warfarin?

   a) Protamine sulfate
   b) Praxbind
   c) Andexxa
   d) Mephyton
   e) Six-Factor Prothrombin Complex Concentrate

2023-2024 Practice NAPLEX® Exam

This section will consist of a 250-question practice exam. You should consider this the real deal and time yourself as if you are taking the actual exam. We have tried our best to ensure this practice exam reflects highly on the actual NAPLEX® exam. It is advised to provide yourself 5 hours to take this exam to allow a 30-minute buffer time. Good luck!

2023-2024 Practice NAPLEX® Exam: 250 Questions, 5 hours

1. Which of the following statements concerning lithium and drug interactions are true? (Select **ALL** that apply.)

   a) Lithium is a relatively safe drug in elderly patients if the serum creatinine is below 1 g/dL
   b) Lithium is not considered serotonergic and can be mixed safely with meperidine, but not with tramadol
   c) Increased salt intake increases serum lithium levels
   d) If a drug has a high degree of nephrotoxicity, it will likely not be a safe option in a patient using chronic lithium therapy
   e) Lithium is not metabolized; it is excreted renally

2. Amiodarone is both a substrate and an inhibitor of CYP450 2C9, 2D6, and 3A4. Which of the following medications must have their doses reduced when prescribed with amiodarone? (Select **ALL** that apply.)

   a) Quinidine
   b) Warfarin
   c) Lithium
   d) Pravastatin
   e) Digoxin

3. Which drugs exhibit sorption issues? (Select **ALL** that apply.)

   a) Regular human insulin
   b) Tacrolimus
   c) Paclitaxel
   d) Nitroglycerin
   e) Etoposide

4. Ash has a history of atrial fibrillation and is picking up moxifloxacin. He is currently taking atorvastatin, amiodarone, Januvia®, Byetta®, and metformin. Which of the following can be caused by potential drug interactions? (Select **ALL** that apply.)

   a) QT prolongation
   b) Impaired absorption of moxifloxacin
   c) Hypoglycemia or hyperglycemia
   d) Peripheral edema, fluid retention due to quinolone addition
   e) Additive nephrotoxicity

5. Which of the following sections of the US Pharmacopoeia (USP) National Formulary includes standards for sterile compounding?

   a) USP 790
   b) USP 795
   c) USP 797
   d) USP 875
   e) USP 890

6. What is the brand for olanzapine?

   a) Zyprexa®
   b) Zygonda®
   c) Zyloprim®
   d) Zylox®
   e) Zyzez®

7. What is the generic for Calan® and its mechanism of action?

   a) Losartan; Angiotensin Receptor Blocker
   b) Lisinopril; Angiotensin Converting Enzyme Inhibitor
   c) Verapamil; Calcium Channel Blocker
   d) Amlodipine; Calcium Channel Blocker
   e) Diltiazem; Calcium Channel Blocker

8. What is the generic name of Tradjenta® and its mechanism of action?

   a) Linagliptin; DPP-4 inhibitor
   b) Saxagliptin; DPP-4 inhibitor
   c) Sitagliptin; DPP-4 inhibitor
   d) Alogliptin; DPP-4 inhibitor
   e) None of the above

9. What is the generic name of Onglyza® and its mechanism of action?

   a) Linagliptin; DPP-4 inhibitor
   b) Saxagliptin; DPP-4 inhibitor
   c) Sitagliptin; DPP-4 inhibitor
   d) Alogliptin; DPP-4 inhibitor
   e) None of the above

10. What is the generic name of Januvia® and its mechanism of action?

   a) Linagliptin; DPP-4 inhibitor
   b) Saxagliptin; DPP-4 inhibitor
   c) Sitagliptin; DPP-4 inhibitor
   d) Alogliptin; DPP-4 inhibitor
   e) None of the above

11. A patient is picking up a prescription for erythromycin ethylsuccinate (E.E.S.) oral suspension. Which of the following statements is correct?

   a) This medication cannot be used if the patient has a penicillin allergy
   b) This medication should not be administered with food
   c) This medication is a major inhibitor of cytochrome P450 2C9
   d) This medication is effective for treating the flu
   e) This medication should be refrigerated

12. Of the following oral suspension antibiotics, which one should not be refrigerated?

   a) Augmentin®
   b) Pen VK
   c) Ceftin®
   d) Keflex®
   e) Biaxin®

13. Which of the following IV agents are not refrigerated? (Select **ALL** that apply.)

   a) Ceftriaxone
   b) Cefazolin
   c) Moxifloxacin
   d) Phenylephrine
   e) Bactrim®

14. Which of the following statements concerning IV medications are correct? (Select **ALL** that apply.)

   a) Furosemide and metronidazole IV bags are not refrigerated
   b) Phenytoin IV requires a filter due to the potential for precipitation
   c) Sulfamethoxazole/trimethoprim and phenytoin IV are diluted with NS only
   d) Phenytoin IV has a maximum infusion rate of 50 mg/min
   e) Metronidazole IV does not require protection from light

15. What is the rationale of combination therapy with hydralazine and isosorbide dinitrate in management of patients with heart failure?

   a) Isosorbide dinitrate relieves chest pain, hydralazine reduces preload
   b) Isosorbide dinitrate decreases afterload, hydralazine reduces preload
   c) Isosorbide dinitrate and hydralazine both decrease preload
   d) Isosorbide dinitrate and hydralazine both decrease afterload
   e) Isosorbide dinitrate decreases preload, hydralazine decreases afterload

16. Which of the following anticonvulsants is the drug of choice for treatment of trigeminal neuralgia?

   a) Valproate
   b) Primidone
   c) Phenobarbital
   d) Diazepam

e) Carbamazepine

17. Which of the following anti-retroviral drugs can be used in pediatric patients?

   a) Amprenavir
   b) Atazanavir
   c) Emtricitabine
   d) Raltegravir
   e) Tipranavir

18. Which is used in a bronchial challenge test (bronchoprovocation)?

   a) Acetylcholine
   b) Bethanechol
   c) Carbachol
   d) Plasma cholinesterase
   e) Methacholine

19. A patient has tested positive for the HLA-B*5701 allele. Which of the following statements is correct?

   a) The patient can receive Epzicom®
   b) The patient cannot be dispensed Ziagen®
   c) The patient can receive Trizivir®
   d) The patient would be expected to launch an aggressive immune response against HIV
   e) The patient is not at risk for hypersensitivity reactions

20. What is the generic of Reyataz® and its mechanism of action?

   a) Abacavir; NRTI
   b) Atazanavir; protease inhibitor
   c) Atonavir; protease inhibitor
   d) Nelfinavir; entry inhibitor
   e) Darunavir; protease inhibitor

21. What is the generic of Complera®?

   a) Efavirenz/emtricitabine/tenofovir DF
   b) Rilpivirine/emtricitabine/tenofovir DF
   c) Elvitegravir/cobicistat/emtricitabine/tenofovir alafenamide
   d) Elvitegravir/cobicistat/emtricitabine/tenofovir DF
   e) Dolutegravir/abacavir/lamivudine

22. Jesse is a 41-year-old male who is HIV positive and has reduced renal function with a CrCl of 24 mL/min who is on hemodialysis. He is currently taking Genvoya® with Prezista®. Which of the following is false? (Select **ALL** that apply.)

   a) The patient cannot take Genvoya® and needs to switch to an alternative agent
   b) The patient can be switched to Truvada®
   c) The patient can continue his Genvoya® and Prezista® regimen

    d) The patient can be switched to Atripla®
    e) Cobicistat in Genvoya® should not be given less than 70 mL/min

23. What is the generic name for Selzentry® and what is the binding target and host?

    a) Maraviroc; CCR4/CXCR4 on Human CD4 cells
    b) Maraviroc; CCR5 on Human CD4 cells
    c) Maraviroc; CCR5 on HIV virus
    d) Maraviroc; CCR4/CXCR4 on HIV virus
    e) Maraviroc; CCR6 on HIV virus

24. What is the benefit of adding Norvir® to an HIV regimen? (Select **ALL** that apply.)

    a) Blocks first pass metabolism
    b) Leads to higher concentrations of other HIV medications in regimen
    c) Blockage of GLUT4 insulin-regulated transporter
    d) At high doses, it can enhance other protease inhibitors
    e) It inhibits the major P450 enzymes 3A4 and 2D6

25. A patient is prescribed Atripla®. What are the components of Atripla®?

    a) Efavirenz, etravirine, delavirdine
    b) Efavirenz, elvitegravir, rilpivirine
    c) Emtricitabine, rilpivirine, tenofovir
    d) Emtricitabine, efavirenz, tenofovir
    e) Emtricitabine, tenofovir

26. Which of the following statements are true about HIV pre-exposure prophylaxis? (Select **ALL** that apply.)

    a) An individual who does not have HIV can take one Truvada® tablet daily to reduce his risk of becoming infected.
    b) An individual who has HIV can take one Atripla® tablet daily to reduce his risk of transmitting the virus
    c) The individual must be at a very high risk for acquiring HIV in order to be a candidate for pre-exposure prophylaxis
    d) The HIV test must be taken weekly when using pre-exposure prophylaxis therapy
    e) Once treatment is initiated, the individual no longer needs to follow safe sex practices

27. Which of the following HIV drugs needs to be refrigerated? (Select **ALL** that apply.)

    a) Fuzeon® once mixed
    b) Norvir® liquid
    c) Epivir® liquid
    d) Aptivus® + Norvir® before opening package
    e) Norvir® capsules

28. A patient in the critical care unit is receiving Precedex® for sedation. Which of the following statements concerning Precedex® is correct?

    a) It is reconstituted in dextrose solutions only
    b) Precedex® should only be given if a patient is also receiving a paralytic
    c) Precedex® is an alpha-2-adrenergic antagonist
    d) The maximum infusion duration is 48 hours
    e) Patients are more easily arousable and alert when stimulated, compared to propofol

29. What is the formulation of propofol?

    a) Oil-in-water emulsion
    b) Water-in-oil emulsion
    c) Suspension
    d) Water-soluble prodrug
    e) Solubilized in Cremophor EL®

30. A pharmacist is preparing an IVIG infusion. Which of the following statements is incorrect?

    a) If the patient experiences side effects such as nausea or a drop in blood pressure during the infusion, slowing the infusion rate may be helpful
    b) IVIG may come already in solution, or it may come as a powder that is reconstituted with diluent
    c) The IVIG dose is based on the Ideal Body Weight (IBW)
    d) If particles are present, the pharmacist should shake well to dissolve the particles prior to the infusion
    e) Certain patients respond to one IVIG brand better than another

31. You have a vial that contains 5 grams of drug and the chart to the right for mixing the drug for use. Nurses want to mix the vial so that it comes out with 200 mg per mL and ask you how much diluent they should add to make that concentration? (Round the answer to the nearest **tenths**.)

Diluent added	Final Concentration
9.6 mL	500 mg per mL
19.6 mL	250 mg per mL
49.6 mL	100 mg per mL

32. A bottle is labeled 0.89 PPM of Drug X. How many liters of this solution will contain 5 mg of Drug X? (Round the answer to the nearest **tenths**.)

33. A patient with recently diagnosed active tuberculosis was prescribed isoniazid, rifampin, pyrazinamide and ethambutol. Which vitamin supplement is recommended with this regimen?

   a) Vitamin B1
   b) Vitamin B12
   c) Vitamin B2
   d) Vitamin B3
   e) Vitamin B6

34. What condition may be caused by a lack of vitamin B12 deficiency? Select all that apply.

   a) Microcytic anemia
   b) Macrocytic anemia
   c) Pernicious anemia
   d) Fanconi anemia
   e) Myelophthisic anemia

35. What is benzyl alcohol used for compounding?

   a) Preservative
   b) Binding agent
   c) Stabilizer
   d) Antioxidant
   e) Distillant

36. Where can a patient apply testosterone gel? Click to select on the following image.

37. A 78-year-old 135-pound male is hospitalized with a deep vein thromboembolism (DVT). He is receiving unfractionated heparin for DVT treatment. What does should he receive?

   a) Administer 4900 units IV bolus, then 1100 units/hour continuous infusion
   b) Administer 5000 units IV bolus, then 1300 units/hour continuous infusion
   c) Administer 5000 units SC every 8 to 12 hours
   d) Administer 7500 units SC every 12 hours
   e) Administer 8000-10,000 units IV initially, then 50-70 units/kg Q4-6 hours

38. Which of the following statements regarding the drug interaction between valproic acid and lamotrigine is correct? (Select **ALL** that apply.)

    a) Valproic acid inhibits lamotrigine metabolism
    b) This interaction increases the risk for a severe lamotrigine-induced rash
    c) This interaction increases the risk for severe valproate-induced pancreatitis
    d) When using these two medications concurrently, the *Lamictal Dose Titration* pack® cannot be used; lower doses will be required
    e) This interaction increases the risk for severe valproate-induced hepatotoxicity

39. Which of the following statements concerning IV medications are correct? (Select **ALL** that apply.)

    a) Flolan® and moxifloxacin IV bags are not refrigerated
    b) Lorazepam IV requires a filter due to the potential for precipitation
    c) Sulfamethoxazole/trimethoprim and phenytoin IV are diluted with NS only
    d) Fosphenytoin IV has a maximum infusion rate of 150 mg/min
    e) Doxycycline IV does not require protection from light

40. What are possible complications with long-term phenytoin therapy? (Select **ALL** that apply.)

    a) Hirsutism
    b) Skin thickening (children)
    c) Shrinkage/atrophy of dental gum tissue
    d) Osteoporosis
    e) Hypertension

41. Which of the following anti-retroviral drugs would need dosage adjustment in patients with renal impairment?

    a) Tipranavir
    b) Raltegravir
    c) Emtricitabine
    d) Atazanavir
    e) Amprenavir

42. Which of the following is the most potent inhibitor of CYP2D6?

    a) Fluoxetine
    b) Paroxetine
    c) Fluvoxamine
    d) Quinidine
    e) Ketoconazole

43. Which of the following enzymes or transporters is implicated in drug interactions with raltegravir?

    a) CYP3A4
    b) UGT1A1
    c) P-GP
    d) N-Acetyltransferase
    e) Glutathione transferase

44. Which of the following antimicrobial agents is a useful alternative to vancomycin in treatment of MRSA infection?

    a) Clindamycin
    b) Metronidazole
    c) Penicillin
    d) Azithromycin
    e) Linezolid

45. Which of the following drugs can be used to reverse apnea and coma in a patient with opioid toxicity?

    a) Codeine
    b) Naloxone
    c) Methadone
    d) Pentazocine
    e) Nucynta

46. Patient AJG arrived amidst a severe depressive episode. Patient self-discontinued use of paroxetine and lithium due to the side effects, as well as the need for therapeutic drug monitoring

    Patient Name: AJG   **Age:** 28 **Sex:** Male   **Race:** Caucasian   **Height:** 5' 10"
    Weight: 76 kg   **Family history**: None   **Allergies:** NKDA

    PMH: 5 year standing diagnosis of bipolar disorder, relapse of bipolar disorder
    MEDICATIONS: None upon admission

    Which of the following is appropriate dosage regimen for each of the listed medications?

    a) Lithium 3000 to 4000 mg per day
    b) Valproic acid 300 to 600 mg per day
    c) Lamotrigine 150 to 400 mg per day
    d) Risperidone 30 to 60 mg per day
    e) Topiramate 1000 to 2000 mg per day

47. A 68-year-old man with chronic lymphocytic leukemia was asymptomatic up until 3 months ago, when he started to develop increasing night sweats, fatigue, and weight loss. He also complains of easy bruising. Current labs include Hgb 8 g/dL and platelets of 50,000/dL. His past medical history is significant for hypertension, which is treated with diltiazem and hydrochlorothiazide, and benign prostatic hypertrophy, which is treated with tamsulosin. His doctor is about to start him on alemtuzumab.

    Which regimen is indicated in prophylaxis of infections caused by this agent?

    a) Trimethoprim/sulfamethoxazole and famciclovir
    b) Trimethoprim/sulfamethoxazole, fluconazole, and acyclovir
    c) No prophylaxis required
    d) Ganciclovir and levofloxacin
    e) Ganciclovir and fluconazole

48. A 23-year-old white female who is sexually active with multiple partners presents after noticing postcoital vaginal bleed. Her last pap smear was performed 3 years ago, and was found to be normal. A mass lesion is visualized on the cervix. Further workup and cone biopsy of this lesion demonstrated locally advanced cervical cancer.

    Which vaccine that is currently available could have prevented this patient's condition?

    a) HSV vaccine
    b) DTaP vaccine
    c) Yellow fever vaccine
    d) HPV vaccine
    e) Flu vaccine

49. Which of the following statements describing pertinent pharmacokinetic and pharmacodynamic measures for different antibacterial agents is true?

    a) AUC:MIC ratio is an appropriate measure for macrolides
    b) Time > MIC is an appropriate measure for beta-lactams
    c) AUC:MIC ratio is an appropriate measure for beta-lactams
    d) Time > MIC is an appropriate measure for aminoglycosides
    e) Time > MIC is an appropriate measure for azalides

50. DS is a 76-year-old male with a prior history of HTN and hyperlipidemia admitted yesterday to the CCU following a large anterior-wall MI. Current medications include: ASA 325 mg po daily, nitroglycerin 0.4 mg SL prn, metoprolol 50 mg po BID, ramipril 5 mg po daily, and atorvastatin 20 mg po daily. Overnight, DS began experiencing runs of PVCs at a ventricular rate of 80 bpm despite his current therapy. A previous echo estimates an LVEF of 50%. The medical intern rotating through the CCU asks if metoprolol should be switched to sotalol to control PVC's.

DS converts to normal sinus rhythm. Approximately 1 hour later the team observes a "party streamer-like" wave-pattern on the EKG. What is now the drug of choice for DS?

a) Magnesium 2 g IV bolus
b) Epinephrine 1 mg IV bolus
c) Warfarin 5 mg PO daily
d) Amiodarone 300 mg IV bolus
e) Sotalol 50 mg PO daily

51. Which of the following is the regimen of choice for treatment of infection caused by *Clostridium difficile*?

a) Intravenous vancomycin 1 g q12h
b) Oral loperamide 4 mg 4 times daily
c) Oral vancomycin 125 mg 4 times daily
d) Oral metronidazole 500 mg 3 times daily
e) Intravenous vancomycin 1 g q6h

52. Which of the following medications can interact with vitamin D?

a) Aspirin
b) Orlistat
c) Vitamin C
d) Digoxin
e) Lidocaine

53. A patient is diagnosed with anxiety disorder and complains of the inability to fall asleep at night. Which hypnotic drug is most appropriate for this patient?

a) Triazolam
b) Zolpidem
c) Flurazepam
d) Ramelteon
e) Diphenhydramine

54. The antifungal agent ketoconazole is sometimes combined with cyclosporine to achieve which of the following therapeutic goals?

a) Increase cyclosporine levels
b) Reduce cyclosporine exposure
c) Reduce white blood cell count
d) Reduce infection potential

e) Reduce cyclosporine-related GI toxicity

55. A patient is receiving high-dose methotrexate and the nurse is about the start administering leucovorin rescue therapy. Which of the following statements is correct regarding the administration of leucovorin?

a) Leucovorin should be administered concurrently with methotrexate
b) Leucovorin should not be administered at a rate >160 mg/min
c) Leucovorin should not be given with high-dose methotrexate (only low dose)
d) Leucovorin can be given with 72 hours of methotrexate
e) Leucovorin may increase the side effects of methotrexate

56. The physician is unable to obtain CSF after multiple attempts. Based on clinical findings, the team believes that the 13-day-old former 35-week gestational age baby may have meningitis. What is the best empirical therapy to begin in this baby before sending her to a pediatric hospital?

a) Ampicillin and gentamicin
b) Ceftriaxone and gentamicin
c) Vancomycin and cefotaxime
d) Ampicillin and ceftriaxone
e) Cephalexin and ampicillin

57. Jamie is a 20-year-old female patient who received kidney transplantation 3 months ago. She fills her prescription for tacrolimus, mycophenolate sodium, and prednisone at your pharmacy.

Which of the following represents two adverse effects specific to corticosteroids Jamie may experience?

a) Diarrhea and leukopenia
b) Alopecia and hyperglycemia
c) Water retention and osteoporosis
d) Hirsutism and nephrotoxicity
e) Blood in urine and bruising

58. A physician decides to start a 66-year-old woman on vancomycin, ampicillin, and ceftriaxone, but the patient has a history of difficult IV access. Which of the following is an appropriate plan for treatment of this patient's bacterial meningitis?

a) Attempt immediate IV-line placement and administer antibiotics IV for the duration of therapy
b) Administer antibiotics orally for the duration of therapy
c) Administer antibiotics intramuscularly for the duration of therapy
d) Immediately insert an external ventricular drain into the brain and administer antibiotics intraventricularly for the duration of therapy
e) Administer antibiotics rectally for the duration of therapy

59. Which of the following medications should be given to a patient before administering paclitaxel?

a) Colony stimulating factors (e.g., filgrastim)
b) Diphenhydramine, dexamethasone, ranitidine
c) Amifostine

    d) Dexrazoxane

    e) Neulasta®

60. Which of the following combinations of antiretrovirals should be **avoided**? (Select **ALL** that apply.)

    a) Rilpivirine and tenofovir

    b) Efavirenz and nevirapine

    c) Lamivudine and zidovudine

    d) Fosamprenavir and ritonavir

    e) Truvada® and Atripla®

61. Which of the following antineoplastics can cause a disulfiram-like reaction when a patient drinks alcohol?

    a) Cisplatin

    b) Methotrexate

    c) Procarbazine

    d) Hydroxyurea

    e) Fluorouracil

62. A treatment experienced patient receiving atazanavir therapy should avoid the addition of which of the following medications? (Select **ALL** that apply.)

    a) Omeprazole

    b) Metronidazole

    c) Pravastatin

    d) Metoprolol

    e) Pantoprazole

63. JL is a 47-year-old Caucasian man who reports to his primary care physician complaining of a 2-week history of fatigue and fever. A CBC with differential reveals an elevated WBC (35,000 U/L) and profound thrombocytopenia (platelets 30,000 U/L). The patient is diagnosed with acute myeloid leukemia (AML-M4). Initial induction therapy should consist which of the following?

    a) Mitoxantrone

    b) Cytarabine + idarubicin

    c) Cytarabine + imatinib

    d) Asparaginase

    e) Avastin®

64. The diagnostic criterion for which of the following opportunistic infections is seropositive for immunoglobulin G (IgG)?

    a) Candidiasis

    b) Toxoplasmosis

    c) MAC

    d) PCP

    e) IgE

65. Ryan is an HIV patient on the following medications: simvastatin, pantoprazole, TMP/SMZ, and as needed ibuprofen. Because his CD4 count has decreased, he is to be placed on MAC primary prophylaxis. Which of the following medications may be utilized for MAC prophylaxis? (Select **ALL** that apply.)

    a) Azithromycin
    b) Clarithromycin
    c) Clindamycin
    d) Clotrimazole
    e) Metronidazole

66. A 4-year-old girl with no significant past medical history is admitted for suspected bacterial meningitis and started on empirical therapy with ceftriaxone and vancomycin. What is the purpose of adding vancomycin to this empirical regimen for bacterial meningitis?

    a) To provide coverage against resistant *Listeria monocytogenes*
    b) To provide coverage against resistant *Neisseria meningitidis*
    c) To provide coverage against resistant *Streptococcus pneumoniae*
    d) Vancomycin is not needed in a 4-year-old with bacterial meningitis because *Staphylococcus aureus* is unlikely
    e) This patient needs *C. difficile* coverage

67. A 70-year-old man presents with fever, nausea, vomiting, severe headache, and extreme photophobia. CSF results: WBC 2500 cells/mm^3, 87% neutrophils, glucose 37 mg/dL, and protein 240 mg/dL. What type of CNS infection is considered based upon the information provided?

    a) Bacterial meningitis
    b) Aseptic meningitis
    c) Viral meningitis
    d) HSV encephalitis
    e) Fungal meningitis

68. A 12-year-old boy presents to his pediatrician for a routine follow-up visit. The patient denies having any complaints. Physical exam, vital signs, and laboratory values are all within normal limits. Which of the following vaccinations should the patient receive today as part of routine care for a healthy adolescent?

    a) PPSV23
    b) PPSV15
    c) MPSV4
    d) MCV4
    e) PCV13

69. A 70-year-old patient with bacterial meningitis has a penicillin allergy but no signs of shortness of breath or respiratory distress. How would you treat this patient?

    a) Vancomycin
    b) Vancomycin and ceftriaxone
    c) Vancomycin, ceftriaxone, and ampicillin

d) Ampicillin and ceftriaxone
e) None of the above

70. BT is a 54-year-old African American man recently diagnosed with non-ischemic cardiomyopathy. His past medical history is notable for moderate asthma since childhood and hypertension. Current medications include salmeterol 50 mcg, one inhalation twice daily; fluticasone 88 mcg, one inhalation twice daily, inhaled twice daily; furosemide 80 mg twice daily; enalapril 20 mg twice daily; and spironolactone 25 mg daily.

Which of the following medication changes may provide further mortality benefit for BT once stabilized on β-blocker therapy?

a) Digoxin 0.125 mg daily
b) Combination hydralazine 25 mg and isosorbide dinitrate 10 mg TID
c) Valsartan 160 mg twice daily
d) Amlodipine 5 mg daily
e) Entresto® 5 mg daily

71. BT is a 54-year-old African American man recently diagnosed with non-ischemic cardiomyopathy. His past medical history is notable for moderate asthma since childhood and hypertension. Current medications include salmeterol 50 mcg, one inhalation twice daily; fluticasone 88 mcg, one inhalation twice daily, inhaled twice daily; furosemide 80 mg twice daily; enalapril 20 mg twice daily; and spironolactone 25 mg daily.

Which of the following β-blockers is the best option to treat BT's heart failure and minimize aggravating his asthma?

a) Carvedilol
b) Metoprolol succinate
c) Propranolol
d) Atenolol
e) Nadolol

72. You want to counsel a patient who is picking up their new prescription of orlistat. Which of the following counseling points do you make? (Select **ALL** that apply.)

a) Take vitamin supplements at least 2 hours before or after orlistat
b) A nutritionally balanced diet should be maintained with 30% of calories from fat
c) Take a multivitamin with fat-soluble vitamins
d) If taking levothyroxine, administer at least 4 hours apart from orlistat
e) The brand name of orlistat is Xeniteel®

73. What is Adcirca® used to treat?

a) Erectile dysfunction
b) Pulmonary arterial hypertension
c) Hyperlipidemia
d) Diabetes
e) Asthma

74. A 48-year-old man comes in with the chief complaint of wheezing in morning that gets better as day progresses. They have had one episode of cough in last month and required three courses of oral steroids within the last year. They have been diagnosed with asthma. Their current FEV1 = 55%. What is the preferred treatment option for this patient?

    a) Medium-dose inhaled corticosteroid (ICS)
    b) Low-dose ICS and LABA
    c) Medium-dose ICS and LABA
    d) Theophylline
    e) Brovana®

75. What are the components of Symbicort®?

    a) Fluticasone/Salmeterol
    b) Budesonide/Formoterol
    c) Fluticasone furoate/Vilanterol
    d) Mometasone/Formoterol
    e) Budesonide/Salmeterol

76. What drugs are used to treat pinworm? (Select **ALL** that apply.)

    a) Pyrantel pamoate
    b) Mebendazole
    c) Metronidazole
    d) Albendazole
    e) Pantoprazole

77. What is another name of phytonadione?

    a) Vitamin K1
    b) Vitamin B12
    c) Vitamin E
    d) Vitamin K3
    e) Vitamin K2

78. Jamie is a 37-year-old female coming into your pharmacy to pick up Pylera®. What condition does Jamie most likely have?

    a) Heartburn
    b) Upset stomach
    c) H. pylori
    d) Flu
    e) Common Cold

79. What are side effects of erythropoiesis-stimulating agents (ESAs)? (Select **ALL** that apply.)

    a) High blood pressure
    b) Swelling
    c) Pyrexia

d) Dizziness
e) Pain at injection site

80. What is the pathophysiology of Alzheimer's disease? (Select **ALL** that apply.)

a) Plaques and tangles are present in the neurons of brain tissue
b) Neuron signaling is interrupted and shortened
c) Neurotransmitters are altered (i.e., decrease acetylcholine)
d) Blood brain barrier presents with gaps and crevices
e) The fluid and white matter in the brain become dry

81. Kara has a presentation coming up soon and she is under a lot of anxiety. Her main complaint is helping her sleep until she is done with the presentation. What benzodiazepine do you recommend helping Kara in the short term for a few days? (Select **ALL** that apply.)

a) Temazepam
b) Triazolam
c) Flurazepam
d) Estazolam
e) Alprazolam

82. RA is taking Risperdal Consta® for his bipolar disorder. How often does his doctor need to administer his medication?

a) Every two weeks
b) Every four weeks
c) Every day
d) Once a week
e) Every other day

83. What is the brand name of ziprasidone and olanzapine, respectively?

a) Zyprexa®, Geodon®
b) Geodon®, Zyprexa®
c) Zyprexa®, Seroquel®
d) Seroquel®, Zyprexa®
e) Seroquel®, Geodon®

84. What is the active ingredient medication in Plan B?

a) Levonorgestrel 1.5 mg
b) Levonorgestrel 5 mg
c) Ulipristal acetate 30 mg
d) Ulipristal acetate 15 mg
e) Mifepristone 5 mg

85. What diagnostics are used to measure thyroid function? (Select **ALL** that apply.)

a) Thyroid-Stimulating Hormone (TSH)
b) Free thyroxine

    c) Free T4
    d) Total or free triiodothyronine
    e) Total or free T3

86. A patient is picking up Synthroid®, which of the following counseling points do you recommend? (Select **ALL** that apply.)

    a) The generic name is levothyroxine and may be cheaper
    b) Take Synthroid® on an empty stomach 30-60 minutes before eating anytime during the day at changing intervals of morning and night
    c) Partial hair loss may occur in the first few months of therapy
    d) Drug should not be administered within 4 hours of iron, calcium supplements or antacids
    e) Notify your doctor if you have a rapid heartbeat, chest pain, or SOB

87. Warfarin doses can be identified by the color of the tablet. Which of the following is a correct match? (Select **ALL** that apply.)

    a) 1 mg - Green
    b) 5 mg - Peach
    c) 10 mg - White
    d) 2 mg - Blue
    e) 7.5 mg - Yellow

88. Amitriptyline is structurally similar to which of the following medications? (Select **ALL** that apply.)

    a) Desipramine
    b) Cyclobenzaprine
    c) Doxepin
    d) Nortriptyline
    e) Imipramine

89. Which of the following counseling points should you give to a patient who is taking ibandronate? (Select **ALL** that apply.)

    a) You must sit upright or stand for at least one full hour after administration
    b) Take ibandronate first thing in the morning 1 hour before eating or drinking or taking any other medication
    c) Take ibandronate with a full glass (6-8 ounces) of mineral water
    d) If you develop signs of bone loss in the jaw, report to your doctor
    e) Ibandronate is used to treat or prevent osteoporosis in woman after menopause

90. Which of the following are prodrugs? (Select **ALL** that apply).

    a) Clopidogrel
    b) Plavix®
    c) Brillinta®
    d) Effient®
    e) Ticagrelor

91. What is a recommended drug reference for immunizations and injectables, respectively?

    a) CDC Pink Book, Trissel's Handbook
    b) CDC Yellow Book, Trissel's Handbook
    c) Briggs Drugs, Remington's
    d) Trissel's Handbook, CDC Pink Book
    e) Sanford Guide, National Library of Medicine (NLM)

92. What is the mechanism of action of pramipexole?

    a) Norepinephrine agonist
    b) Serotonin agonist
    c) Norepinephrine and dopamine agonist
    d) Dopamine agonist
    e) Dopamine antagonist

93. Which of the following medications can be used to treat relapsing-emitting multiple sclerosis? (Select **ALL** that apply.)

    a) Fingolimod
    b) Teriflunomide
    c) Amantadine
    d) Pemoline
    e) Glatiramer acetate

94. CR is a 1-year-old boy who was recently prescribed montelukast. What is the recommended dose, mechanism of action, and brand name respectively?

    a) Montelukast 4 mg, leukotriene receptor antagonist, Singulair®
    b) Montelukast 10 mg, leukotriene receptor antagonist, Singulair®
    c) Montelukast 5 mg, leukotriene receptor antagonist, Accolate®
    d) Montelukast 1 mg, 5-lipoxygenase inhibitor, Zyflo®
    e) Montelukast 4 mg, 5-lipoxygenase inhibitor, Zyflo®

95. JR is a new patient in your pharmacy. He brings in a few notes from his doctor stating, "ADHD with aggressive behavior" and is taking risperidone. What is risperidone used to treat? (Select **ALL** that apply.)

    a) ADHD
    b) Aggressive behavior
    c) Schizophrenia
    d) Bipolar I disorder
    e) Irritability with autistic disorder

96. A 72-year-old male comes into your pharmacy asking about the vaccinations he needs to get to be "up to date". You review his profile and see that he received a shingles vaccine five years ago. Which of the following vaccines do you recommend? (Select **ALL** that apply).

    a) Influenza
    b) Td/Tdap
    c) PCV20
    d) PPSV23
    e) Zoster

97. A 26-year-old female comes into your pharmacy. She has a past medical history of HIV and is immunocompromised with a CD4 count < 200. Which of the following vaccines should she avoid? (Select **ALL** that apply.)

    a) Zoster
    b) Td/Tdap
    c) MMR
    d) Varicella
    e) LAIV

98. Natalie comes into your pharmacy with her first born 18-month infant, Jeffe. She asks you what vaccines her Jeffe needs and states she never gave a vaccine to her child. What do you recommend? (Select **ALL** that apply.)

    a) HepB
    b) DTaP
    c) HiB
    d) PCV13
    e) MMR

99. Natalie comes back in with Jeffe again, her 18-month infant. She sees that your pharmacy is advertising for flu season, so she decides it would be best for Jeffe to get a flu shot. However, she is concerned about his egg allergy. She asks you which flu vaccine Jeffe can receive. What do you recommend?

    a) FluMist® Quadrivalent vaccine
    b) Flublok® Quadrivalent vaccine
    c) Flucelvax® Quadrivalent vaccine
    d) Fluzone® Quadrivalent vaccine
    e) FLUAD® Quadrivalent vaccine

100. James is a 64-year-old male who has end stage renal disease on dialysis three times weekly. His provider ran some labs, and it has shown the following:

   Calcium: 12.5 mg/dL
   Phosphate: 6.5 mg/dL

   What medication(s) do you recommend to the attending for Mr. James and for what condition, respectively? (Select **ALL** that apply.)

   a) Sevelamer; hyperphosphatemia
   b) Renagel®; hypercalcemia
   c) Pamidronate; hyperphosphatemia
   d) Fosamax®; hyperphosphatemia
   e) Sensipar®; hypercalcemia

101. Which of the following affects the steady-state plasma drug concentration for a constant infusion drug? (Select **ALL** that apply.)

   a) Half-life
   b) Clearance
   c) V_d
   d) Infusion rate
   e) Dose

102. JR is an African American 64-year-old female with a past medical history of diabetes. She is currently taking metformin 500 mg twice daily and glyburide 5 mg once daily. Her labs are as follows: CrCl 59 mL/min, SCr 1.4 mg/dL, eGFR 45 mL/min/1.73 m² and A1c 8.5%. She does not want insulin and refuses needle sticks. What would you recommend to JR's primary care physician? (Select **ALL** that apply.)

   a) Discontinue metformin
   b) Double metformin from 500 mg to 1000 mg by mouth twice daily
   c) Increase glyburide frequency to glyburide 5 mg by mouth twice daily
   d) Recommend Novolin N/R
   e) Switch from glyburide to glimepiride 4 mg by mouth twice daily

103. Sammy is a 46-year-old male who was recently diagnosed with MRSA. What drugs listed below do NOT treat for MRSA?

   a) Doxycycline
   b) Vancomycin
   c) Cefepime
   d) Oxacillin
   e) Daptomycin

104. Kelly is a 22-year-old pregnant female who comes into your pharmacy with her allergies acting up again. She asks you what she can take that would be non-drowsy as she has to get to work quickly. What do you recommend?

    a) Allegra
    b) Claritin
    c) Desloratadine
    d) Zyrtec
    e) Chlorpheniramine

105. Which insulin(s) can be stored outside of the refrigerator for only up to 28 days? (Select **ALL** that apply.)

    a) Levemir®
    b) Novolin N®
    c) Lantus®
    d) Toujeo®
    e) Novolin R®

106. Which insulin provides a long, non-peak release?
    a) Glargine
    b) Levemir®
    c) Novolin N®
    d) Apidra®
    e) Novolin R®

107. Which anti-convulsant comes in a sprinkle capsule formulation release?

    a) Topiramate
    b) Carbamazepine
    c) Lamotrigine
    d) Levetiracetam
    e) Primidone

108. You perform a medication therapy management call for a 67-year-old female patient. She has a part medical history of congestive heart failure (CHF), hypertension, depression, and COPD. Her current medication regimen is lisinopril, Nitrostat® PRN, ProAir®, and Symbicort®. She says her doctor wants to start her on a beta-blocker and was wondering if she should avoid any due to her history of depression. What do you recommend that she avoids?

    a) Propranolol
    b) Labetalol
    c) Carvedilol
    d) Atenolol
    e) Nadolol

109. JR is a 12-year-old male with a past medical history of bipolar disorder and ADHD. He recently tried Concerta® but is failing treatment and doesn't like taking pills. His parents are requesting any recommendations to try something else. What do you recommend?

    a) Ritalin®
    b) Focalin®
    c) Adderall®
    d) Daytrana®
    e) Intuniv®

110. What is the benefit of digoxin in patients with atrial fibrillation?

    a) Increased mortality benefit
    b) Restoring normal heart rate control
    c) Restoring normal sinus rhythm control
    d) Repairing leaky heart valves
    e) Increased mortality benefit in ventricular fibrillation

111. MC is a 45-year-old male with schizophrenia and bipolar disorder. He also has congestive heart failure and atrial fibrillation. He asks you what medications he should avoid for something his doctor called, "QT prolonging". What medications should you advise this patient to avoid? (Select **ALL** that apply.)

    a) Abilify®
    b) Seroquel®
    c) Risperdal®
    d) Zyprexa®
    e) Invega®

112. MR is a 54-year-old male with a history of Hepatitis C. He has lots of anxiety in starting his new Harvoni® treatment and hoping it "cures" him from his Hepatitis C. He asks you if he should try Kava. What do you recommend?

    a) Kava has shown benefit for anxiety and MR can take this herb
    b) Kava is like a benzodiazepine so it should provide fast relief
    c) Kava is safe and has not been linked to deaths for long-term use
    d) Kava is not safe due to hepatotoxicity and should be avoided
    e) Try Valerian instead of Kava due to less liver toxicity

113. MS is a 33-year-old nurse who complains of migraines. She is looking for an herb to help her with her migraines. What do you recommend?

    a) Kava
    b) Valerian
    c) Ginger
    d) Feverfew
    e) Coenzyme Q10

114. A frantic mother bursts into your pharmacy with her 4-year-old son who is autistic. Her doctor keeps asking her to get her son up to date on vaccinations, but she wants to consult you as her trusty pharmacist for the evidence. What do you say to her?

    a) MMR vaccines have shown to cause autism
    b) Thimerosal-containing vaccines cause autism
    c) There is no association between vaccines and autism
    d) The antigens from vaccines cause autism
    e) Preservatives in vaccines cause autism

115. Brock, a 25-year-old male, suffered from a car accident recently, and is otherwise a healthy young adult. His current medical history is severe back pain and has no history of taking any medications. The prescriber prescribed Brock a fentanyl patch to help with the pain. What recommendations do you make regarding this patient's treatment?

    a) Fentanyl is a strong pain medication that will help provide relief
    b) Fentanyl should not be dispensed as Brock is opioid naïve and be at a high risk of respiratory depression and possibly death
    c) Fentanyl is a safe non-addictive choice for long-term pain relief
    d) Fentanyl should be dispensed as Brock is opioid naïve and will be at a low risk of respiratory depression and possibly death
    e) Fentanyl should be dispensed as it is a patch and Brock hates taking pills

116. Where can enoxaparin be administered to a patient? Click to select on the following image.

117. Which antipsychotics have the lowest potential to worsen movement disorders? (Select **ALL** that apply.)

    a) Chlorpromazine
    b) Fluphenazine
    c) Haloperidol
    d) Perphenazine
    e) Quetiapine

118. Timmy is a 64-year-old male who gets readmitted to your hospital and is on a tracheostomy. The nurse asks what she should use to clean his intra-tracheal tube to prevent pneumonia. What medication do you recommend?

    a) Bactrim
    b) Metronidazole
    c) Chlorhexidine
    d) Normal saline and hydrogen peroxide
    e) Normal saline

119. What is a major side effect of sorbitol?

    a) Diarrhea
    b) Constipation
    c) Bleeding
    d) Bruising
    e) Sore throat

120. James had a recent heart attack and is started on clopidogrel. His current medication history includes clopidogrel, aspirin, metoprolol, Nitrostat®, pantoprazole, and fish oil. He presents a prescription with omeprazole. What counseling point do you recommend for Mr. James?

    a) It is safer to take omeprazole with your clopidogrel versus pantoprazole
    b) Evidence has shown it is safe to co-administer clopidogrel and PPIs
    c) Clopidogrel does interact with PPIs, but it only applies to pantoprazole
    d) Clopidogrel does interact with PPIs, but it only applies to omeprazole
    e) Pantoprazole has a major inhibitory effect on CYP2C19

121. A patient is a 67-year-old man weighing 246 lbs and standing 5' 9" tall. What is this patient's body surface area? (Round the answer to the nearest **hundredths**.)

122. A patient is a 23-year-old woman weighing 146 lbs and standing 5' 3" tall. What is this patient's body surface area? (Round the answer to the nearest **hundredths**.)

123. Kate, a recent pharmacist grad, is trying to find a good resource where she can find drug recalls. What resource do you recommend?

    a) CDC
    b) NIH
    c) FDA
    d) CMS
    e) NLM

124. Samantha is a 27-year-old female who comes into your pharmacy to pick up amoxicillin and fluticasone nasal spray. Her past medication history is Zyrtec® and pseudoephedrine. What is the possible condition this patient has?

   a) Acute sinusitis
   b) Allergic rhinitis
   c) Bronchitis
   d) Lower respiratory tract infection
   e) Sleep apnea

125. Jaris was recently diagnosed with gonorrhea. He was prescribed aqueous procaine penicillin G 5 M units IM. What other condition do you suspect he has?

   a) Herpes
   b) Chlamydia
   c) Syphilis
   d) Urethritis
   e) HIV

126. Which of the following agents is a surfactant?

   a) Psyllium
   b) Docusate
   c) Senna
   d) Bisacodyl
   e) Milk of magnesia

127. What HIV medication can also be used to treat for Hepatitis B?

   a) Lamivudine
   b) Efavirenz
   c) Abacavir
   d) Dolutegravir
   e) Rilpivirine

128. What medication can also be used to treat for Hepatitis C and HIV co-infection without regard for drug interactions?

   a) Daclatasvir
   b) Ledipasvir-Sofosbuvir
   c) Ombitasvir-Paritaprevir-Ritonavir
   d) Tenofovir alafenamide
   e) Ribavirin

129. How are interferons such as Pegasys® administered in a patient?

   a) SQ
   b) IM
   c) IV
   d) Oral
   e) Rectal

130. TF is a 10-year-old female recently diagnosed with active tuberculosis. Her other medications include methylphenidate 10 mg twice daily. She is HIV negative. Which medication should not be included in her regimen for TB?

   a) Isoniazid
   b) Rifampin
   c) Pyrazinamide
   d) Ethambutol
   e) Ribavirin

131. JK is a 32-year-old HIV-negative patient presenting to your clinic. He receives a Mantoux skin test that returns positive 2 days later. He was born in the United States and works as a prison guard. He injects heroin on a regular basis. His chest x-ray comes back normal, he has no symptoms of tuberculosis, and his smear culture is negative. What type of drug therapy would be appropriate for this patient?

   a) Isoniazid 300 mg daily x 9 months
   b) Rifampin 100 mg daily x 4 months
   c) No drug therapy needed
   d) Isoniazid 300 mg and rifampin 600 mg x 6 months
   e) Isoniazid, rifampin, ethambutol, and pyrazinamide

132. Which of the following is true regarding acid-fast bacteria?

   a) They retain their stained color even with acid-alcohol washes
   b) Cultures of acid-fast bacteria grow faster than other bacteria
   c) Mycobacterium tuberculosis is the only type of acid-fast bacteria
   d) They cause the majority of bacterial infectious diseases in the US
   e) They do not retain their stained color with acid-alcohol washes

133. SF is a 57-year-old male patient with a latent TB infection. He had a positive IGRA result and TST reaction of greater than 5 millimeters. He also has a past medical history of HIV but wants to wait before getting treated. How long can SF wait before getting treatment for his latent TB infection?

   a) 6 months
   b) 9 months
   c) 12 months
   d) Immediately, do not wait for treatment
   e) 3 months

134. Jamie is a 46-year-old female weighing 246 lbs and is 5' 3". She has congestive heart failure, hypertension, and hyperlipidemia. She recently experienced a deep vein thrombosis in her left arm and was discharged on warfarin 5 mg daily. What is her INR target?

    a) INR 2.0 - 3.0
    b) INR 1.5 - 2.5
    c) INR 2.5
    d) INR 2.0
    e) INR 1.0 - 2.0

135. Jamie is a 46-year-old female weighing 246 lbs and is 5' 3". She has congestive heart failure, hypertension, and hyperlipidemia. She comes back into the ER with another DVT in her left leg. What is the emergent treatment?

    a) Enoxaparin SQ 112 mg every 12 hours
    b) Enoxaparin SQ 52 mg every 12 hours
    c) Enoxaparin SQ 76 mg every 12 hours
    d) Xarelto® 20 mg twice daily with food for 21 days
    e) Pradaxa® 150 mg daily after parenteral anticoagulation

136. What is the mechanism of action of ropinirole?

    a) Direct replacement of dopamine in the central nervous system
    b) Inhibition of the enzymatic breakdown of dopamine in the CNS
    c) Inhibition of the enzymatic breakdown of dopamine in the periphery
    d) Direct stimulation of postsynaptic dopamine receptors
    e) Activation of enzymatic breakdown of dopamine in the periphery

137. Your long-term patient with Parkinson's disease, WO, is complaining of hallucinations. She has no recent additions to her medication regimen or changes in medication doses. Her symptoms include visual hallucinations which are frightening to her. The decision is to initiate antipsychotic therapy. Which is the best initial treatment of her Parkinson's disease–associated psychosis?

    a) Chlorpromazine
    b) Haloperidol
    c) Olanzapine
    d) Alprazolam
    e) Quetiapine

138. SP was diagnosed with Parkinson's disease 7 years ago. Originally, she was taking carbidopa/levodopa 25/100 mg TID, which has since been increased to 50/250 mg 4 times daily. Nonmotor symptoms include constipation and insomnia. She also has arthritis for which she takes acetaminophen 650 mg TID. Assuming another medication is to be added at this time, which medication would you suggest avoiding based on her history of present illness?

    a) Selegiline
    b) Ropinirole
    c) Rasagiline
    d) Pramipexole

e) Sinemet

139. Which drug should be dosed simultaneously with levodopa?

a) Rasagiline
b) Pramipexole
c) Entacapone
d) Amantadine
e) Selegiline

140. TS lives in a rural community where there is no neurology practice nearby. For the last several years, he has been experiencing tremors, rigidity, and bradykinesia that began on his left side, but has since migrated and become bilateral, though his left side is still affected more than his right. He is diagnosed with Parkinson's disease, and his motor symptoms are graded as moderate (tremor and bradykinesia) and moderate to severe (rigidity). What is the most appropriate order for the initiation and progression for his treatment?

a) Carbidopa/levodopa, rotigotine, rasagiline
b) Ropinirole, levodopa/carbidopa, tolcapone
c) Pramipexole, entacapone, carbidopa/levodopa
d) Benztropine, rasagiline, carbidopa/levodopa
e) Rasagiline, rotigotine, carbidopa/levodopa

141. What is the concern of using Sinemet® long-term?

a) Taking Sinemet® over time loses its efficacy
b) Sinemet® is effective for many years and its loss of efficacy is due to the progression of the disease than with duration of treatment
c) Taking Sinemet® over time increases side effects and will cause more nausea
d) Carbidopa will shift from blocking levodopa breakdown inside the CNS
e) Taking Sinemet® over times increases its efficacy

142. JR is a 45-year-old male with a history of an MI back in 2015. He had a bare metal stent placed to help prevent more blockages. He is also taking atorvastatin 40 mg daily and metoprolol 25 mg daily. What other medications should JR be on to help his stents last longer? (Select **ALL** that apply.)

a) Warfarin
b) Aspirin
c) Clopidogrel
d) Xarelto
e) Pradaxa

143. Rank in order the correct donning procedures per USP 797 for sterile compounding. (**ALL** options must be used.) Left click the mouse to highlight, drag, and order the answer options.

    a) Perform hand hygiene, Wash hands
    b) Sanitize the gloves with 70% isopropyl alcohol and allow gloves to dry
    c) Don sterile powder-free gloves
    d) Place surgical scrub solution into palm and rub nails then work way to elbows. Pump again into other hand and repeat until both hands are sanitized. Ensure to sanitize hands using an alcohol-based hand rub and allow hands to dry
    e) Don shoe covers, hair and beard covers, and a face mask
    f) Don gown, fastened securely at the neck and wrists

144. Sammie is a 67-year-old male who has recently been diagnosed with osteoarthritis. His kidney function is poor, with a CrCl of 30 mL/min. He comes to your pharmacy asking what he should take to help with the pain. What do you recommend?

    a) Ibuprofen
    b) Excedrin®
    c) Advil®
    d) Tylenol®
    e) Naproxen

145. Sovanie is a 69-year-old female who has terrible GERD and heartburn. She is considering an NSAID to help with her pain. What NSAID would have the lowest risk of worsening her GERD?

    a) Etodolac
    b) Celebrex®
    c) Mobic®
    d) Nabumetone
    e) Indomethacin

146. Nancy is a 59-year-old female who has a past medical history of diabetes. Her most recent HbA1c is 7.1%. She has terrible foot callouses and is wondering how to treat them. What do you recommend?

    a) Use a butter knife to gentle remove the callus
    b) Use well-fitted walking shoes and inserts in addition to a pumice stone
    c) Use hydrogen peroxide and bleach to flake off the dead cells
    d) Use a callus chemical remover and soak foot in isopropyl alcohol
    e) Use Dr. Scholl's Salicylic Acid® and don't wear 100% cotton socks

147. DeeDee is a 57-year-old female with Sjogren's syndrome. She is complaining of dry mouth and hasn't tried anything yet to treat it. What do you suggest as an initial option?

    a) Artificial Saliva
    b) Pilocarpine
    c) Cevimeline
    d) Chewing gum
    e) Tea

148. Celebe is a 29-year-old female who is taking paroxetine, mirtazapine, and Adderall®. She comes to your pharmacy concerned about serotonin syndrome. The nurse stated that she should be cautious to report these symptoms. What medications increase the risk of developing serotonin syndrome?

   a) Tramadol
   b) Percocet®
   c) Mirtazapine
   d) Bupropion
   e) Cyproheptadine

149. What is the mechanism of action of how risperidone causes gynecomastia?

   a) Histaminergic receptor antagonist
   b) Norepinephrine receptor antagonist
   c) Serotonin receptor antagonist
   d) GABA receptor antagonist
   e) Dopamine receptor antagonist

150. What is aluminum acetate used for in compounding medications?

   a) Surfactant
   b) Preservative
   c) Topical astringent and antiseptic
   d) Wetting agent
   e) Plasticizer

151. Which inhalers need to be washed and how often? (Select **ALL** that apply.)

   a) HFA inhalers, once a week
   b) Asthmanefrin®, once a week
   c) Dry powder inhalers, once a month
   d) CFC inhalers, once a month
   e) Actuator, once a week

152. What is the generic of Cardura® and its mechanism of action?

   a) Terazosin, alpha-1 adrenergic receptor blocker
   b) Prazosin, alpha-2 adrenergic receptor blocker
   c) Tamsulosin, alpha-2 adrenergic receptor blocker
   d) Alfuzosin, alpha-2 adrenergic receptor blocker
   e) Doxazosin, alpha-1 adrenergic receptor blocker

153. A woman would like you to make a product selection to help her in case she experiences motion sickness and nausea on a deep-sea fishing trip she plans to take during her summer vacation. What herbal do you recommend?

   a) Kava
   b) Valerian
   c) Ginger
   d) Emetrol
   e) Chocolate

154. A 17-year-old male cocaine addict develops substernal chest pain and is rushed to the emergency room by his friends. They reveal that he had been smoking 'crack' when the symptoms developed. An ECG is consistent with anterior wall myocardial ischemia. This effect on the heart is attributed to the drug. What is the mechanism of this effect?

   a) Direct inhibition of beta-adrenergic receptors
   b) Indirect stimulation of alpha-adrenergic receptors
   c) Direct stimulation of adenosine receptors
   d) Direct stimulation of beta-adrenergic receptors
   e) Indirect inhibition of alpha-adrenergic receptors

155. Ondansetron is commonly given to patients who exhibit nausea and vomiting associated with chemotherapy. The mechanism of the antiemetic effect of ondansetron is blocking which of the following central receptors?

   a) Dopamine receptors
   b) Histamine receptors
   c) Muscarinic cholinergic receptors
   d) Serotonin receptors
   e) Norepinephrine receptors

156. Which of the following are genitourinary adverse reactions associated with cyclophosphamide?

   a) Cardiomyopathy
   b) Myelosuppression
   c) Ototoxicity
   d) Xerostomia
   e) Hemorrhagic cystitis

157. Which of the following chemoprotectants can be used to prevent nephrotoxicity and xerostomia?

   a) Leucovorin
   b) Mesna
   c) Amifostine
   d) Dexrazoxane
   e) Folic Acid

158. Which antineoplastic is associated with causing tinnitus?

   a) Cytarabine
   b) Cisplatin
   c) Cyclophosphamide
   d) Dactinomycin
   e) Ifosfamide

159. Which of the following antineoplastics can cause a disulfiram-like reaction when a patient drinks alcohol?

   a) Allopurinol
   b) Methotrexate
   c) Cisplatin
   d) Metronidazole
   e) Carbamazepine

160. Using the diagram below, identify where in the HIV life cycle maraviroc exerts its mechanism of action. (Select the **text** response and left click the mouse. To change your answer, move the cursor, select alternate **text** response, and click.)

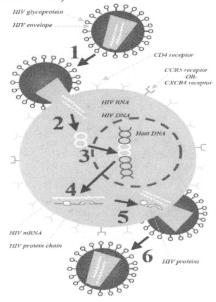

161. A patient is receiving doxorubicin. What common side effect should this patient be aware of that is not harmful?

   a) Nails turning bright orange or red
   b) Urine may appear red, dark brown, or orange
   c) Eyes drying
   d) Hirsutism
   e) Diarrhea

162. Using the diagram below, identify in the HIV life cycle where efavirenz exerts its mechanism of action. (Select the **text** response and left click the mouse. To change your answer, move the cursor, select alternate **text** response, and click.)

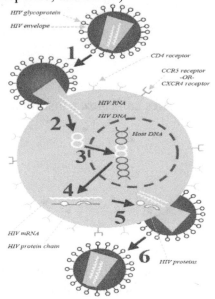

163. Using the diagram below, identify in the HIV life cycle where raltegravir exerts its mechanism of action. (Select the **text** response and left click the mouse. To change your answer, move the cursor, select alternate **text** response, and click.)

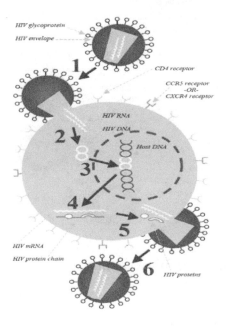

164. Using the diagram below, identify on the cell platelet below where clopidogrel exerts its mechanism of action. (Select the **text** response and left click the mouse. To change your answer, move the cursor, select alternate **text** response, and click.)

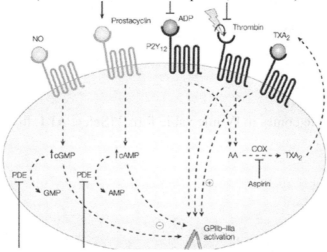

165. Using the diagram below, identify on the cell platelet where eptifibatide exerts its mechanism of action. (Select the **text** response and left click the mouse. To change your answer, move the cursor, select alternate **text** response, and click.)

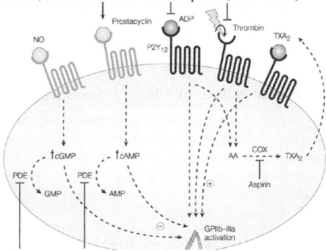

166. What is the maximum dose of Imodium® per day?

a) 5 mg
b) 10 mg
c) 16 mg
d) 15 mg
e) 20 mg

167. What type of device is albuterol HFA?

a) Autohaler
b) Handihaler
c) Flexhaler
d) Inhaler

e) Nebulizer

168. What are the types of Risperdal® formulations? (Select **ALL** that apply.)

   a) Tablet
   b) Orally Dissolving Tablet
   c) Oral Solution
   d) Suspension IM Injection
   e) IV injection

169. Which bisphosphonate comes in IV injectable form? (Select **ALL** that apply.)

   a) Boniva®
   b) Fosamax®
   c) Actonel®
   d) Reclast®
   e) Prolia®

170. Which of the following has intrinsic sympathomimetic activity? (Select **ALL** that apply.)

   a) Pindolol
   b) Nadolol
   c) Labetalol
   d) Acebutolol
   e) Metoprolol

171. What are the current market tablet doses of Allegra®? (Select **ALL** that apply.)

   a) 30 mg
   b) 60 mg
   c) 180 mg
   d) 50 mg
   e) 20 mg

172. Simps is a 36-year-old male picking up Welchol® from your pharmacy. What are some counseling points for this medication? (Select **ALL** that apply.)

   a) Welchol® should be separated by 4 hours from other medications such as calcium, iron, and cholestyramine
   b) This medication is recommended for patients with greater than 500 mg/dL of serum triglyceride concentrations and patients using insulin
   c) Take a multivitamin at least 4 hours before Welchol®
   d) Take fat-soluble vitamins A, D, E, and K at least 4 hours before Welchol®
   e) A major side effect of Welchol® is diarrhea

173. Which of the following are category X drugs? (Select **ALL** that apply.)

   a) Warfarin
   b) Xanax®
   c) Crestor®

    d) Trexall®
    e) Allegra®

174. What are the side effects of Trexall®? (Select **ALL** that apply.)

    a) Hirsutism
    b) Alopecia
    c) Thrombocytopenia
    d) Stomatitis
    e) Bleeding

175. What can be taken with Colyte®? (Select **ALL** that apply.)

    a) Pepsi®
    b) Orange juice
    c) Clear broth
    d) Apple juice
    e) White grape juice

176. IO is a 31-year-old woman starting a new job in a dental clinic. In addition to wishing to quit for health reasons, her new job also does not allow employees to smoke during their shift. She smokes approximately 15 cigarettes daily and has her first one in the car on the way to work (about 95 minutes after waking). She wishes to use the lozenges for her quit attempt. What product would you suggest that IO use?

    a) Nicotrol® 4 mg
    b) Commit® 2 mg
    c) Commit® 4 mg
    d) Nicotrol® 2 mg
    e) Commit® 5 mg

177. LK is a 62-year-old woman with osteoporosis, chronic allergic rhinitis, and a 50-pack-year history of smoking cigarettes. At a recent trip to the dentist, she was told that due to poor oral hygiene and tooth decay, she needs her teeth removed and fitted for dentures. The dentist also recommended that she quit smoking as it most likely contributed to her current predicament. Which agent listed below would be the best agent for LK to choose?

    a) Nicotine transdermal patch
    b) Nicotine nasal spray
    c) Nicotine lozenge
    d) Nicotine polacrilex gum
    e) Vapor cigarettes

178. JE is a 72-year-old man who has smoked one pack per day for the last 40 years. He has never attempted to quit smoking previously but wants to try quitting after his recent hospitalization for pneumonia. While he was in the hospital, he was given a nicotine patch to wear and change daily until discharge. Upon discharge, he was not given the nicotine patch, but wants to continue using it. What dose of the patch should JE start?

    a) 7 mg/d patch
    b) 14 mg/d patch
    c) 21 mg/d patch
    d) 30 mg/d patch
    e) He does not smoke enough to qualify for NRT with a patch

179. TY is a 40-year-old man with a medical history significant for hypertension, dyslipidemia, and obesity. He also smokes cigarettes and has smoked 1.5 packs per day for the last 16 years. His most recent blood pressure was 161/94 mmHg. His physician is convinced that if TY were to lose weight and quit smoking, many of his medical issues would be easier to manage. Which of the following medications would be the best choice for TY?

    a) Bupropion
    b) Catapres®
    c) Nicotine polacrilex gum
    d) Nicotine patch
    e) Varenicline

180. Wernicke-Korsakoff syndrome is caused by what vitamin deficiency?

    a) Vitamin B1
    b) Vitamin B2
    c) Vitamin B12
    d) Riboflavin
    e) Pyridoxine

181. Dr. Smith calls your pharmacy and wants to know what to prescribe for his patient with primary early Lyme disease. The patient is a 33-year-old male. Which of the following agents would you recommend?

    a) Amoxicillin 500 mg PO TID x 14 days
    b) Itraconazole 400 mg PO BID x 14 days
    c) Fluconazole 400 mg PO daily x 14 days
    d) Ciprofloxacin 500 mg PO BID x 14 days
    e) Doxycycline 100 mg PO BID x 14 days

182. Dr. Smith calls your pharmacy again and wants to know what to prescribe for his patient with late Lyme neurologic disease. The patient is a 23-year-old female who got a tick bite a year ago. Which of the following agents would you recommend?

    a) Ceftriaxone 2 grams IV twice daily x 28 days
    b) Cefuroxime 500 mg PO daily x 14 days
    c) Ceftriaxone 2 grams IV once daily x 28 days
    d) Ciprofloxacin 500 mg PO BID x 14 days
    e) Doxycycline 100 mg PO BID x 14 days

183. Which of the following are drugs with high emetogenicity? (Select **ALL** that apply.)

    a) Cisplatin
    b) Bleomycin
    c) Anthracycline
    d) Lomustine
    e) Bortezomib

184. What are the major side effects and toxicity of cisplatin? (Select **ALL** that apply.)

    a) Peripheral neuropathy
    b) Chemotherapy-induced nausea and vomiting
    c) Nephrotoxicity
    d) Ototoxicity
    e) Anemia

185. Mary comes into your pharmacy with a prescription for amiodarone. She states how her friends say this is a "scary" drug and what her doctor needs to check to make sure she will be okay. What monitoring labs do you recommend? (Select **ALL** that apply.)

    a) Hearing exams
    b) Ophthalmic exams
    c) Thyroid panel tests
    d) ECG and rhythm monitoring
    e) Liver function tests

186. JR is a frequent flyer in your pharmacy. He is taking amiodarone 800 mg daily and presents new prescriptions for simvastatin and lovastatin from two different prescribers. What are the max doses of simvastatin and lovastatin respectively when taken with amiodarone?

    a) Simvastatin 80 mg/day, lovastatin 20 mg/day
    b) Simvastatin 40 mg/day, lovastatin 40 mg/day
    c) Simvastatin 20 mg/day, lovastatin 20 mg/day
    d) Simvastatin 20 mg/day, lovastatin 40 mg/day
    e) Simvastatin 40 mg/day, lovastatin 80 mg/day

187. The American College of Cardiology (ACC) and American Heart Association (AHA) developed a staging classification of heart failure based on disease progression and risk factors. An asymptomatic patient with structural heart disease would be classified into which of the following stages?

    a) Stage A
    b) Stage B
    c) Stage C
    d) Stage D
    e) Stage E

188. Which of the following medical terms refers to the time until maximal level of anticancer drug-related toxicity on white blood cells or absolute neutrophil counts?

    a) Threshold
    b) Onset of effect
    c) Nadir
    d) Suppression time
    e) Time to maximum concentration

189. When differentiating Cushing's syndrome and idiopathic Addison's disease, both can exhibit elevated levels of adrenocorticotropic hormone (ACTH). Additionally, Cushing's syndrome exhibits _____ levels of cortisol and Addison's disease exhibits _____ levels of cortisol.

    a) Elevated; decreased
    b) Elevated; elevated
    c) Decreased; elevated
    d) Decreased; decreased
    e) Cushing syndrome usually has a reduced level of ACTH

190.

Patient Name: Sal		**Height:** 5' 10" **Weight:** 75 kg	
Age: 66 **Sex:** Male **Race:** Caucasian		**Family history:** None	
		Allergies: None	
DIAGNOSES: Seizure, diabetes, mild obesity		**LAB/DIAGNOSTIC TESTS**	
		Na	138	Phenobarbital	25

Patient Name: Sal
Age: 66   **Sex:** Male   **Race:** Caucasian

DIAGNOSES: Seizure, diabetes, mild obesity

MEDICATIONS: Phenytoin 400 mg q hs, Phenobarbital 120 mg q hs, Insulin NPH/Reg 20U/10U q am and 10U/10U q pm

Gen: Mildly obese WM complaining of swelling and drainage from left foot
VS: 150/96, 85(regular), 38°C, 14
HEENT: Nystagmus on lateral gaze
Neuro: Alert and oriented x 3, slight gait ataxia

Height: 5' 10"   **Weight:** 75 kg
Family history: None
Allergies: None
LAB/DIAGNOSTIC TESTS

Na	138	Phenobarbital	25
BUN	22	Cl	99
WBC	17K	Hgb	15
Phenytoin	16	FBS	140
K	4.5	HCO3	24
SCr	1.5	Hct	45
Plt	300K	Alb	2.5

Based on the information provided, what is the primary medical problem with respect to the phenytoin regimen?

a) Phenytoin-induced renal dysfunction
b) Phenytoin-induced hyperglycemia
c) Phenytoin-induced obesity
d) Phenytoin toxicity
e) Phenytoin-induced infection

191. Patients with heart failure have been traditionally classified into different New York Heart Association (NYHA) classes based on their presenting symptoms. A patient with symptoms associated with ordinary exertion would be classified into which NYHA category?

a) Class I
b) Class II
c) Class III
d) Class IV
e) Class V

192. A patient's arterial blood gas results are as follows:

pH = 7.6
pCO$_2$ = normal
HCO$_3$ = 39 mEq/L

Which of the following interpretations is correct?

a) Metabolic acidosis
b) Mixed acidosis
c) Respiratory alkalosis
d) Respiratory acidosis
e) Metabolic alkalosis

193. What class of organisms appears purple on a Gram stain?

    a) Gram-positive organisms
    b) Gram-negative organisms
    c) Fungal organisms
    d) Atypical organisms
    e) Viral organisms

194. A TPN solution contains 750 mL of D5W. If each gram of dextrose provides 3.4 kcal, how many kcals would the TPN solution provide? (Round the answer to the nearest **tenths**.)

195. How many 60 mg tablets of codeine sulfate should be used to make this cough syrup? (Round the answer to the nearest **whole number**.)

    Codeine SO$_4$ 30 mg/teaspoon
    Cherry Syrup qs ad 150 mL
    Sig: 1 teaspoonful every 6 hours as needed for cough

196. If 10 mL of a diluent is added to an injectable containing 0.5 g of a drug with a final volume of 7.3 mL, what is the final concentration of the parenteral solution in mg/mL? (Round the answer to the nearest **tenths**.)

197. An inhalant solution contains 0.025% w/v of a drug in 5 mL. What is the number of milligrams in this solution? (Round the answer to the nearest **hundredths**.)

198. How many milliequivalents of potassium are in 240 mL of a 10% solution of KCL? (MW: KCl = 74.5, K = 39, Cl = 35.5) (Round the answer to the nearest **whole number**.)

199. How many millimoles of HCl are contained in 130 mL of a 10% solution? (MW: HCl = 36.5). (Round the answer to the nearest **whole number**.)

200. A medication order of a drug calls for a dose of 0.6 mg/kg to be administered to a child weighing 31 lb. The drug is to be supplied from a solution containing 0.25 g in 50 mL bottles. How many milliliters of this solution are required to fill this order? (Round the answer to the nearest **hundredths**.)

201. How many milliliters of a 17% solution of benzalkonium chloride are required to prepare 350 mL of a 1:750 w/v solution? (Round the answer to the nearest **hundredths**.)

202. A solution contains 2 mEq of KCl/mL. If a TPN order calls for the addition of 180 mg of K+, how many milliliters of this solution should be used to provide the potassium required? (MW: K = 39, Cl = 35.5) (Round the answer to the nearest **tenths**.)

203. How many milliosmoles of sodium chloride are there in 1 L of a 0.9% solution of normal saline solution? (MW: NaCl = 58.5) (Round the answer to the nearest **whole number**.)

204. If 120 mL of a cough syrup contains 0.4 g of dextromethorphan, how many milligrams are contained in 1 teaspoonful? (Round the answer to the nearest **whole number**.)

205. How many milligrams of a drug would be contained in a 10 mL container of a 0.65% w/v solution of a drug? (Round the answer to the nearest **whole number**.)

206. Interferon injection contains 5 million U/mL. How many units are in 0.65 mL? (Round the answer to the nearest **whole number**.)

207. What is the percentage concentration (w/v) of a 250 mL solution containing 100 mEq of ammonium chloride? (MW: $NH_4Cl = 53.5$) (Round the answer to the nearest **hundredths**.)

208. 437.5 grains is equal to how many ounces? (Round the answer to the nearest **whole number**.)

209. A study is evaluating the cost associated with anxiety due to an illness. What type of cost would anxiety represent? (Select **ALL** that apply.)

    a) Direct medical
    b) Direct nonmedical
    c) Indirect
    d) Intangible
    e) Indirect nonmedical

210. What type of pharmacoeconomic analysis assumes the outcomes are equal?

    a) Epidemiologic study
    b) Parametric analysis
    c) Cost-minimization
    d) Retrospective study
    e) Cost-effectiveness

211. A medical center located in the Northeast part of the United States is dealing with resistant bacterial organisms at their institution. Specifically, they are overwhelmed with cases of extended spectrum β-lactamase gram-negative rods. The medical center director charges pharmacy service with comparing different types of treatment to optimize clinical cure outcomes. Which of the following types of pharmacoeconomic evaluations should be conducted?

    a) Cost-minimization analysis
    b) Cost-benefit analysis
    c) Cost-effectiveness analysis
    d) Cost-utility analysis
    e) Cost-maximization analysis

212. Which of the following pharmacoeconomic models evaluated adjusted life years?

    a) Cost-minimization analysis
    b) Cost-benefit analysis
    c) Cost-effectiveness analysis
    d) Cost-utility analysis
    e) Cost-maximization analysis

213. The infusion rate of theophylline established for an infant is 0.08 mg/kg/h. How many milligrams of drug is needed for a 12-hour infusion bottle if the body weight is 16 lb? (Round the answer to the nearest **whole number**.)

214. What flow rate must be programmed into the PCA unit to obtain the desired amount of morphine per minute? (Round the answer to the nearest **hundredths**.)

   Dosing to start at 08:00 AM tomorrow
   Morphine sulfate 500 mg in a 100-mL PCA unit to deliver 0.05 mg/min

215. You prepare a solution of ^{99m}Tc (40 mCi/mL) at 06:00 AM. If the solution is for administration at 12:00 PM at a dose of 20 mCi, how many milliliters of the original solution is needed? The half-life of the radioisotope is 6 hrs. (Round the answer to the nearest **whole number**.)

216. Based on the below values, what is the **sensitivity** of this test? (Round the answer to the nearest **whole number**.)

Number of subjects ($n = 910$)

Results	Disease Present	Disease Not Present
Testing positive	80	20
Testing negative	10	800

217. Dopamine 200 mg in 500 mL normal saline at 5 mg/kg/min is ordered for a 155-lb patient. At what rate (mL/min) should the solution be infused to deliver the desired dose of 5 mg/kg/min? (Round the answer to the nearest **whole number**.)

218. How many milliliters of normal saline should be mixed in a syringe with 1 mL of a 1:1,000 strength solution in order to obtain a 1:2,500 dilution? (Round the answer to the nearest **tenths**.)

219. What is the decay constant (k) of the radioisotope ^{32}P if its half-life is 14.3 days? Assume that radiopharmaceutical decay follows first-order kinetics. (Round the answer to the nearest **thousandths**.)

220. View case below:

Parenteral admixture order	For: Alex Sanders, Room: M 704
Cefazolin sodium 400 mg in 100 mL NS	Infuse over 20 min q6h ATC for 3 days

Available in the pharmacy are cefazolin sodium 1-g vials with reconstitution directions of "addition of 2.5 mL SWFI will give 3.0 mL of solution." What infusion rate in mL/min should the nurse establish for each bottle? (Round the answer to the nearest **whole number**.)

221. A vial containing 1,000 units of an expensive drug powder is labeled "add 9 mL SWFI to obtain 100 units/mL." How many milliliters of diluent is needed if the nursing staff requests a concentration of 120 units/mL? (Round the answer to the nearest **tenths**.)

222. Based on the below values, what is the **prevalence** of disease in population tested? (Round the answer to the nearest **whole number**.)

Number of subjects ($n = 910$)

Results	Disease Present	Disease Not Present
Testing positive	80	20
Testing negative	10	800

223. If a Lantus® insulin pen contains 100 units/mL, how many mL would you need for a 20-unit dose?

a) 2 mL
b) 0.2 mL
c) 0.5 mL

d) 2.5 mL

e) 3.0 mL

224. What is the minimum amount of a potent drug that may be weighed on a prescription balance with a sensitivity requirement of 6 mg if at least 95% accuracy is required?

a) 6 mg

b) 120 mg

c) 180 mg

d) 200 mg

e) 300 mg

225. An ICU order reads "KCl 40 mEq in 1-liter NS. Infuse at 0.5 mEq/min". How many minutes will this bottle last on the patient?

a) 20

b) 500

c) 1000

d) 80

e) 2000

226. The usual dose of sulfamethoxazole/trimethoprim (Bactrim®) is 150 mg TMP/m²/day in divided doses every 12 hours for PCP prophylaxis. What would be the usual dose for SG who is a 2-year-old male (Wt = 12 kg, Ht = 34")?

a) 5 mg

b) 10 mg

c) 40 mg

d) 80 mg

e) 20 mg

227. After 1 month of therapy, all of the patients listed using the following data had a systolic blood pressure reduction of 10 mm with a standard deviation (SD) of ± 5 mm. What percentage of patients had a reduction between 5 and 15 mm? (Round the answer to the nearest **whole number**.)

Patient	1	2	3	4	5
B.P.	140/70	160/84	180/88	190/90	150/70

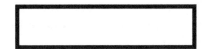

228. A hospital pharmacy technician adds by syringe 20 mL of a concentrated sterile 2% w/v dye solution to a 250-mL commercial bag of sterile normal saline. A very accurate assay of the solution will probably result in the solution being which of the following?

a) Slightly stronger than calculated

b) Significantly stronger than calculated

c) Exactly as calculated

d) Significantly lower than desired

e) Slightly weaker than desired

229. What is the following structure?

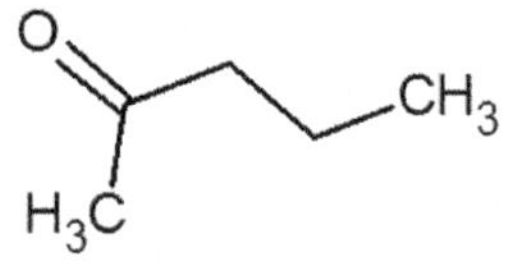

a) Carboxylic acid
b) Ester
c) Ether
d) Alcohol
e) Ketone

230. What is the following drug?

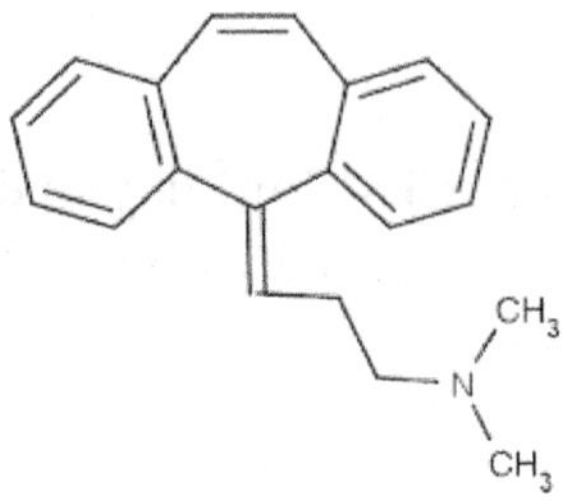

a) Cyclobenzaprine
b) Sildenafil
c) Tadalafil
d) Methotrexate
e) Isosorbide mononitrate

231. LM is a 20-year-old woman who is leaving for her first semester of college next month. She would like to know what vaccinations she needs before going to college. Her vaccination record shows the following: DTaP at 2, 4, 6, and 15 months, and 5 years; Hib (ActHIB) at 2, 4, and 6 months; PCV at 2, 4, 6, and 15 months; IPV at 2, 4, and 6 months, and 5 years; MMR at 15 months and 5 years; Varicella at 15 months and 5 years; Hep A at 12 and 18 months; Hep B at 11 years, 11 years 2 months, and 11 years 6 months; Tdap at 15 years. LM does not have any medical conditions and is not allergic to any medications or vaccines. What vaccines should LM receive today?

a) MPSV and HPV
b) Tdap and MCV
c) MCV and HPV
d) Tdap, MCV, and HPV
e) HPV, Varicella, MMR

232. Kaly, a 5-year-old girl, has an appointment today with her pediatrician to receive vaccines. Her vaccination record shows the following: Hep B at birth, 2 months, and 6 months; RV at 2, 4, and 6 months; DTaP at 2, 4, 6, and 15 months; Hib (ActHIB) at 2, 4, 6, and 15 months; PCV at 2, 4, 6, and 15 months; IPV at 2, 4, and 6 months; MMR at 15 months; Varicella at 15 months; and Hep A at 15 months. What vaccines should she receive today?

   a) DTaP, IPV, MMR, Varicella, and Hep A
   b) DT, PPSV, IPV, MMR, MCV, and Hep A
   c) DTaP, PPSV, IPV, MMR, Varicella, and Hep A
   d) Tdap, IPV, MMR, Varicella, and Hep A
   e) DT, IPV, MMR, Hep A, HPV

233. TR is a 54-year-old man with HCV genotype 2 infection, he is treatment naïve. Which of the following would be the best treatment option for TR?

   a) Peginterferon and ribavirin for 24 weeks
   b) Sofosbuvir and ribavirin for 12 weeks
   c) Sofosbuvir and daclatasvir for 12 weeks
   d) Sofosbuvir and daclatasvir for 24 weeks
   e) Sofosbuvir and velpatasvir for 12 weeks

234. Which of the following drugs has the highest incidence of hemolytic anemia?

   a) Ribavirin
   b) Peginterferon alfa-2a
   c) Lamivudine
   d) Tenofovir
   e) Efavirenz

235. MJ is a 55-year-old African American man newly diagnosed with acute lymphoblastic leukemia (ALL). His physician has recommended part A hyper-CVAD regimen (cyclophosphamide, vincristine, doxorubicin, and dexamethasone).

   Patient's specifics: Height 5′8″, weight 180 lb
   Notable laboratory test results: SCr 1 mg/dL, total bilirubin 2.5 mg/dL
   Dosing recommendations: CrCl <50 mL/min: No dosage adjustment necessary; serum bilirubin 1.2 to 3 mg/dL: Administer 50% of dose; serum bilirubin 3.1 to 5 mg/dL: Administer 25% of dose

   Regimen:
   Cyclophosphamide 300 mg/m^2 IV q12h days 1 to 3
   Mesna 600 mg/m^2 CIVI days 1 to 3
   Vincristine 2 mg IV days 4 and 11
   Doxorubicin 50 mg/m^2 IV over 24 hours day 4
   Dexamethasone 40 mg po days 1 to 4 and days 11 to 14

   Why is MJ receiving Mesna given continuously with cyclophosphamide on days 1 to 3?

   a) Prevention of renal toxicity associated with cyclophosphamide
   b) Neutropenic fever prophylaxis
   c) Prevention of chemotherapy-induced nausea and vomiting

d) Reduction in incidence of cyclophosphamide-induced hemorrhagic cystitis

e) Prevention of hypocalcemia, hypouricemia, and hyperkalemia

236. RJ, a 70-kg male, comes into your emergency department with diabetic ketoacidosis (DKA). His blood glucose is down to 250 mL/dL with an anion gap of 32 mEq/L. Which of the following do you suggest as initial treatment?

a) Stop insulin infusion 0.1 units/kg/hour drip when the glucose normalizes, and the anion gap is 12 mEq/L

b) Continue insulin drip and add dextrose

c) Continue insulin drip and add fluids while monitoring potassium levels

d) Monitor potassium and serum ketones

e) Add dextrose only

237. Your outpatient clinic wants to improve safety with vitamin K. What would you recommend to your safety officer to prevent vitamin K overdose and ensure safe use?

a) Ensure vitamin K is not available in-patient care areas and restrict to guideline recommendations

b) Place vitamin K in kits in all patient care areas

c) Place vitamin K only in crash carts in the ER

d) Educate the staff on appropriate vitamin K use

e) Educate the patient only on appropriate vitamin K use

238. RJ is an HIV-positive male who comes into your clinic for follow-up. His current medication regimen includes abacavir, lamivudine, and ritonavir-lopinavir combination. He is also taking simvastatin. Which of the following treatment changes would you recommend for RJ?

a) Change abacavir and lamivudine to tenofovir DF and emtricitabine

b) Change ritonavir and lopinavir to raltegravir and efavirenz

c) Change ritonavir and lopinavir to darunavir and cobicistat

d) Change abacavir and lamivudine to tenofovir disoproxil fumarate

e) Adjust abacavir to lopinavir

239. MJ is a 30-year-old female who is HIV-positive and in her second trimester of pregnancy. Her HIV is well-controlled, and her current medication regimen include raltegravir 400 mg BID, emtricitabine, and tenofovir disoproxil fumarate. She has GERD and wants to take an OTC antacid to treat. What do you recommend?

a) Advise her to take pantoprazole

b) Advise her to take an H2 antagonist blocker such as famotidine and use standard twice daily

c) Advise she may use H2 antagonist or calcium carbonate antacids

d) Recommend aluminum/magnesium antacid for quick relief

e) Recommend daily antacids and proton pump inhibitors

240. RJ is a 46-year-old man taking carbidopa and levodopa. He was recently started on ephedrine OTC and metoclopramide. He complains of experiencing Parkinson's-like symptoms. Which drug likely caused the symptoms, and by what mechanism?

a) The symptoms are likely due to ephedrine and its dopamine receptor antagonism

b) The symptoms are likely due to metoclopramide and its dopamine receptor antagonism
c) The symptoms are likely due to metoclopramide and its dopamine receptor agonism
d) The symptoms are likely due to ephedrine and its dopamine receptor agonism
e) None of the above

241. MK comes into your clinic complaining of tingling fingers and extremities. You run labs and get the following: Hgb 8 g/dL, Vitamin B12 of 90 pg/mL, and a TSH level of 3 mIU/L. She currently takes metformin 1000 mg twice daily, Synthroid® 75 mcg once daily, and a multivitamin. What do you recommend for MK?

a) Decrease her metformin dose to 1000 mg once daily
b) Increase her Synthroid® dose to 95 mcg once daily
c) Start her on Vitamin B12 2mg once daily
d) Start her on thiamine 2 mg once daily
e) Start her on thiamine 5 mg once daily

242. PT is a 75-year-old female who has heart failure with a left ejection fraction of 25%, which lands her a diagnosis of HFrEF. PT is currently taking spironolactone 25 mg once daily, carvedilol 25 mg twice daily, lisinopril 10 mg once daily, furosemide 12.5 mg once daily. She comes into your clinic with BP 145/95 mmHg, HR 85, and pulmonary capillary wedge pressure (PCWP) of 16 mmHg. To further reduce her morbidity/mortality, what do you recommend?

a) Stop lisinopril and start sacubitril/valsartan 24 mg/26 mg twice daily
b) Continue lisinopril and start sacubitril/valsartan 24 mg/26 mg twice daily
c) Stop carvedilol and start metoprolol succinate 100 mg once daily
d) Continue carvedilol and start metoprolol succinate 100 mg once daily
e) Stop furosemide and start on metoprolol succinate 100 mg once daily

243. FJ is suffering from rheumatoid arthritis that is uncontrolled on his DMARD therapy, and his doctor would like to start him on infliximab. His past medical history includes congestive heart failure, diabetes, rheumatoid arthritis, and hypertension. His current medications are metformin 1000 mg BID, lisinopril 10 mg daily, naproxen 250 mg daily, folic acid 2 mg daily, furosemide 12.5 mg daily, and methotrexate 25 mg daily. Radiographic evaluation of his foot shows progression of joint space narrowing and bone erosion. Should his provider start him on infliximab, why or why not?

a) Yes, infliximab would be the next therapy of choice
b) No, infliximab has a worsening effect on heart failure
c) No, infliximab is the wrong therapy choice. The patient should be changed to leflunomide
d) No, infliximab will have a worsening effect on her hypertension due to tumor necrosis factor (TNF) induction
e) The patient should stay on current therapy

244. PJ is being treated in the hospital for an infection with vancomycin. You notice the patient starts developing a fever and a maculopapular rash. Your medical resident screams, "Red Man Syndrome!" and is not sure what to do for treatment. She rushes to you asking desperately how to treat. What should you recommend?

a) Start ceftriaxone as the infection is getting worst and not being treated
b) Increase the infusion time

c) Stop vancomycin and give a corticosteroid and fluids
d) Stop vancomycin and give diphenhydramine with fluids
e) Decrease the infusion time

245. SnoFlow comes into your clinic complaining of pain in his leg when he walks that is relieved when he rests. He describes the pain as a deep-seated muscle ache in his calf and complains of cramping. He says after 2-5 minutes his pain is relieved upon rest. He denies osteoarthritis or neurospinal compression. His doctor diagnoses him with intermittent claudication. What treatment would you recommend to SnoFlow?

a) Start SnoFlow on L-arginine
b) Start SnoFlow on cilostazol
c) Start SnoFlow on pentoxifylline
d) Tell SnoFlow he needs to exercise more
e) Stop SnoFlow from walking

246. You work at the Food and Drug Administration (FDA), and you get a new investigational drug application (IND). In the application, it states that newborns will be studied along with children the age of 5-16 years of age. Who is allowed to give consent for the children to be in the study?

a) The IRB board of the study
b) FDA needs to give consent
c) The newborn and children's guardian or parent
d) The children over the age of 12 years can give their own consent
e) The sponsor-investigator of the study

247. You pull a voriconazole level 12 hours after the last dose on a patient and it comes back at a drug level of 2 mg/L. The patient has been on the drug for 5 days. What should you do?

a) Wait, because it takes 7 days to reach steady state with voriconazole
b) Continue with the current dose, because current levels are therapeutic
c) Increase the voriconazole dose, because the current levels are subtherapeutic
d) Switch to fluconazole
e) Switch to esomeprazole

248. Frank is a patient in your hospital that has started on total parenteral nutrition (TPN). He is extremely ill with cancer, poor nutritional intake for the past 3 weeks, weight loss, and malnourished so the provider started him on parenteral nutrition. You notice on his labs that his phosphate levels are low along with his magnesium levels. You are not sure why as his TPN should have provided sufficient levels. What should you do?

a) Increase his phosphate and magnesium in his TPN to increase his levels
b) Increase his caloric requirements
c) Increase his albumin
d) Provide less than 50% of caloric requirements then slowly taper up to goal
e) Decrease his albumin

249. Sissy is a sickle cell patient who comes to your pharmacy after a recent hospital admission due to pain. She current takes hydroxyurea, clozapine, naproxen, and a multivitamin. You pull up her current medication profile and she asks you what medication helps her with pain. What do you counsel Sissy on?

   a) Speak with your doctor to change your clozapine to another antipsychotic as hydroxyurea increases the effect of clozapine, potentially causing agranulocytosis
   b) Speak with your doctor to change your naproxen to another NSAID as hydroxyurea increases the effect of naproxen, potentially causing Stevens-Johnson syndrome
   c) Speak with your doctor to change your hydroxyurea to an opioid as hydroxyurea decreases the effect of clozapine
   d) Ask your doctor to increase your dose of hydroxyurea
   e) Ask your doctor to decrease your dose of hydroxyurea

250. Which agency provides incentives for hospitals to use the electronic health record (EHR)?

   a) AHRQ
   b) CMS
   c) HRSA
   d) NCQA
   e) FDA

Section 1 Calculations: Answers and Explanations

1. **1095**

   Ratio strengths are expressed in g/mL (or g/g) and are represented as 1:[value].

   $$54 \, mg \, \times 8 = 432 \, mg$$

   $$\frac{432 \, mg}{1000} = 0.432 \, g$$

   Recall that the conversion factor for a pint is 1 pt = 473 mL

   $$\frac{0.432 \, g}{473 \, mL} = \frac{1}{x}$$

   $$x = \mathbf{1095}$$

2. **1069**

   $$KCl \; volume = 18 \, mEq \; \times \frac{1 \, mL}{2 \, mEq} = 9 \, mL$$

   $$NaCl \; volume = 25 \, mEq \; \times \frac{1 \, mL}{4 \, mEq} = 6.25 \, mL$$

   $$Mg \; sulfate \; volume = 10 \, mEq \; \times \frac{1 \, mL}{4.08 \, mEq} = 2.45 \, mL$$

   $$calcium \; gluconate \; volume = 15 \, mEq \; \times \frac{1 \, mL}{0.465 \, mEq} = 32.26 \, mL$$

   $$potassium \; phosphate \; volume = 17 \, mEq \; \times \frac{1 \, mL}{3 \, mmol} = 5.67 \, mL$$

   $$500 \, mL \, (AA) + 500 \, mL \, (dextrose) + 6.25 \, mL \, (NaCl) + 9 \, mL \, (KCl) + 2.45 \, mL \, (Mg \; sulfate)$$
   $$+ \, 32.26 \, mL \, (calcium \; gluconate) + 5.67 \, mL \, (potassium \; phosphate) + 10 \, mL \, (MVI)$$
   $$+ \, 3 \, mL \, (TE) = 1068.83 \, mL \sim \mathbf{1069 \, mL}$$

3. **C. 2.82 kg**

   $$MW = \frac{grams}{1 \, mole}$$

   Calculate the MW of calcium gluconate: $40(1) + 1(11) + 16(7) = 235 \frac{g}{mole}$

   Multiply by the number of moles present: $235 \frac{g}{mole} \times 12 \, moles = 2820 \, g$

   Convert to kilograms: $2820 \, g \times \frac{1 \, kg}{1000 \, g} = \mathbf{2.82 \, kg}$

2023-2024 NAPLEX® Practice Questions | RxPharmacist, LLC © 2023

4. **B. 39 mL**

   Specific gravity is a useful tool to convert between weight and volume. Remember the formula:

   $$specific\ gravity = \frac{mass\ (g)}{volume\ (mL)}$$

   $$0.92 = \frac{36\ g}{X} \qquad x = \mathbf{39\ mL}$$

5. **E. Give 0.8 mL by mouth every 6 to 8 hours**

   Pharmacists are routinely expected to help parents evaluate appropriate doses of over-the-counter products for their children. In this case the following steps should be followed.

   Convert 15 pounds to kilograms: $15\ lb \times \frac{1\ kg}{2.2\ lb} = 6.8\ kg$

   Multiply the child's weight by the dose range for acetaminophen:

   $$6.8\ kg \times \frac{10\ mg}{kg} = 68\ mg \qquad to \qquad 6.8\ kg \times \frac{15\ mg}{kg} = 102\ mg$$

   The dose range for the child for acetaminophen is from 68 mg to 102 mg. Finally convert the dose to a volume of medication:

   $$68\ mg \times \frac{0.8\ mL}{80\ mg} = 0.7\ mL \qquad to \qquad 102\ mg \times \frac{0.8\ mL}{80\ mg} = 1\ mL$$

   The infant's dose of acetaminophen should be **between 0.7 mL and 1 mL**.

   An answer of 3.3 mL or 5 mL would be reached if the weight in pounds was multiplied by 2.2 instead of dividing appropriately. 1.5 mL occurs if using 15 pounds without converting to kilograms. 0.8 mL is a 2-fold error on the higher end of the dosing range.

6. **24**

   Determine the molecular weight for calcium carbonate: $MW = 40 + 12 + 16(3) = 100$

   Then, calculate mEq using the following formula:

   $$mg = \frac{mEq}{valence}, \quad where\ valence = \#\ of\ ions \times net\ charge$$

   $CaCO_3 \rightarrow 1\ Ca^{+2} + 1\ [CO_3]^{-2}$ therefore: $valence = 1 \times 2 = 2$

   $$\frac{600\ mg\ CaCO_3}{dose} \times \frac{2\ doses}{day} = 1200\ \frac{mg}{day}$$

$$1200 \ mg \ CaCO_3 = \frac{x \ mEq(100)}{2} \qquad x = \textbf{24 \ mEq}$$

7. 139

Determine the weight, in mg, of Drug X and Drug Y:

$$Drug \ X: \quad \frac{0.004g}{100 \ mL} = \frac{x \ g}{30 \ mL} \qquad x = 0.0012 \ g = 1.2 \ mg$$

$$Drug \ Y: \quad \frac{1.2 \ g}{100 \ mL} = \frac{x \ g}{30 \ mL} \qquad x = 0.36 \ g = 360 \ mg$$

Determine the sodium chloride equivalents of Drug X and Y by multiplying weight by the E-value, and add them together:

$$Drug \ X: \quad 1.2 \ mg \ \times 0.92 = 1.104 \ mg$$

$$Drug \ Y: \quad 360 \ mg \ \times 0.36 = 129.6 \ mg$$

$$1.104 + 129.6 = 130.7 \ mg \ NaCl \ equivalents$$

Determine how much sodium chloride would be necessary to make the solution isotonic, assuming no other compounds are present:

$$\frac{0.9 \ g}{100 \ mL} = \frac{x \ g}{30 \ mL} \qquad x = 0.27 \ g = 270 \ mg$$

Subtract the NaCl equivalents from the total NaCl needed to determine how much NaCl should be added:

$$270 - 130.7 = \textbf{139.3 \ mg \ NaCl}$$

8. B. 5.91 grams

Calculate this patient's ideal body weight: $\quad IBW = 45.5 \ kg + (2.3 \times 7) = 61.6 \ kg$

Calculate the maintenance dose:

$$\frac{2 \ mg}{IBW} = \frac{x \ mg}{61.6 \ kg} \qquad x = 123.2 \frac{mg}{kr}$$

$$\frac{123.2 \ mg}{hr} = \frac{x \ g}{48 \ hr} \qquad x = 5913.6 \ mg$$

Convert the answer to grams:

$$5913.6 \ mg \ \times \frac{1 \ g}{1000 \ mg} = \textbf{5.91 \ g}$$

9. B. 1.2 L

Determine the number of parts of high and low concentrations needed by setting up an alligation:

Available Strengths (%)	Desired Strength (%)	Parts
25%		$12 - 3 = 9 \; parts \; of \; 25\%$
	12%	
3%		$25 - 12 = 13 \; parts \; of \; 3\%$
		$9 + 13 = 22 \; parts \; total \; (12\%)$

Use the ratio to determine how much solution you can make with the 500 mL of high (25%) concentration solution:

$$\frac{9 \; parts \; of \; 25\%}{22 \; parts \; of \; 12\%} = \frac{500 \; mL \; of \; 25\%}{x \; mL \; of \; 12\%} \qquad x = 1222 \; mL = \mathbf{1.2 \; L}$$

10. 54 mg

Determine the patient's body surface area:

$$BSA = \sqrt{\frac{height(cm) \times weight(kg)}{3600}} = \sqrt{\frac{180.34 \; cm \times 112 \; kg}{3600}} = 2.37 \; m^2$$

Multiply the dose during the second phase by the BSA to obtain a daily dose:

$$45 \; ^{mg}/_{m^2} \times 2.37 \; m^2 = 106.7 \; mg \quad {\sim}107 \; mg$$

Divide the dose in half to determine the morning dose: $\quad 107 \; mg \div 2 = 54 \; mg$

11. B. 0.09 L

Density is the weight of a substance divided by volume, usually in grams/mL:

$$density = \frac{mass}{volume}$$

$$\frac{0.62 \; g}{1 \; mL} = \frac{56 \; g}{x \; mL} \qquad x = 90.3 \; mL \times \frac{1 \; L}{1000 \; mL} = \mathbf{0.09 \; L}$$

12. B. 639 grams

The best way to solve this concentration problem is by setting up an alligation.

Available Strengths (%)	Desired Strength (%)	Parts
10.7		$4.6 - 2.9 = 1.7\ parts\ of\ 10.7\%$
	4.6	
2.9		$10.7 - 4.6 = 6.1\ parts\ of\ 2.9\%$
		$1.7 + 6.1 = 7.8\ total\ parts\ (of\ 4.6\%)$

If we know the final concentration is 4.6% and the total parts of the ointment are 7.8, we can use the ratio between parts of high/low concentration and total parts to determine how much ointment to prepare. Since we have a smaller amount of the 2.9% ointment, we can calculate the total amount prepared by assuming we will use all of it to prepare the 4.6% ointment.

$$\frac{6.1\ parts\ of\ 2.9\%\ ointment}{7.8\ parts\ of\ 4.6\%\ ointment} = \frac{500\ g\ of\ 2.9\%\ ointment}{x} \qquad x = \boldsymbol{639\ g\ of\ 4.6\%\ ointment}$$

13. 14 bags

$$\frac{50\ mL}{1\ g} \times 1.5\ g = \frac{75\ mL}{dose} \times \frac{3\ doses}{day} = \frac{225\ mL}{day} \times 3\ days = 675\ mL$$

$$675\ mL \times \frac{1\ bag}{50\ mL} = 13.5\ bags$$

14. D. 302 mg

Gentamycin is an aminoglycoside, so we need to compare ideal body weight (IBW) vs. total body weight (TBW). If the patient is obese (TBW ≥ 120% IBW), then dosing will be based on adjusted body weight.

Calculate this patient's ideal body weight: $IBW = 45.5\ kg + 2.3(4) = 54.7\ kg$

Compare patient's IBW vs. total body weight: $145\ lb \times \frac{1\ kg}{2.2\ lb} = 66\ kg$

Since this is > 120% IBW, we need to calculate adjusted body weight:

$$54.7\ kg + 0.4(66 - 54.7)\ kg = 59.22\ kg$$

Calculate the daily dose using adjusted body weight:

$$\frac{1.7\ mg}{kg} \times 59.22\ kg = \frac{100.7\ mg}{dose} \times \frac{3\ doses}{day} = \boldsymbol{302\ mg\ daily}$$

15. C. 31 mL

Specific gravity refers to the weight of a substance relative to the weight of an equal volume of water. At atmospheric pressure and room temperature this value is similar to the density of a substances, which is weight per volume:

$$\frac{0.84\ mg}{1\ mL} = \frac{26\ g}{x\ mL} \qquad x = 31\ mL$$

16. 2.5

Final dilution: (quantity₁)(concentration₁) = (quantity₂)(concentration₂)

$$(250\ mL)(20\%) = (2000mL)(X\%) \qquad X = \mathbf{2.5\%}$$

17. 774,000

To solve equations involving moles, it is important to remember the formula: $MW = \frac{grams}{1 mole}$

Calculate the molecular weight of sodium citrate: $23(3) + 12(6) + 1(5) + 16(7) = 258\frac{g}{mole}$

Multiply by the number of moles present: $258\frac{g}{mole} \times 3\ moles = 774\ g$

Convert to milligrams: $774\ g \times \frac{1000mg}{g} = 774,000\ mg$

18. B. 2.05 mg

Convert his weight in pounds to kg: $258\ lb \times \frac{1\ kg}{2.2lb} = 117.3\ kg$

Calculate the dose in mcg/kg: $\frac{17.5\ mcg}{kg} = \frac{x\ mcg}{117.3\ kg} \qquad x = 2052.75\ mcg$

Convert mcg to mg: $2052.75\ mcg \times \frac{1\ mg}{1000\ mcg} = \mathbf{2.05\ mg}$

19. 605

To make things easier, first convert lb to kg, and inches to cm:

$$W = 156\ lb \times \frac{1\ kg}{2.2\ lb} = 70.91\ kg$$
$$H = 5\ ft\ 3\ inches = 63\ in \times \frac{2.54\ cm}{in} = 160.02\ cm$$
$$A = 31\ years\ old$$

Insert these values into the given equation for BEE: Female = 655 + (9.6 × W) + (1.8 × H) - (4.7 × A)

Multiply that value by the stress factor 1.2 (given) to determine total daily calories:

$$1478.08 \frac{kcal}{day} \times 1.2 = 1773.69 \text{ kcal/day}$$

Assuming that the daily amino acids (aka protein) requirement is 0.75 g per kg of body weight:

$$\frac{0.75 \, g \, protein}{kg} \times 70.91 \, kg = 53.18 \, gram \, protein$$

Assuming that amino acids provide 4 kcal per gram:

$$53.18 \, g \, protein \times 4 \frac{kcal}{g} = 212.72 \, kcal \, from \, protein$$

Convert grams to mL amino acids:

$$53.18 \, g \times \frac{100 \, mL}{7g} = 759.71 \, mL \, of \, amino \, acids$$

Assuming that the daily lipid requirement is 30% of one's total daily calories:

$$1773.69 \frac{kcal}{day} \times 0.3 = 532.11 \, kcal \, of \, lipids/day$$

Now that we know the amount of kcal contributed by proteins and lipids, we can figure out the rest of total daily calories that should be provided by dextrose.
$Total \, Daily \, Calories = kcal \, protein + kcal \, lipids + kcal \, dextrose$

Rearrange that to get: $Total \, Daily \, Calories - kcal \, protein - kcal \, lipids = kcal \, dextrose$

$$1773.69 \, kcal - 212.72 \, kcal - 532.11 \, kcal = 1028.86 \, kcal \, dextrose$$

Assuming that dextrose provides 3.4 kcal per gram:

$$1028.86 \, kcal \, dextrose \times \frac{g}{3.4 \, kcal} = 3021.61 \, g \, dextrose$$

Convert grams to mL dextrose:

$$3021.61 \, g \, dextrose \times \frac{100 \, mL}{50 \, g} = \mathbf{605.22 \, mL \, dextrose}$$

20. E. 333

$$flow \, rate \, (\frac{ml}{hr}) = \frac{total \, volume \, (mL)}{infusion \, time \, (hr)}$$

$$flow \, rate = \frac{1000 \, mL}{3 \, hr} = \mathbf{333.33 \frac{ml}{hr}}$$

2023-2024 NAPLEX® Practice Questions | RxPharmacist, LLC © 2023

21. B. 24 mL

Percentage volume-in-volume indicates the number of parts by volume of the active ingredient contained in the total volume of the liquid preparation considered as 100 parts by volume. The answer to this problem can be found by multiplying the volume (in mL) by the percent (expressed as a decimal) to get the mL of active ingredient: $300 \, mL \times 0.08 = 24 \, mL$

22. D. 0.15 mg

50 mcg per mL would be equal to 150 mcg per 3 mL, which is the same as 0.15 mg in 3 mL

$$\frac{50 \, mcg}{mL} \times 3 \, mL = 150 \, mcg \times \frac{1 \, mg}{1000 \, mcg} = 0.15 \, mg$$

23. C. 5.4 L

Convert tablespoons to mL: $\quad 4 \, tbsp \times \frac{15 \, mL}{1 \, tbsp} = 60 \, mL \, per \, dose$

Determine how many mL the patient would receive in a day: $\quad \frac{60 \, mL}{dose} \times \frac{3 \, doses}{day} = 180 \, mL \, per \, day$

Determine how many mL in a 30 day supply: $\frac{180 mL}{day} \times 30 \, days = 5400 \, mL$

Convert to liters: $\quad 5400 \, mL \times \frac{1 \, L}{1000 \, mL} = \mathbf{5.4 \, L}$

24. D. 34 grams

$2 \, oz \times \frac{28.35 \, g}{oz} = 56.7 \, g; \qquad$ Conversion factor: $\frac{56.7 \, g}{1000 \, g} \times 600 \, g = 34.02 \, g$

25. 280

Calculate the number of grams of each component in 8 oz, or 240 mL (30 mL/fl oz), of liquid:

$Protein: \quad \frac{6.9 \, g}{100 \, mL} = \frac{x}{240 \, mL} \qquad x = 16.56 \, g \qquad Carb: \quad \frac{15 \, g}{100 \, mL} = \frac{x}{240 \, mL} \qquad x = 36 \, g$

$Fat: \quad \frac{3.2 \, g}{100 \, mL} = \frac{x}{240 \, mL} \qquad x = 7.68 \, g$

Calculate the number of calories. There are 9 calories/gram of fat and 4 calories/gram of carbohydrate and protein.

$Protein: \quad 16.56 \, g \times \frac{4 \, kcal}{g} = 66.24 \, kcal \qquad Carb: \quad 36 \, g \times \frac{4 \, kcal}{g} = 144 \, kcal$

$Fat: \quad 7.68 \, g \times \frac{9 \, kcal}{g} = 69.12 \, kcal$

Add the number of calories from each component to determine the total calorie intake.

$$66.24 \text{ kcal} + 144 \text{ kcal} + 69.12 \text{ kcal} = \textbf{279 kcal}$$

26. 35 drops

Determine how many mg of gentamicin solution will be added to the IV bag:

$$\frac{40 \, mg}{mL} = \frac{127.5 \, mg}{x \, mL} \qquad x = 3.2 \, mL$$

Add the volume of the solution to the volume of gentamicin to obtain your total volume:

$$50 \, mL \, NS + 3.2 \, mL \, gentamicin \, solution = 53.2 \, mL \, total \, volume$$

Set up a chain of ratios to determine drops per minute:

$$\frac{53.2 \, mL}{30 \, min} \times \frac{20 \, drops}{mL} = \textbf{35.46 drops/min}$$

27. D. 1:25 (w/v)

$$\frac{40 \, mg}{mL} \times \frac{1 \, g}{1000 \, mg} = \frac{40 \, g}{1000 \, mL} = \frac{0.04g}{mL} = \frac{1 \, mL}{0.04g} = 25, thus \, \textbf{1:25} \, (\boldsymbol{w/v})$$

28. A. 800 mg/day

At first, you may think the answer would be 40 mg/hr x 24 hr = 960 mg/day; however, aminophylline contains about <u>80% theophylline</u>, which is the moiety measured in therapeutic drug monitoring. The appropriate conversion is: $960 \, mg/day \, x \, 0.8 = 768 \, mg/day$

Theo-24 is available in 100 mg, 200 mg, 300 mg and 400 mg strength capsules. Round up to the appropriate unit dose available which would be 4 x 200 mg capsules/day or, more conveniently, 2 x 400 mg capsules/day.

29. C. 1:316

Ratio strength is expressed as 1:x (g:mL for solid in liquid preparations). The easiest way to solve the problem is to set up an equation to solve for x:

$$\frac{0.380 \, g}{120 \, mL} = \frac{1}{x} \qquad x = \textbf{316 } mL, or \, \textbf{1:316}$$

The same concentration expressed as a percentage strength would be 0.32% (0.32 g/100 mL)

30. C. 26.25 mL/hr

The patient weighs 70 kg: $70 \, kg \times 10 \mu g/kg/minute = 700 \, \mu g/minute$

$$\frac{700\mu g}{minute} \cdot \frac{60\ minutes}{hour} = 42,000\frac{\mu g}{hr} \qquad \rightarrow \qquad 42,000\frac{\mu g}{hr} \times \frac{250ml}{400mg} \times \frac{1000\mu g}{mg}$$

$$= 26.25\frac{mL}{hr}$$

31. 15.6

Determine the weight of the active ingredient in each product:

12.2% w/w: $\quad \dfrac{12.2\ g}{100\ g} = \dfrac{x\ g}{37.5\ g} \qquad x = 4.575\ g$

17.6% w/w: $\quad \dfrac{17.6\ g}{100\ g} = \dfrac{x\ g}{62.5\ g} \qquad x = 11\ g$

Add the weights together to determine the final weight: $4.575\ g\ +\ 11\ g\ =\ 15.575g$

Divide the weight of the active ingredient by the final weight to determine the final concentration:

$$\frac{15.75}{37.5 + 62.5} = 15.575\%\ w/w$$

32. 7

The formula to calculate mEq is: $\quad mg = \dfrac{mEq}{valence}$, where $valence = \#\ of\ ions \times net\ charge$

$KCl = 1[K]^{+1} + 1[Cl]^{-1}$; therefore, $valence = 1 \times 1 = 1$

$$500\ mg\ KCl = \frac{(x\ mEq)74.5}{1} \qquad x = 6.7\ \sim 7mEq$$

33. 360

Calculate the molecular weight of potassium chloride (KCl) and sodium chloride (NaCl):

$KCl = 1[K]^{+1} + 1[Cl]^{-1}$ $\qquad\qquad$ MW = 39 + 35.5 = 74.5
Number of species formed = 2 (1 K + 1 Cl)

$NaCl = 1[Na]^{+1} + 1[Cl]^{-1}$ $\qquad\qquad$ MW = 23 + 35.5 = 58.5
Number of species formed = 2 (1 Na + 1 Cl)

Determine mOsm, for each, using the formula: $\quad mOsm = \dfrac{weight(g)}{MW} \times 1000 \times number\ of\ species$

$$KCl\ mOsm = \frac{0.5\ g}{74.5\ g} \times 1000 \times 2 = 13\ mOsm\ in\ 250\ mL$$

$$NaCl\ mOsm = \frac{2.25\ g}{58.5\ g} \times 1000 \times 2 = 77\ mOsm\ in\ 250\ mL$$

Normal saline is 0.9% w/v sodium chloride. Determine the weight of sodium chloride in 250 mL, you must set up a ratio using the 0.9% w/v and solve for the grams of sodium chloride:

$$\frac{x \; mg}{250 \; mL} = \frac{0.9 \; g}{100 \; mL} \qquad x = 2.25 \; g$$

If there are 2 products, you need to figure out each one separately and add mOsm together:

$$13 \; mOsm \; KCl \; + \; 77 \; mOsm \; NaCl \; = \; 90 \; mOsm \; in \; 250 \; mL$$

Convert to liters, since osmolarity is reported as the number of milliosmoles in 1 liter of solution:

$$\frac{90 \; mOsm}{250 \; mL} = \frac{x \; mOsm}{1000 \; mL} \qquad x = 360 \; mOsm/L$$

34. 8.7

$$MW = \frac{mg}{mmol}$$

Calculate the total amount of potassium consumed: $\frac{680 \; mg}{serving} \times 0.5 \; servings = 340 \; mg \; K$

Use the formula to determine millimoles of potassium using the atomic weight of K (not KCl):

$$\frac{39 \; mg}{mmol} = \frac{340}{x \; mmol} \qquad x = \boldsymbol{8.7 \; mmol}$$

35. A. 2.2 g/mL

Density is determined by dividing mass by volume. Density is usually reported in g/mL

$$Density \; of \; Drug \; Z: \quad \frac{55,020 \; g}{25,000 \; mL} = \boldsymbol{2.2 \; g/mL}$$

36. B. 1 g in 10,000 mL

The abbreviation ppm stands for parts per million, or a concentration in grams per 1,000,000 mL of water. Therefore, 100 ppm would be equal to 100 grams in 1,000,000 mL of water, or 1 gram in 10,000 mL, or 1 gram in 10 L

37. C. 170 kcal

1 gram of dextrose provides 3.4 kilocalories (kcal). A 5% dextrose solution provides 5 gram/100 mL, or 50 gram in 1000 mL (1 L). The calories provided by the solution would be 50 $gram \; x \; 3.4 \; kcal/ gram \; = \; 170 \; kcal$

38. 5.3 mg/gtt/day

$$\frac{0.8 \; g}{10 \; mL} \times \frac{1 \; mL}{15 \; gtt} = \frac{0.00533 \; g}{gtt} \times \frac{1000 \; mg}{g} = \boldsymbol{5.33 \; mg/gtt/day}$$

39. A. 10 days

The patient is to receive 100 mL of a 500 mg/5 mL ciprofloxacin suspension. The directions are for the patient to take 1 teaspoon (5 mL) twice daily (Q12H and BID) till all is taken (tat):

$$2\ tsp \times \frac{5\ mL}{tsp} = 10\ mL\ per\ day \qquad 100\ mL \times \frac{10\ mL}{day} = \boldsymbol{10\ days}$$

40. B. 30 mL

$$3\ g \times \frac{1\ mL}{0.5\ g} = 6\ mL\ per\ bag \times 5\ bags = \boldsymbol{30\ mL}$$

41. 1% (w/v)

$$\frac{10\ mg}{mL} \times \frac{1\ g}{1000\ mg} = \frac{10\ g}{1000\ mL} = \frac{1\ g}{100\ mL} = \boldsymbol{1\%\ (w/v)}$$

42. 0.08 mL

Insulins are dosed in terms of units of activity rather than milligrams or grams. "U-100" refers to a potency of 100 Units/mL of activity, while "U-500" refers to a potency of 500 Units/mL. The U-500 product is 5-times more concentrated. To convert dosing volumes the equation $C_1V_1 = C_2V_2$ is used:

$$(0.4\ mL)(100\ Units/mL) = (X)(500\ Units/mL) \qquad X = \boldsymbol{0.08\ mL\ of\ insulin}$$

43. 11.6 mL

Specific gravity refers to the weight of a substance relative to the weight of an equal volume of water. At atmospheric pressure and room temperature this value is similar to the density of a substances, which is weight per volume:

$$\frac{0.43\ g}{1\ mL} = \frac{5\ g}{x\ mL} \qquad x = \boldsymbol{11.6\ mL}$$

44. D. 18.5 mmol

Millimoles formula:
$$MW = \frac{mg}{mmol}$$

Calculate the total amount of potassium consumed: $240\ mg \times 3\ servings = 720\ mg\ potassium$

Use the formula above to determine millimoles of potassium using the atomic weight of K (not KCl):

$$\frac{39\ mg}{1\ mmol} = \frac{720\ mg}{x\ mmol} \qquad x = \boldsymbol{18.5\ mmol}$$

45. A. 1907 kcal

First, convert lb to kg, and inches to cm.

$$W = 198 \; lb \times \frac{1 \; kg}{2.2 \; lb} = 90 \; kg$$

$$H = 73 \; in \times \frac{2.54 \; cm}{1 \; in} = 185.42 \; cm$$

$$A = 47 \; years \; old$$

Insert into the equation for BEE:

$$66 + (13.7 \times 90) + (5 \times 185.42) - (6.8 \times 47) = \mathbf{1906.50 \; kcal}$$

46. B. 0.37 kg

$$MW = \frac{g}{mol}$$

Calculate the molecular weight of potassium chloride (KCl): $39 + 35.5 = 74.5 \; g/mole$

Multiply by the number of moles present: $74.5 \frac{g}{mole} \times 5 \; moles = 372.5 \; g$

Convert to kilograms: $372.5 \; grams \times \frac{1 \; kg}{1000 \; g} = \mathbf{0.37 \; kg}$

47. 30 gtt/min

$$\frac{50 \; g}{hr} \times \frac{50 \; mL}{1 \; g} = 100 \frac{mL}{hr} \times 18 \frac{gtt}{mL} = \frac{1800 \; gtt}{hr} \times \frac{1 \; hr}{60 \; minutes} = \mathbf{30 \; gtt/min}$$

48. A. 1.3 kg

$$MW = \frac{g}{mol}$$

Calculate the MW of ferrous gluconate: $56(1) + 12(12) + 22(1) + 16(14) = 446 \; g/mole$

Multiply by the number of moles present: $446 \frac{g}{mole} \times 3 \; moles = 1338 \; g$

Convert to kilograms: $1338 \; g \; x \; \frac{1 \; kg}{1000 \; g} = \mathbf{1.3 \; kg}$

49. A. 119

$C_1Q_1 = C_2Q_2$, where Q = quantity and C = concentration

$$(2.7\%)(x \; mL) = (10.7\%)(30 \; mL) \qquad x = 119 \; mL$$

50. A. 0.000154

It's important to know metric system:
    1 gram = 1000 mg
    1 mg = 1000 mcg
    1 mcg = 1000 ng

To solve this problem: $154 \, ng \times \dfrac{1 \, mg}{1,000,000 \, ng} = \boldsymbol{0.000154 \, mg}$

Section 2 Calculations: Answers and Explanations

1. **C. 210 mg**

   The patient has been diagnosed with chronic kidney disease (CKD). Ferric citrate ($Fe^{3+}[C_3O_7]x$? y H2O (x = 0.7 – 0.87; y = 1.9 – 3.3) has an approximate average molecular weight of 265.93 g/mol; it is available as a 1 gram (1000 mg) oral tablet. Ferric chloride is used to treat hyperphosphatemia by formation of insoluble precipitates. According to the package insert, each gram of ferric citrate provides 210 milligrams of ferric iron:

   $$\frac{1000 \; mg \; ferric \; citrate}{265.93 g/mol} = \frac{X \; mg \; Fe^{3+}}{55.85 \; g/mol} \qquad X = \mathbf{210 \; mg}$$

2. **1000**

   Mega (M) is **1000 times bigger** than kilo. It's important to know the metric system.

3. **C. 32.36 mL**

   $$\text{Calcium Gluconate volume} = 15 \; mEq \times \frac{mL}{0.465 \; mEq} = \mathbf{32.26 \; mL}$$

4. **0.4**

   Determine the weight, in g, of Drug Z and Drug X:

   $$\frac{0.05 \; g}{100 \; mL} = \frac{Z \; g}{60 \; mL} \qquad Z = 0.03 \; g \qquad\qquad \frac{2.7 \; g}{100 \; mL} = \frac{X \; g}{60 \; mL} \qquad X = 1.62 \; g$$

   Determine the sodium chloride equivalents of Drug Z and X and add them together:

   $$Drug \; Z: 0.03 \; g \times 0.82 = 0.0246 \; g \qquad Drug \; X: 1.62 \; g \times 0.07 = 0.1134 \; g$$

   $$0.0246 + 0.1134 = 0.138 \; g \; NaCl \; equivalents$$

   Determine how much NaCl would be necessary to make the solution isotonic, assuming no other compounds are present:

   $$\frac{0.9 g}{100 mL} = \frac{x \; g}{60 mL} \qquad x = 0.54 \; g$$

   Subtract the NaCl equivalents from the total NaCl needed to determine how much NaCl should be added:

   $$0.540 - 0.138 = \mathbf{0.402 \; g \; NaCl}$$

5. D. 2.7 L

Convert tablespoons to mL:

$$\frac{2\ tbsp}{x\ mL} = \frac{1\ tbsp}{15\ mL} \qquad x = 30\ mL\ per\ dose$$

Determine how many mL the patient would receive in a day:

$$\frac{30\ mL}{dose} \times 3\ doses = 90\ mL\ per\ day$$

Determine how many mL in a 30 day supply:

$$\frac{90\ mL}{day} \times 30\ days = 2700\ mL$$

Double check the question for the requested units. In this case, we need to convert to liters:

$$2700\ mL \times \frac{1\ L}{1000\ mL} = \mathbf{2.7\ L}$$

6. E. 9 mL

$$KCl\ volume:\ \ 18\ mEq \times \frac{mL}{2\ mEq} = \mathbf{9\ mL}$$

7. 18

Specific gravity refers to the weight of a substance relative to the weight of an equal volume of water. At atmospheric pressure and room temperature this value is similar to the density of a substances, which is weight per volume:

$$\frac{0.84\ g}{1\ mL} = \frac{15\ g}{x\ mL} \qquad x = 17.9\ mL\ \sim\mathbf{18\ mL}$$

8. B. 1:1,666 (w/v), 0.06%

$$30\ mg \times \frac{1\ g}{1000\ mg} = 0.03\ g \qquad \frac{0.03\ g}{50\ mL} = \frac{x\ g}{100\ mL} \qquad x = \frac{0.06\ g}{100\ mL} = 0.0006\frac{g}{mL}$$

$$\frac{0.0006\ g}{mL} = \frac{1\ g}{x\ mL} \qquad x = 1,666\ mL$$

$$Ratio\ strength = \mathbf{1{:}1,666\ (w/v)}$$

$$Percent\ strength = \frac{0.06\ g}{100\ mL} \times 100 = \mathbf{0.06\%\ (w/v)}$$

9. 198

Determine the weight, in mg, of Drug A and Drug B:

$$Drug\ A:\quad \frac{0.05\ g}{100\ mL} = \frac{x\ g}{180\ mL}\qquad x = 0.9\ g = 900\ mg$$

$$Drug\ B:\quad \frac{2\ g}{100\ mL} = \frac{x\ g}{180\ mL}\qquad x = 3.6\ g = 3600\ mg$$

Determine the sodium chloride equivalents of Drug A and B, then add them together:

$$Drug\ A:\quad 900\ mg \times 0.54 = 486\ mg$$

$$Drug\ B:\quad 3600\ mg \times 0.26 = 936\ mg$$

$$486\ +\ 936\ =\ 1422\ mg\ NaCl\ equivalents$$

Determine how much sodium chloride to make the solution isotonic (normal saline solution):

$$\frac{0.9\ g}{100\ mL} = \frac{x\ g}{180\ mL}\qquad x = 1.62\ g = 1620\ mg$$

Subtract the NaCl equivalents from the total NaCl needed to determine how much NaCl should be added:

$$1620\ -\ 1422\ =\ \mathbf{198\ mg\ NaCl}$$

10. C. 180 mg/L

Valence of Mg is +2 and molecular weight is 24.

$$mEq = \frac{MW}{valence},\qquad where\ valence = \ of\ ions \times net\ charge$$

$$1\ mEq = \frac{24\ mg}{2} = 12\ mg \qquad\qquad \frac{1\ mEq}{12\ mg} = \frac{1.5m\ Eq}{x\ mg}\qquad x = 18\ mg$$

$$\frac{18\ mg}{100\ mL} \times \frac{1000\ mL}{1L} = \mathbf{180\ mg/L}$$

11. B. 2.45 mL

$$Mg\ Sulfate\ volume:\ 10\ mEq \times \frac{mL}{4.08\ mEq} = 2.45\ mL$$

12. D. 588,000 mg

$$MW = \frac{grams}{1\ mole}$$

Calculate the MW of sodium bicarbonate: $23(1) + 1(1) + 12(1) + 16(3) = 84 \ g/mole$

Multiply by the number of moles present: $84 \ \frac{g}{mole} \times 7 \ moles = 588 \ grams$

Convert to milligrams: $588 \ g \times 1000 \ \frac{mg}{g} = \mathbf{588,000 \ mg}$

13. 855

Determine the number of parts of high and low concentrations needed by setting up an alligation:

Available Strengths (%)	Desired Strength (%)	Parts
12.5		$7 - 3 = 4 \ parts \ of \ 12.5\%$
	7	
3		$12.5 - 7 = 5.5 \ parts \ of \ 3\%$
		$4 + 5.5 = 9.5 \ parts \ total \ of \ 7\%$

Use the ratio to determine how much solution you can make with the 360 mL of 12.5%:

$High$: $\dfrac{4 \ parts \ of \ 12.5\%}{9.5 \ parts \ of \ 7\%} = \dfrac{360 \ mL \ of \ 12.5\%}{x \ mL}$ $\qquad x = \mathbf{855 \ mL \ of \ 7\%}$

14. 1.7

To maintain the buffer capacity of a buffer used in the compounding of ophthalmic products, it is recommended that approximately 1/3 of the final volume contains buffer.

For this product: $5 \ mL \div 3 = \mathbf{1.7 \ mL}$ **of Sorensen's Phosphate Buffer.**

15. A. 50 drops/minute

The total volume (100 mL) will be infused over 30 minutes, a rate of 3.33 mL/minute. If the administration set delivers 15 drops/mL, set up a ratio to solve for drops per minute:

$\dfrac{15 \ drops}{1 \ mL} = \dfrac{x \ drops}{3.33 \ mL/min}$ $\qquad x = 50 \ drops/minute$

16. C. 28

$$BMI = \frac{weight(kg)}{\left(height \ (m)\right)^2}$$

Calculate the patient's weight in kg: $185 \ lb \times \dfrac{1 \ kg}{2.2 \ lbs} = 84.1 \ kg$

Calculate the patient's height in meters: $68 \ inches \times \dfrac{2.54 \ cm}{1 \ in} \times \dfrac{1 \ m}{100 \ cm} = 1.72 \ m$

Calculate the BMI: $BMI = \dfrac{84.1}{(1.72)^2} = \mathbf{28 \ kg/m^2}$

This patient's BMI indicates that he is overweight, and lifestyle modifications should be encouraged to help him reach a normal BMI (<25).

17. 75 tablets

30 mg daily/5 mg/tab = 6 tabs per day x 5 days =	30 tabs
25 mg daily/5 mg/tab = 5 tabs per day x 3 days =	15 tabs
20 mg daily/5 mg/tab = 4 tabs per day x 3 days =	12 tabs
15 mg daily/5 mg/tab = 3 tabs per day x 3 days =	9 tabs
10 mg daily/5 mg/tab = 2 tabs per day x 3 days =	6 tabs
5 mg daily/5 mg/tab = 1 tab per day x 3 days =	3 tabs
End of taper	75 tabs

18. A. 0.38 g

Convert her weight in pounds to kg: $\frac{140\ lb}{x\ kg} = \frac{2.2\ lb}{1\ kg}$ $x = 63.6\ kg$

Calculate the dose in mg/kg: $\frac{6\ mg}{kg} = \frac{x\ mg}{63.6\ kg}$ $x = 381.6\ mg$

Convert mg to g: $381.6\ mg \times \frac{1\ g}{1000\ mg} = 0.38\ g$

19. A. 1:10

Ratio strength is the expression of concentration of a pharmaceutical formulation by using a ratio. A 1% (w/v) percentage strength would indicate a ratio of 1 gram per 100 mL. The conversion from a 10% solution to x ratio strength would be 10 g/100 mL:

$$\frac{10g}{100mL} = \frac{x\ parts}{100\ parts}$$ $x = 10, so\ the\ ratio\ strength\ is\ \textbf{1:10}$

20. 4628

$Dextrose: 500\ mL \times \frac{70\ g}{100\ mL} = 350\ g \times 3.4\frac{kcal}{g} = 1190\ kcal;\ 170\ kcal\ +\ 1190\ kcal\ =\ 1360\ kcal$

$KCl\ volume: 15\ mEq \times \frac{mL}{2\ mEq} = 7.5mL$

$NaCl\ volume: 20\ mEq \times \frac{mL}{4\ mEq} = 5\ mL$

$Mg\ sulfate\ volume: 8\ mEq \times \frac{x\ mL}{4.08\ mEq} = 1.96\ mL$

$Calcium\ gluconate\ volume: 12\ mEq \times \frac{mL}{0.465\ mEq} = 25.81\ mL$

$$Potassium\ phosphate\ volume: 23\ mmol \times \frac{mL}{3\ mmol} = 7.67\ mL$$
$$500\ mL\ (AA) + 500\ mL\ (Dextrose) + 5\ mL\ (NaCl) + 7.5\ mL\ (KCl)$$
$$+ 1.96\ mL\ (Mg\ Sulfate) + 25.81\ mL\ (Ca\ Gluconate)$$
$$+ 7.67\ mL\ (Potassium\ Phosphate) + 10\ mL\ (MVI) = 1057.94\ mL$$

$$\frac{1360\ kcal}{1058\ mL} \times \frac{150\ mL}{hr} = \frac{192.82\ kcal}{hr} \times \frac{24\ hr}{day} = \mathbf{4,627.6\ kcal/day}$$

21. 390

$$120\ lbs \times \frac{1\ kg}{2.2\ lb} = 54.54\ kg \times \frac{5\ g}{kg} = 272.73\ g \times \frac{100\ mL}{70\ g} = 389.6\ mL\ \sim\mathbf{390\ mL}$$

22. E. 0.04 L

Specific gravity refers to the weight of a substance relative to the weight of an equal volume of water. At atmospheric pressure and room temperature this value is similar to the density of a substances, which is weight per volume:

$$\frac{0.62\ g}{1\ mL} = \frac{24\ g}{x\ mL} \qquad x = 38.7\ mL \times \frac{1\ L}{1000\ mL} = 0.0387\ L\ \sim\mathbf{0.04\ L}$$

23. 0.38

Triamcinolone acetonide 0.025% ointment contains 0.25 mg of API per gram of total mixture.

$$0.025\% = \frac{0.025\ g}{100\ g} \rightarrow \frac{0.025\ mg\ TA}{100\ g\ ointment} \times \frac{1000\ mg}{1\ g} = 0.25\ mg\ TA\ per\ g\ total\ mixture$$

The prescription is written for 60 grams of ointment.

$$\frac{x\ mg\ TA}{60\ g\ ointment} \times \frac{0.25\ mg\ TA}{1\ g\ ointment} \qquad x = 15\ mg\ triamcinolone\ acetonide$$

Each vial contains 40 mg/mL.

$$\frac{40\ mg}{mL} = \frac{15\ mg}{x\ mL} \qquad x = 0.375\ mL\ \sim\mathbf{0.38\ mL}$$

It is rounded up to 0.38 mL to accommodate the fact that 1 mL syringes are graduated only in 1/100 mL measurement.

24. C. Amoxicillin 250 mg/5 mL sig: 2 teaspoons PO Q12hr x 10 days

The patient weighs 33.3 kg. The doctor wants him to receive 30 mg/kg per day, and he wants it divided into 2 doses.

$$33.3\ kg \times 30\ mg/kg/day = 999\ mg\ \sim 1000\ mg\ daily \div 2\ doses = 500\ mg$$

To get approximately 500 mg in each dose, you would give 2 teaspoonfuls of Amoxicillin 250 mg/5 mL q 12 hours for 10 days. An alternative is trying Amoxicillin 250 mg chewable tablets that the patient may also take, take 2 tablets by mouth twice daily for 10 days. The patient should be counseled on taking a probiotic after the antibiotic course to help replenish the gut flora and lessen concerns for GI upset.

25. 0.99

Density is determined by dividing mass by volume. Density is usually reported in g/mL.

$$\frac{775\ g}{785\ mL} = 0.99\ g/mL$$

26. A. 348 mOsm/L

Calculate the molecular weight of potassium chloride (KCl) and sodium chloride (NaCl):

KCl: MW = 39 + 35.5 = 74.5   NaCl: MW = 23 + 35.5 = 58.5

Determine mOsm, for each, using the formula: $mOsmol = \frac{weight\ (g)}{MW} \times 1000 \times number\ of\ species$

$KCl\ mOsmol$: $\frac{0.75}{74.5} \times 1000 \times 2 = 20\ mOsm\ in\ 500\ mL$

$NaCl\ mOsmol$: $\frac{4.5}{58.5} \times 1000 \times 2 = 154\ mOsm\ in\ 500\ mL$

If there are 2 products, you need to figure out each one separately and add mOsm together:

$20\ mOsm\ KCl\ +\ 154\ mOsm\ NaCl\ =\ 174\ mOsm\ in\ 500\ mL$

Convert to mOsm per liter:

$$\frac{174\ mOsm}{500\ mL} = \frac{x\ mOsm}{1000\ mL} \qquad x = 348\ mOsm/L$$

27. 25

Rx #889 is ProAir inhaler. With each fill, the patient receives 1 inhaler containing 200 puffs. The patient can use up to 2 puffs 4 times per day, which comes to a total of 8 puffs per day. $200\ puffs\ total \div 8\ puffs\ per\ day = 25\ days.$ The patient's prescription will last of 25 days. If a patient is filling for ProAir every month, then it is a sign their asthma is not well-controlled.

28. C. 5% dextrose in water

Dextrose at 5% concentration is isotonic and has the same osmotic pressure as blood. To determine the tonicity of the solution, convert the concentration of dextrose to an equivalent concentration of sodium chloride using the E-value ($E_{dextrose} = 0.18$):

$$\frac{5\ g\ dextrose}{100\ mL} \times 0.18 = \frac{0.9\ g\ NaCl}{100\ mL}$$

29. 36

To calculate CrCl, first calculate ideal body weight (IBW): $IBW = 45.5\ kg + 2.3\ kg\ (6) = 59.3\ kg$

Cockcroft-Gault equation for a <u>female</u>:

$$CrCl = \frac{\left(140 - age\ (yrs)\right) \times weight(kg)}{72 \times SCr}(\times\ 0.85\ if\ female)$$

$$CrCl = \frac{(140 - 41) \times 59.3}{72 \times 1.9}(\times\ 0.85) = 36.47\ mL/min \quad \boldsymbol{\sim 36\ mL/min}$$

30. A. 100 drops/minute

The prescribed dose is 50 mg and the drug is available as a 25 mg/mL solution. Calculate the volume of drug that should be injected into the 100 mL NSS bag: $50\ mg \times \frac{1\ mL}{25\ mg} = 2\ mL$.

The total volume of the infusion is therefore: $100\ mL + 2\ mL = 102\ mL$.

Calculate the appropriate infusion rate for over 20 minutes: $\frac{102\ mL}{20\ minutes} = 5.1\ mL/min$.

Convert this value to drops/min for IV administration: $\frac{5.1\ mL}{minute} \times \frac{20\ drops}{mL} = 102\ drops/min$.

Remember, the volume of drug being added to the IV bag is < 10% of the initial bag volume; it would be ignored in the calculation of the infusion rate:

$$\frac{100\ mL}{20\ minute} = \frac{5\ mL}{minute} \times \frac{20\ drops}{mL} = 100\ drops/min$$

31. D. 5 mL PO daily for 10 days

Convert lb to kg: $39\ lb \times \frac{1\ kg}{2.2\ lb} = 17.73\ kg$

To calculate the daily dose: $17.73\ kg \times \frac{14\ mg}{kg} = 248.2\ mg \quad \sim 250\ mg\ every\ 24\ hours$

The strength is given (250 mg/5 mL). You want to give the patient 250 mg, so give them 5 mL daily.

32. 0.58

Use the sodium chloride equivalent (E-value) method. First, determine the weight (g), of the drugs:

$Drug\ A: \frac{0.75\ g}{100\ mL} = \frac{x\ g}{480\ mL} \qquad x = 3.6\ g \qquad Drug\ B: \frac{3\ g}{100\ mL} = \frac{x\ g}{480\ mL} \qquad x = 14.4\ g$

Determine the sodium chloride equivalents of Drug A and B and add them together:

Drug A: $3.6\ g \times 0.52 = 1.872\ g$ Drug B: $14.4\ g \times 0.13 = 1.872\ g$
$1.872 + 1.872 = 3,744\ g\ NaCl\ equivalents$

Determine how much sodium chloride would be necessary to make the solution isotonic, assuming no other compounds are present (normal saline solution):

$$\frac{0.9\ g}{100\ mL} = \frac{x}{480\ mL} \qquad x = 4.32\ g$$

Subtract the NaCl equivalents from the total NaCl needed to see how much NaCl to add:
$4.320 - 3.744 = 0.576\ g\ NaCl \quad \sim \textbf{0.58 g NaCl}$

33. 3

Calculate conversion factor: $45\ mL/10\ mL = 4.5$
Multiply amount of cherry flavor by conversion factor: $10\ gtt \times 4.5 = 45\ gtt$
Multiply total drops by drop factor: $45\ gtt \times \frac{mL}{15\ gtt} = \textbf{3 mL}$

34. 2

$$\frac{1\ L}{8.5\ hr} \times \frac{1000\ mL}{1\ L} = 117.64\ \frac{mL}{hr} \times \frac{1hr}{60\ minutes} = 1.96\ mL/min \quad \sim \textbf{2 mL/min}$$

35. C. 26 mL

Calcium Gluconate volume: $12\ mEq\ x\ \frac{mL}{0.465\ mEq} = 25.81\ mL \sim \textbf{26 mL}$

36. E. 39 kcal

Calculate the number of grams of fat in 4 ounces, or 120 mL (30 mL/fl oz), of liquid:

$$\frac{3.6\ g}{100\ mL} = \frac{x\ g}{120\ mL} \qquad x = 4.32\ g$$

Calculate the number of calories from fat. There are 9 kcal/g of fat:

$$4.32\ g \times 9\ \frac{kcal}{g} = 38.9\ kcal \quad \sim \textbf{39 kcal}$$

37. 1657

$W = 136\ lb \times \frac{1\ kg}{2.2\ lb} = 61.82\ kg$ \qquad $H = 65\ in \times \frac{2.54\ cm}{in} = 165.1\ cm$ \qquad $A = 35\ years\ old$

$$655 + (9.6 \times 61.82) + (1.8 \times 165.1) - (4.7 \times 35) = 1,381.2\ \frac{kcal}{day} \times 1.2 = \textbf{1657 kcal/day}$$

38. C. 630 mL

Convert teaspoons to mL:

$$\frac{3\ tsp}{x\ mL} = \frac{tsp}{5\ mL} \quad x = 15\ mL\ per\ dose$$

Determine how many mL the patient would receive in a day:

$$\frac{15\ mL}{dose} \times 3\ doses = 45\ mL\ per\ day$$

Determine how many mL in a 14 day supply:

$$\frac{45\ mL}{day} \times 14\ days = \mathbf{630\ mL}$$

39. E. 100 mg TID

The patient should be given a gentamicin dose of 1.5 mg/kg IBW every 8-12 hours depending on renal function (CrCl).

Calculate IBW: $IBW = 50 + (2.3)(7) = 66.1\ kg$

Creatinine clearance (CrCl; mL/min) can be estimated using the Cockcroft-Gault equation as follows:

$$CrCl = \frac{\big(140 - age\ (yrs)\big) \times weight(kg)}{72 \times SCr} \quad \rightarrow \quad CrCl = \frac{(140 - 37) \times 66.1}{72 \times 0.8} = 118.2\ mL/min$$

Calculate final dosing:

$$66.1\ kg \times \frac{1.5\ mg}{kg} = 99.15\ mg\ every\ 8\ hours \quad \sim\mathbf{100\ mg\ every\ 8\ hours}$$

40. A. 197

C1Q1 = C2Q2, where Q = quantity and C = concentration   1 pint = 473 mL

Determine the volume of a 0.12% solution needed to prepare 1 pint of a 0.07% solution:

$$0.12\%(X\ mL) = 473\ mL\ (0.07\%) \qquad X\ mL = \frac{473(0.07)}{0.12} = 276\ mL\ of\ 0.12\%\ solution$$

Determine the amount of water to be added to the 0.12% solution by subtracting the volume of the 0.12% solution from the final volume: $473\ mL - 276\ mL = 197\ mL$

41. A. 1058 mL

$$KCl \; volume: \quad 15 \; mEq \times \frac{mL}{2 \; mEq} = 7.5 \; mL$$

$$NaCl \; volume: \quad 20 \; mEq \times \frac{mL}{4 \; mEq} = 5 \; mL$$

$$Mg \; Sulfate \; volume: \quad 8 \; mEq \times \frac{mL}{4.08 \; mEq} = 1.96 \; mL$$

$$Calcium \; Gluconate \; volume: \quad 12 \; mEq \times \frac{1 \; mL}{0.465 \; mEq} = 25.81 \; mL$$

$$Potassium \; Phosphate \; volume: \quad 23 \; mmol \times \frac{1 \; mL}{3 \; mmol} = 7.67 \; mL$$

$$500 \; mL \; (AA) + 500 \; mL \; (Dextrose) + 5 \; mL \; (NaCl) + 7.5 \; mL \; (KCl) + 1.96 \; mL \; (Mg \; Sulfate)$$
$$+ \; 25.81 \; mL \; (Ca \; Gluconate) + 7.67 \; mL \; (Potassium \; Phosphate) + 10 \; mL \; (MVI)$$
$$= \mathbf{1057.94 \; mL}$$

42. 2.5

Calculate conversion factor: $\quad 50 \; mL / 20 \; mL \; = \; 2.5$
Multiply amount of cherry flavor by conversion factor: $\quad 15 \; gtt \times 2.5 \; = \; 37.5 \; gtt$
Multiply total drops by drop factor: $\quad 37.5 \; gtt \times \frac{mL}{15 \; gtt} = \mathbf{2.5 \; mL}$

43. B. 93.8 kg

$Females: \quad IBW = 45.5 \; kg \; + \; 2.3 \; kg \; for \; each \; inch \; over \; 5 \; feet$

$$IBW \; = \; 45.5 \; kg + 2.3(21) \; = \mathbf{93.8 \; kg}$$

44. 800

Note this is a trick question as lots of unnecessary information (like BEE) is given to test student's knowledge. The important information given is that the amino acids makes up 0.75 g/kg body weight and provides 4 kcal/g of energy. 7% amino acid solution is 7 g/100 mL.

Convert lb to kg: $166 \; lb \times \frac{1 kg}{2.2 lb} = 75.45 \; kg$

$$56.6 \; kg \times \frac{100 \; mL}{7 \; g} \; = \; 808.6 \; mL \; of \; amino \; acids$$

$$daily \; protein \; (g): \quad \frac{0.75 \; g \; protein}{kg} \times 75.45 \; kg = 56.6 \; g$$

$$kcal \; from \; protein: \quad 56.6 g \times \frac{4 \; kcal}{g} = 226.4 \; kcal$$

$$56.6 \; g \times \frac{100 \; mL}{7 \; g} = 808.6 \; mL \; amino \; acids \quad \mathbf{\sim 800 \; mL}$$

45. B. 2.54 mg/kg/dose

$$13 \; lbs \times \frac{2.2 \; kg}{1 \; lb} = 5.91 \; kg \qquad\qquad 15 \; mg \; \div 5.91 \; kg = \boldsymbol{2.54 \; mg/kg/dose}$$

If the amount of mg/kg/*day*, rather than per dose, is calculated, then 5.1 mg/kg/dose is the result.

46. 372

Calculate BSA:

$$BSA \; (m^2) = \sqrt{\frac{height \; (in) \times weight \; (lb)}{3131}} \qquad \rightarrow \qquad BSA \; (m^2) = \sqrt{\frac{44 \; in \times 70 \; lb}{3131}} = 0.99 \; m^2$$

Calculate the dose:

$$\frac{375 \; mg}{m^2} = \frac{x \; mg}{m^2} \qquad x = \boldsymbol{372 \; mg}$$

47. 8.3

$$Potassium \; phosphate \; volume: \;\; 25 \; mmol \times \frac{mL}{3 \; mmol} = \boldsymbol{8.3 \; mL}$$

48. D. 0.06 mol

$$MW = \frac{grams}{1 \; mole}$$

Calculate the total amount of sodium consumed:

$$2(171 \; mg) \times 3(192 \; mg) \times 2(148 \; mg) \times 4(27 \; mg) = 1322 \; mg \; sodium$$
$$1322 \; mg \; sodium \times \frac{1 \; g}{1000 \; mg} = 1.322 \; g \; sodium$$

Use the formula above to determine millimoles of sodium using the atomic weight of Na (not NaCl):

$$23 \; g \; Na = \frac{1.322}{x \; mol} \qquad x = 0.058 \; mol \quad \boldsymbol{\sim 0.06 \; mol}$$

49. E. 360 mL

Convert tablespoons to mL: $\qquad \frac{1 \; tbsp}{15 \; mL} \times 4 \; tbsp = 60 \; mL \; per \; dose$

Determine how many mL the patient would receive in a day: $\frac{60 \; ml}{dose} \times 3 \; doses = 180 \; mL \; per \; day$

Determine how many mL in a 2-day supply: $\qquad \frac{180 \; mL}{day} \times 2 \; days = \boldsymbol{360 \; mL}$

50. C. 250 mL/hr

$$flow\ rate\ \left(\frac{ml}{hr}\right) = \frac{total\ volume\ (mL)}{infusion\ time\ (hr)} \quad \rightarrow \quad \frac{500\ mg}{hr} \times \frac{200\ mL}{400\ mg} = \boldsymbol{250\ mL/hr}$$

Section 3 Calculations: Answers and Explanations

1. **0.23**

   The prescription calls for 15 mL of a 0.35 % solution of cefazolin sodium:

   $$(0.35\%)(15\,mL) = 0.0525\,g \times 1000\,mg/g = 52.5\,mg\ of\ cefazolin.$$

   The vial contains 500 mg of cefazolin in a total reconstituted volume of 2.2 mL.

   $$\frac{2.2\,mL}{500\,mg} \times 52.5\,mg = \boldsymbol{0.23\,mL\ total}$$

2. **A. 80**

   Set up an alligation to determine the number of parts of high and low concentrations needed.

Available Strengths (%)	Desired Strength (%)	Parts
25		$15 - 10 = 5\ parts\ of\ 25\%$
	15	
10		$25 - 15 = 10\ parts\ of\ 10\%$
		$5 + 10 = 15\ parts\ total\ (15\%)$

   Use the ratio to determine the number of mL needed:

   $$\frac{5\ parts\ of\ 25\%}{15\ parts\ of\ 15\%} = \frac{x\ mL\ of\ 25\%}{240\ mL\ of\ 15\%} \qquad x = \boldsymbol{80\,mL\ of\ 25\%}$$

3. **C. 3 g**

   Conversion Factor: $10\ g/1000g = 0.03$ $\qquad 100\,g \times 0.03 = 3\,g$

4. **26**

   Calculate the molecular weight of calcium chloride, or $CaCl_2$: $MW = 40 + 35.5(2) = 111$

   Determine the osmolarity (mOsm/L), using the formula below:

   $$\frac{mOsm}{L} = \frac{weight(g)}{MW} \times 1000 \times number\ of\ species$$

   $$\frac{mOsm}{L} = \frac{0.95}{111} \times 1000 \times 3 = 25.68\,mOsm/L \quad \sim \boldsymbol{26\,mOsm/L}$$

5. **D. 4.9%**

Determine the weight of the drug:

$$\frac{x \ g}{480 \ mL} = \frac{15 \ g}{100 \ mL} \qquad x = 72 \ g$$

Determine the final volume: $480 \ mL \ + \ 1000 \ mL \ = \ 1480 \ mL$

Determine the concentration:

$$\frac{72 \ g}{1480 \ mL} = \frac{x \ g}{100 \ mL} \qquad x = 4.9 \ g \ or \ 4.9\%$$

Alternative to use C1V1 = C2V2 → (15%)(480mL) = (C2)(1480 mL) → C2 = 4.9%

6. **3**

Calculate BSA with the following formula:

$$BSA = \sqrt{\frac{height \ (cm) \times weight \ (kg)}{3600}} \rightarrow BSA = \sqrt{\frac{210.8 \times 157.3}{3600}} = 3.03 \ m^2$$

7. **B. 450 mL**

According to the medication order, the patient is to receive 180 mmoles of sodium bicarbonate per liter of solution; 2.5 liters of solution is ordered. Sodium bicarbonate is available as an 8.4% solution (8.4 g/100 mL). First, using the molecular weight of the drug, convert the dose of sodium bicarbonate from mmoles to grams:

$$\frac{180 \ mole}{L} \times \frac{84 \ g}{mole} \times \frac{1 \ mole}{1000 \ mmol} \times 2.5 \ L = 37.8 \ g$$

Determine the volume of 8.4% sodium bicarbonate solution that will provide 37.8 g of the drug:

$$\frac{8.4 \ g}{100 \ mL} = \frac{37.8 \ g}{x \ mL} \qquad x = \textbf{450 } \textbf{\textit{mL}}$$

8. **60 mL**

Convert teaspoons to mL: $\frac{1 \ tsp}{5 \ mL} \times 2 \ tsp = 10 \ mL \ per \ dose$

Determine how many mL the patient would receive in a day: $\frac{10 mL}{dose} \times 3 \ doses = 30 \ mL \ per \ day$

Determine how many mL in a 2-day supply: $\frac{30 \ mL}{day} \times 2 \ days = 60 \ mL$

9. D. 50 gtt/min

$$\frac{0.5g}{hr} \times \frac{1000 \ mL}{3 \ g} = \frac{166.67 \ mL}{hr} \times \frac{18 \ gtt}{mL} = \frac{3000 \ gtt}{mL} \times \frac{1hr}{60 \ minutes} = \boldsymbol{50 \ gtt/minute}$$

10. A. 384 mL

Set up an alligation:

Available Strengths (%)	Desired Strength (%)	Parts
17.5%		$15 - 5 = 10 \ parts \ of \ 17.5\%$
	15%	
5%		$17.5 - 15 = 2.5 \ parts \ of \ 5\%$
		$10 + 2.5 = 12.5 \ parts \ total \ (15\%)$

Use the ratio to determine the number of mL needed:

$$\frac{10 \ parts \ of \ 17.5\%}{12.5 \ parts \ of \ 15\%} = \frac{x \ mL \ of \ 17.5\%}{480 \ mL \ of \ 15\%} \qquad x = 384 \ mL$$

11. B. 15 mOsm

Calculate the molecular weight of calcium chloride ($CaCl_2$): $\quad MW = 40 + 35.5(2) = 111$

Number of species formed upon ionization (1 Ca2+ + 2 Cl-) = 3

Determine mOsm, using the following formula: $\quad mOsm = \frac{weight(g)}{MW} \times 1000 \times number \ of \ species$

$$mOsm = \frac{0.55}{111} \times 1000 \times 3 = 14.86 \ mOsm \quad \boldsymbol{\sim 15 \ mOsm}$$

12. C. 285 mg

Calculate this patient's ideal body weight: $\quad IBW = 45.5 \ kg + 2.3 \ kg \ (inches \ over \ 5')$

$$IBW = 45.5 \ kg + 2.3(5) = 57 \ kg$$

Calculate the dose for the patient based on IBW:

$$\frac{5 \ mg}{IBW} = \frac{x \ mg}{57 \ kg} \qquad x = 285 \ mg$$

13. 10 g

$$\frac{250 \ mg}{5 \ mL} = \frac{x \ mg}{200 \ mL} \qquad x = 10,000 \ mg$$

$$10,000 \ mg \times \frac{g}{1000 \ mL} = \boldsymbol{10 \ g}$$

14. 50 gtt/min

$$flow\ rate\ \left(\frac{ml}{hr}\right) = \frac{total\ volume\ (mL)}{infusion\ time\ (hr)} \rightarrow \frac{200\ mL}{hr} \times \frac{1\ hr}{60\ minutes} \times \frac{15\ gtt}{mL} = \mathbf{50\ gtt/min}$$

15. 2.6

The dose for Vincristine sulfate is $1.4mg/m^2$. In order to calculate the dose for this patient, you need to calculate first the patient's body surface area (BSA):

$$BSA = \sqrt{\frac{height\ (cm) \times weight\ (kg)}{3600}} \rightarrow BSA = \sqrt{\frac{172.72 \times 72.7}{3600}} = 1.87\ m^2$$

The dose for this patient is then calculated as 1.4mg/m2 x 1.87 m2 = 2.61 mg.

$$\frac{1.4mg}{m^2} \times 1.87\ m^2 = 2.61\ mg$$

Vincristine is available as a 2 mg/2 mL solution for injection:

$$(2.61\ mg)/(2\ mg/2\ mL) = 2.61\ mL \quad \sim\mathbf{2.6\ mL}$$

16. D. 213 kcal

Convert lb to kg: $156\ lb \times \frac{1\ kg}{2.2\ lb} = 70.9\ kg$

$$Daily\ protein\ requirement\ (grams) = \frac{0.75\ g\ protein}{kg} \times body\ weigh$$
$$= 0.75\ g\ protein \times 70.9\ kg = 51.18\ gram\ protein$$

$$kcal\ from\ protein = 4\frac{kcal}{g} \quad \rightarrow \quad 53.18\ g \times 4\frac{kcal}{g} = \mathbf{212.72\ kcal\ from\ protein}$$

17. A. 3.6 g

Conversion factor: 45 mL/10 mL = 4.5
Multiply amount of progesterone by conversion factor: $0.8\ g \times 4.5 = \mathbf{3.6\ g}$

18. 192.4 mL

$$BSA = \sqrt{\frac{height\ (cm) \times weight\ (kg)}{3600}} \rightarrow BSA = \sqrt{\frac{180.34 \times 112}{3600}} = 2.37\ m^2$$

Determine the daily dose of prednisolone during every phase of the taper:
Phase 1: 60 mg/m^2 x 2.37 m^2 x 14 days = 1990.8 mg
Phase 2: 45 mg/m^2 x 2.37 m^2 x 14 days = 1493.1 mg
Phase 3: 30 mg/m^2 x 2.37 m^2 x 14 days = 995.4 mg
Phase 4: 20 mg/m^2 x 2.37 m^2 x 7 days (dose is every other day) = 331.8 mg
Total amount: 4811.1 mg

Set up a ratio to determine the volume needed:
$$\frac{125\ mg}{5\ mL} = \frac{4811.1\ mg}{x\ mL} \qquad x = 192.4\ mL$$

19. C. 1:605

Ratio strength is expressed as 1:x (g:mL for solid in liquid preparations).

$$\frac{0.826\ g}{500\ mL} = \frac{1}{x} \qquad x = 605.33\ mL, or\ \mathbf{1:605}$$

20. 1445

$$W = 156\ lb\ \times \frac{1\ kg}{2.2\ kg} = 70.9\ kg \qquad H = 63\ in \times= 160.02\ cm \qquad A = 38\ years\ old$$

$$655 + (9.6 \times 70.9) + (1.8 \times 160.02) - (4 \times 38) = \mathbf{1,445.08}$$

21. E. 1.27 mL

The dose for fentanyl citrate sulfate is 100 mcg. Fentanyl citrate is available as a solution for injection containing 50 mcg/ mL of fentanyl base, the dose of fentanyl citrate needs to be converted to the equivalent dose of fentanyl base. This can be done using the molecular weights of the 2 drug forms:

Volume to inject into the infusion bag is:

$$\frac{336.5\ \frac{g}{mol}\ fentanyl\ base}{528.6\ \frac{g}{mol}\ fentanyl\ citrate} \times 100\ mcg\ fentanyl\ citrate = 63.7\ mcg\ fentanyl\ base$$

Volume of solution to be withdrawn from the vial to obtain the dose is:

$$\frac{63.7\ mcg\ fentanyl\ base}{50\ \frac{mcg}{mL}\ fentanyl\ base} = \mathbf{1.27\ mL\ fentanyl\ citrate\ injection, USP}$$

22. B. 9%

$$\frac{x\ g}{300\ mL} = \frac{15\ g}{100\ mL} \qquad x = 45\ g$$

Determine the final volume prepared by combining the 15% solution and water:

$$200\ mL\ +\ 300\ mL\ =\ 500\ mL$$

Determine the final concentration of solute:

$$\frac{45\ g}{500\ mL} = \frac{x\ g}{100\ mL} \qquad x = 9\ g\ in\ 100\ mL, or\ 9\%$$

23. 7.2 L

$$\frac{1\ tbsp}{15\ mL} \times 4\ tbsp = 60\ mL\ per\ dose$$

Determine how many mL the patient would receive in a day:

$$\frac{60\ mL}{dose} \times 4\ doses = 240\ mL\ per\ day$$

Determine how many mL in a 30-day supply:

$$\frac{240\ mL}{day} \times 30\ days = 7200\ mL$$

Double check the question for the requested units. Convert to liters: $7200\ mL \times \frac{1\ L}{1000\ mL} = 7.2\ L$

24. 75

The total volume (150 mL) will be infused over 60 minutes, a rate of 2.5 mL/minute. If the administration set delivers 30 drops/mL, set up a ratio to solve for drops per minute:

$$\frac{30\ drops}{1\ mL} = \frac{x\ drops}{2.5\ mL/min} \qquad x = \textbf{75 drops/min}$$

25. 225

The sig in the patient's profile calls for prednisone 60 mg daily for 3 days, then taper by 5 mg every 3 days to 10 mg daily. For the first 30 days:

$$60\ mg/5\ mg\ =\ 12\ tablets\ daily\ for\ 3\ days\ =\ 36\ tablets$$
$$55\ mg/5\ mg\ =\ 11\ tablets\ daily\ for\ 3\ days\ =\ 33\ tablets$$
$$50\ mg/5\ mg\ =\ 10\ tablets\ daily\ for\ 3\ days\ =\ 30\ tablets$$
$$45\ mg/5\ mg\ =\ 9\ tablets\ daily\ for\ 3\ days\ =\ 27\ tablets$$
$$40\ mg/5\ mg\ =\ 8\ tablets\ daily\ for\ 3\ days\ =\ 24\ tablets$$
$$35\ mg/5\ mg\ =\ 7\ tablets\ daily\ for\ 3\ days\ =\ 21\ tablets$$

$$30 \, mg/5 \, mg \; = \; 6 \, tablets \; daily \; for \; 3 \, days \; = \; 18 \, tablets$$
$$25 \, mg/5 \, mg \; = \; 5 \, tablets \; daily \; for \; 3 \, days \; = \; 15 \, tablets$$
$$20 \, mg/5 \, mg \; = \; 4 \, tablets \; daily \; for \; 3 \, days \; = \; 12 \, tablets$$
$$15 \, mg/5 \, mg \; = \; 3 \, tablets \; daily \; for \; 3 \, days \; = \; 9 \, tablets$$

Total number of tablets needed: $36 + 33 + 30 + 27 + 24 + 21 + 18 + 15 + 12 + 9 = 225 \, tablets$

26. B. 25 days

This patient takes 5 mg per day, which is the equivalent of $\dfrac{5 \, mg}{0.5 \, mg/mL} = 10 \, mL \, per \, day$

If a total volume of 250 mL: $250 \, mL \div 10 \, mL \, per \, day \; = \; \mathbf{25 \, days}$

27. A. 1:625

Ratio strengths are expressed in g/mL for a solid dissolved in a liquid, such as the solution prepared in this problem, and are usually represented as 1:X.

$$100 \, mg \times 4 \; = \; 400 \, mg \times \frac{1 \, g}{1000 \, mg} = 0.4 \, g$$

$$\frac{0.4 \, g}{250 \, mL} = \frac{1}{x} \quad x = 625 \, mL, \quad or \; \mathbf{1:625}$$

28. D. 0.518 g

Convert lb to kg: $190 \, lb \times \dfrac{1 \, kg}{2.2 \, lb} = 86.4 \, kg$

Calculate the dose in mg/kg: $\dfrac{6 \, mg}{kg} = \dfrac{x \, mg}{86.4 \, kg} \quad x = 518.4 \, mg \times \dfrac{1 \, g}{1000 \, mg} = \mathbf{0.518 \, g}$

29. 90

According to the medication order, the patient is to receive 90 mmoles of sodium chloride per liter of solution; 2.5 liters of solution is ordered. Sodium chloride is available as a 14.6% solution (14.6 g/100 mL). Using the molecular weight of the drug, convert the dose of sodium chloride from mmoles to grams:

$$\frac{90 \, mmol}{L} \times \frac{58.5 \, g}{mole} \times \frac{1 \, mol}{1000 \, mmol} \times 2.5 \, L = 13.16 \, g$$

Determine the volume of 14.6% sodium chloride solution that will provide 13.16 g of the drug:

$$\frac{14.6 g}{100 mL} = \frac{13.16 g}{x} \quad x = 90.1 \, mL \quad \mathbf{\sim 90 \, mL}$$

30. 40 kg/m²

Body Mass Index (BMI) is calculated by dividing the patient's weight in kg by the patient's height in meters squared. To accomplish this, first convert the weight from lbs to kg.

$$250 \; lb \times \frac{1 \; kg}{2.2 \; lb} = 113.4 \; kg$$

Convert the height (5' 6") to meters.

$$\frac{1 \; foot}{12 \; inches} \times 5 \; feet = 60 + 6 = 66 \; inches \times \frac{1 \; meter}{39.37 \; inches} = 1.68 \; m$$

Calculate BMI:

$$\frac{113.4 \; kg}{(1.68 \; m)^2} = 40.2 \; \frac{kg}{m^2} \quad \sim \mathbf{40 \frac{kg}{m^2}}$$

31. B. 74.5 mL

Conversion Factor = $240 \; mL \; / \; 5.8 \; parts \; = \; 41.38$
Multiply 1.8 part Nystatin by conversion factor: $1.8 \times 41.38 \; = \; 74.5$

32. C. 25

Determine how many mg of gentamicin solution will be added to the IV bag:

$$1.7 \; mg \times 75 \; kg = 127.5 \; mg$$

Determine how many mL are needed to prepare each dose:

$$\frac{40 \; mg}{mL} = \frac{127.5 \; mg}{x \; mL} \quad x = 3.2 \; mL$$

Determine how many vials are needed per day:

$$3.2 \; mL \times 3 \; doses \; = \; 9.6 \; mL / 2 \; mL \; per \; vial$$

If 1 day requires 4.8 vials, and all doses for each day are made together, 5 vials are needed to prepare 1 days' worth of doses. Multiply the number of vials needed per day by the duration of therapy:
$5 \; vials \; per \; day \times 5 \; days \; = \; 25 \; vials$

The order in which this calculation is solved is very important. If you calculate the total amount (in mg) needed and divide by 5, your number is 23.9 or 24 vials. This is not correct because the vials are single use; partial vials cannot be carried over to the next day.

33. B. Volume of Distribution

The volume of distribution of a drug multiplied by the desirable target concentration (or desirable change in concentration) will provide the numerical value of the amount of drug required for administration as a single dose. Clearance is useful for calculating the maintenance dose to be administered chronically. The protein binding of a drug can affect the distribution space but will not be useful in determining the dose required. The elimination half-life refers to the time interval for 50% of the dose to be eliminated. The oral bioavailability refers to the percent of an orally administered drug that reaches the systemic circulation.

34. E. 7 mL every 12 hours for 7 days

Find the patient's weight in kilograms: $\quad 56 \, lb \, \times \frac{1 \, kg}{2.2 \, lb} = 25.5 \, kg$

The sig for this cefdinir prescription requires 7 mg/kg every 12 hours for 7 days:

$$25.5 \, kg \times \frac{7 \, mg}{kg} = 178.2 \, mg \, cefdinir \, q \, 12 \, hours$$

From a 125 mg/5 mL oral suspension of cefdinir:

$$178.2 \, mg \times \frac{5}{125 \, mg} = 7.13 \, mL, \text{ or approximately } \textbf{7 mL every 12 hours for 7 days}$$

35. 47

To solve the question for this patient, start by determining the patient's ideal body weight:

$$162 \, cm \, \times \, 1 \, inch/2.54 \, cm \, = \, 64 \, inches \rightarrow 64 - 60 \, = \, 4 \, inches \, above \, 5 \, feet$$

The body weight used in the Cockcroft Gault equation is either the ideal body weight (IBW) of the patient (in kg) or the actual body weight (in kg) of the patient, whichever is less. For obese patients, an adjusted body weight is conventionally used.

$$IBW \, = \, 45.5 \, kg \, + \, (2.3 \times 4) = \, 54.7 \, kg$$

Their ACTUAL body weight is 79 kg, which is significantly higher than the ideal body weight. We can determine if this patient can be categorized as obese by calculating this patient's BMI:

$$BMI \, = \frac{79 \, kg}{(1.62 \, m)^2} = 30.1 \, kg/m^2$$

This patient is considered to be obese. Since their actual body weight is 44% greater than ideal body weight, an ADJUSTED body weight should be used:

$$Adjusted \, Body \, Weight = 54.7 \, kg + 0.4[79 - 54.7 \,] \, = \, 64.4 \, kg$$

Now use the Cockcroft-Gault equation:

$$CrCl = \frac{(140 - age \, (yrs)) \times weight(kg)}{72 \times SCr} \times 0.85 \rightarrow CrCl = \frac{(140 - 76) \times 64.4}{72 \times 1.03} \times 0.85$$

$$= 47.2 \, mL/minute \quad \textbf{\textasciitilde47 mL/minute}$$

36. C. 1,203 mL

Convert lb to kg: $150\ lb \times \frac{1\ kg}{2.2\ lb} = 68.2\ kg$

$1.5 \frac{g}{kg} \times 68.2\ kg = 102.3\ grams\ needed$

$102.3\ g \times \frac{100}{8.5\ g} = 1,203.5\ mL$

37. 41.38

Conversion factor: $240\ mL\ /\ 5.8\ parts = 41.38$
Multiply 1 part viscous lidocaine by conversion factor: $1 \times 41.38 = \mathbf{41.38}$

38. 82.8

Conversion factor: $240\ mL\ /\ 5.8\ parts = 41.38$
Multiply 2 parts Maalox by conversion factor: $2 \times 41.38 = \mathbf{82.8}$

39. 11.25

NaCl volume: $45\ mEq \times mL/4\ mEq = \mathbf{11.25\ mL}$

40. 3.33

$$\frac{0.5\ g\ progesterone}{10\ mL} \times \frac{1\ mL}{15\ gtt} = \frac{0.00333\ g}{gtt} \times \frac{1000\ mg}{g} = \mathbf{3.33\ mg/gtt/day}$$

41. 17

Solve for k_e first using the equation:

$$k_e = \frac{Cl}{V_d} = \frac{\ln\left(\frac{C_1}{C_2}\right)}{(t_2 - t_1)} = \frac{\ln(C_1) - \ln(C_2)}{(t_2 - t_1)} \quad \rightarrow \quad \frac{\ln\left(\frac{28}{24.7}\right)}{(3)} = 0.042\ hr^{-1}$$

Solve for half life using the equation:

$$t_{1/2} = \frac{0.693}{k} = \frac{0.693}{0.042\ hr^{-1}} = 16.5 \quad \mathbf{\sim 17\ hr}$$

42. B. 6

$$t_{1/2} = \frac{0.693 \times V_d}{Cl} = \frac{0.693 \times 80\ L}{9.37\ L/hr} = 5.92 \quad \mathbf{\sim 6\ hr}$$

43. C. 100%

$$Bioavailability\ (F\%) = 100 \times \frac{AUC\ extravascular}{AUC\ intravenous} \times \frac{dose\ intravenous}{dose\ extravascular}$$

As the dosing for IV and PO are the same, 675 mg, it is safe to assume 100% bioavailability. The IV route provides 100% bioavailability as the drug is injected directly into the bloodstream.

44. 2.16

$$Cl = \frac{dose \times F}{AUC} \quad \rightarrow \quad \frac{225\ mg \times 0.5}{52\ mg * hr/mL} = \mathbf{2.16\ mL/hr}$$

45. 1.8

$$t_{1/2} = \frac{0.693}{k} = \frac{0.693}{0.38\ hr^{-1}} = 1.82 \quad \sim\mathbf{1.8\ hr}$$

46. 10

$$t_{1/2} = \frac{0.693 \times V_d}{Cl} = \frac{0.693 \times 65\ L}{4.5\ L/hr} = 10.01 \quad \sim\mathbf{10\ hr}$$

47. 11

Convert the 38 mcg*hr/mL to L:

$$\left(38\ mcg * \frac{hr}{mL}\right) \times \frac{1000\ mL}{1\ L} \times \frac{1\ mg}{1000\ mcg} = 38\ mg * \frac{hr}{mL}$$

$$Cl = \frac{dose \times F}{AUC} \quad \rightarrow \quad \frac{400\ mg \times 100\%}{38\ mg * hr/mL} = \mathbf{11\ mL/hr}$$

48. 42

$$V_d = \frac{dose}{k_e \times AUC} \quad \rightarrow \quad \frac{400mg}{0.38\ hr^{-1} \times 25.18\ mg * hr/L} = 42\ L$$

49. D. 4.13

Use the Henderson-Hasselbalch equation: $\quad pH = pKa + log\ [salt/acid]$

$$pH = 3.13 + log\left[\frac{0.5\ M}{0.05\ M}\right] = 3.13 + log[10] = 3.13 + 1 = \mathbf{4.13}$$

50. E. Aminophylline x 0.8 = theophylline dose

Section 4 Calculations: Answers and Explanations

1. **21.6**

   Convert lb to kg: $45\ lb \times \frac{1\ kg}{2.2\ lb} = 20.45\ kg$

   Convert inches to cm: $36\ inches \times \frac{2.54\ cm}{in} = 91.44\ cm$

   To calculate BSA of the child: $\text{BSA} = \frac{\sqrt{Height\ (cm)x\ weight\ (kg)}}{60} = \frac{\sqrt{20.45\ kg\ x\ 91\ cm}}{60} = 0.72\ \text{m}^2$

   $10\ mcg/m^2 \times 0.72\ m^2 = 7.2\ mcg$

   Since the child will take three times daily, the total daily dose will be:

   $7.2\ mcg \times three\ times\ daily = \textbf{21.6}\ \textbf{mcg}$

2. **14**

   Patient takes 1 tablet with every meal and 2 tablets at bedtime, so patient takes 5 tablets per day.

   $70\ tablets \times \frac{1\ day}{5\ tablets} = \textbf{14}\ \textbf{days}$

3. **50**

   Recall 1:400 (w/v) = 1 g: 400 mL

   $C_1V_1 = C_2V_2$

   $\frac{5\ g}{100\ mL} \times V_1 = \frac{1\ g}{400\ mL} \times 1000\ mL$

   $V1 = \textbf{50 mL}$

4. **D. 42.5 g**

   Weight of zinc oxide, talc powder, and lanolin is: $5\ g + 5\ g + 5\ g = 15\ g$

   The prescription was prescribed:
   Lanolin cream
   Petrolatum ointment aa qs ad 100 g

   It means that lanolin cream and petrolatum ointment are added into the compound with the same amount to make a 100 g product (aa = of each, ad = up to; and qs = a sufficient quantity).

   The amount of lanolin cream + petrolatum ointment = $100\ g\ (total) - 15\ g = 85\ g$

   $\rightarrow lanolin\ cream = 85g/2 = \textbf{42.5}\ \textbf{g}$

5. **B. 1:30**

Zinc oxide of 20 grams of the 2.5% zinc oxide ointment:

$$20 \; g \; ointment \; \times \frac{2.5 \; g \; zinc \; oxide}{100 \; g \; ointment} = 0.5 \; g \; zinc \; oxide$$

Zinc oxide of 10 grams of the 5% zinc oxide ointment:

$$10 \; g \; ointment \; \times \frac{5 \; g \; zinc \; oxide}{100 \; g \; ointment} = 0.5 \; g \; zinc \; oxide$$

Total weight of the final product after mixing them: $20 \; g + 10 \; g = 30 \; grams$

Ratio strength $= \frac{0.5 + 0.5 \; g \; zinc \; oxide}{30 \; g \; ointment} = \textbf{1:30}$

6. **154 mg**

Sodium chloride is needed for making 30 mL isotonicity: $\quad 30 \; mL \times \frac{0.9 \; g}{100 \; mL} = 0.27 \; g$

NaCl is equivalent of ephedrine sulfate: $\quad 0.2 \; g \times E_{ephedrine \; sulfate} = 0.2 \; g \times 0.23 = 0.046 \; g$

NaCl is equivalent of tetracycline HCl: $\quad 0.5 \; g \times E_{tetracycline \; HCl} = 0.5 \; g \times 0.14 = 0.07 \; g$

NaCl is needed to be added to make the 30 mL isotonic eye drops:

$$0.27 \; g - (ephedrine \; equivalence \; + \; tetracycline \; equivalence)$$
$$= 0.27 \; g - (0.046 \; g + 0.07 \; g) = 0.154 \; g \; \times \frac{1000 \; mg}{1 \; g} = \textbf{154 mg}$$

7. **2320 kcal**

Recall:
    Amino acids = 4 kcal/gram
    D5W = 3.4 kcal/gram
    20% fat emulsion = 2 kcal/mL

$$Amino \; acid \; = \; 1500 \; mL \times \frac{5 \; gram}{100 \; mL} \times \frac{4 \; kcal}{1 \; gram} = 300 \; kcal$$

$$Dextrose \; = \; 1500 \; mL \times \frac{20 \; gram}{100 \; mL} \times \frac{3.4 \; kcal}{1 \; gram} = 1020 \; kcal$$

$$Fat \; = \; 500 \; mL \; \times \frac{2 \; kcal}{1 \; mL} = 1000 \; kcal$$

$$Total \; daily \; calories \; = \; 300 \; kcal + 1020 \; kcal + 1000 \; kcal = \textbf{2320 kcal}$$

8. E. 168

First of all, we have to calculate non-protein calories:
    Non-protein calories = dextrose + fat
    Non-protein calories: $1020\ kcal\ +\ 1000\ kcal\ =\ 2020\ kcal$

Secondly, we calculate nitrogen content (**Recall: 6.25 gram of amino acids = 1 gram of nitrogen**)

Amino acid 5% content: $1500\ mL \times \frac{5\ gram}{100\ mL} = 75\ g$

Nitrogen content: $75\ g\ amino\ acids \times \frac{1\ g\ nitrogen}{6.25\ g\ amino\ acids} = 12\ g$

Therefore, non-protein calories to nitrogen ratio $\rightarrow \frac{non-protein\ calories}{nitrogen\ content} = \frac{2020\ kcal}{12\ gram} = 168.3$ kcal/gram
    $\rightarrow$ **ratio: 1:168**

9. 429

$C_1V_1=C_2V_2 \rightarrow\ (70\ g/100\ mL) \times V1 = (20\ g/100\ mL) \times 1500\ mL$

$V_1 =$ **429 mL**

10. A. Isotonic

First of all, we will need to calculate how much NaCl is equivalent of 750 mL of D5W:

$D5W: 750\ mL \times \frac{5\ g}{100\ mL} = 37.5\ g\ dextrose$

$37.5\ g\ dextrose\ \times E_{dextrose} = 37.5\ g \times 0.18 = 6.75\ g\ NaCl\ equivalents$

Then we calculate how much NaCl is needed to make a 750 mL of isotonic solution:

$750\ mL\ \times \frac{0.9\ gram}{100\ mL} = 6.75\ g$

6.75 g equivalent NaCl = 6.75 g needed NaCl $\rightarrow$ the solution is **ISOTONIC**

11. B. 25.6 mL/hour

Convert lb to kg: $176\ lb \times \frac{1\ kg}{2.2\ lb} = 80\ kg$

Step 1: calculate total units of heparin that the patient will receive:

$80\ kg \times \frac{16\ units}{kg\ per\ hour}\ =\ 1280\ units/hour$

Step 2: Convert units/hour to mL/hour:

$\frac{1280\ units}{hour} \times \frac{500\ mL}{25000\ units} = \textbf{25.6 mL/hour}$

12. E. 83 mL of 25% dextrose, and 417 mL of 10% dextrose

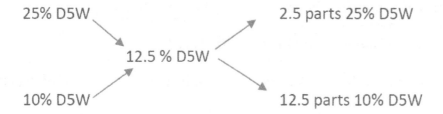

Total parts of the 500 mL solution = 2.5 parts + 12.5 parts = 15 parts.
→15 parts is equal to 500 mL of the final solution.

We need to calculate the volume of each part: $V = 500 \ mL/ \ 15 \ parts = 33.3 \ mL/part$

$25\% \ \boldsymbol{dextrose} = 2.5 \ parts \times 33.3 \ mL = \boldsymbol{83 \ mL}$
$10\% \ \boldsymbol{dextrose} = 12.5 \ parts \times 33.3 \ mL = \boldsymbol{417 \ mL}$
$(or \ 10\% \ dextrose = 500 \ mL \ (total) - 83 \ mL \ (25\% \ dextrose))$

13. 3.3%

Total weight = salicylic acid + benzoic acid + lanolin cream = 1.7 + 4.3 + 45 = 51 g

$$Salicylic \ acid = \frac{1.7 \ g \ salicyclic \ acid}{51 \ g \ final \ product} = 0.033 \times 100\% = \boldsymbol{3.3\% \ (w/w)}$$

14. A. 3230 mcg

Recall: $1 \ ppm = \frac{1 \ gram}{1,000,000 \ mL}$

$$3.4 \ ppm = 3.4 \times \frac{1 \ g}{1,000,000 \ mL} = \frac{3.4 \ g}{1,000,000 \ mL} \times \frac{1,000,000 \ mcg}{1 \ g} = \frac{3.4 \ mcg}{1 \ mL}$$

$$950 \ mL \times \frac{3.4 \ mcg}{1 \ mL} = \boldsymbol{3230 \ mcg}$$

15. 682.5

Convert lb to kg: $154 \ lb \times \frac{1 \ kg}{2.2 \ lb} = 70 \ kg$

Step 1: Calculate how much NaCl is needed (in mEq): $70 \ kg \times \frac{1.5 \ mEq}{1 \ kg} = 105 \ mEq$

Step 2: Find how much (in gram) NaCl is equal to 105 mEq (valence of NaCl = 1)

$$mEq = \frac{Weight}{MW} \times valence \rightarrow weight = \frac{mEq \times MW \ of \ NaCl}{valence}$$

$$Weight = \frac{105 \ mEq \times 58.5}{1} = 6142.5 \ mg \times \frac{1 \ g}{1000 \ mg} = 6.14 \ g$$

Step 3: Find the volume of normal saline contains 6.14 grams sodium chloride:

$$6.14 \, g \times \frac{100 \, mL}{0.9 \, g} = \boldsymbol{682.5 \, mL}$$

16. D. 11.7 mL

Convert lb to kg: $28 \, lb \times \frac{1 \, kg}{2.2 \, lb} = 12.73 \, kg$

Step 1: Volume occupied by the powder: $20 - 16 = 4 \, mL$

Step 2: Calculate how much (in mg) per dose the infant needs: $12.73 \, kg \times \frac{2.5 \, mg}{1 \, kg} = 31.82 \, mg$

Step 3: Volume of the product to contain the dose (10 drops per dose):

$$\frac{10 \, drops}{dose} \times \frac{1 \, mL}{15 \, drops} = 0.667 \, mL \rightarrow \text{for each 0.667 mL contains 31.82 mg (per dose)}$$

Step 4: Calculate the amount of the product (in mL) containing desired dose:

$$750 \, mg \times \frac{0.667 \, mL}{31.82 \, mg} = 15.7 \, mL$$

Step 5: Calculate how much (in mL) of water should be added:

$$V_{water} + V_{powder} = 15.7 \text{ mL} \rightarrow V_{water} = 15.7 \text{ mL} - V_{powder} = 15.7 \text{ mL} - 4 \text{ mL} = \boldsymbol{11.7 \text{ mL}}$$

17. 31.3

$N = N_0 \times e^{-\lambda t}$; where N is the number of radioactive molecules at any time (t); N_0 is defined as the initial number of radioactive atoms presents; e is the base of natural logarithms; λ is a rate constant that depends on the identity of the particular substance

Half-life $= \frac{0.693}{\lambda} = 73$ days $\rightarrow \lambda = 9.49 \times 10^{-3}$ days^{-1}

$$N = N_0 \times e^{-\lambda t} = 1 \, mCi \times e^{-(9.49 \times 10^{-3}) \times 365 \, days} = 1 \, mCi \times e^{-3.465}$$
$$= 0.0313 \, mCi \times \frac{(1000 \, microCi)}{1 \, mCi} = \boldsymbol{31.3 \, microCi}$$

18. C. 13 units of glargine and 4 units of Lispro® with each meal

Total daily dose: $65 \, kg \times \frac{0.4 \, units}{1 \, kg} = 26 \, units$

Since she is eating, TDD will be divided into 50% glargine and 50% short-acting insulin (e.g., Lispro®) → 13 units glargine and 13 units of Lispro® per day.

For Lispro®, we need to divide it by 3 because 13 units are for entire day, and short-acting insulin is given with meal. Therefore, each meal, patient will need 4 units

Answer: 13 units of glargine and 4 units of Lispro® with meal

19. 30

$$60,000 \; units \; heparin \times \frac{hour}{2,000 \; units} = 30 \; hours$$

20. D. 0.37 units/kg/min

Convert lb to kg: $\quad 200 \; lb \times \frac{1 \; kg}{2.2 \; lb} = 91 \; kg$

$$\frac{2,000 \; units}{1 \; hour} \times \frac{1 \; hour}{60 \; minutes} = 33.3 \; units/min$$

$$\frac{33.3 \; units/min}{91 \; kg} = \boldsymbol{0.37 \; units/kg/min}$$

2023-2024 NAPLEX® Practice Questions |RxPharmacist, LLC © 2023

Pharmacotherapy and Case Questions

Practice Test 1 Answers and Explanations

1. **B. Etanercept**

   Etanercept is a dimeric fusion protein consisting of the extracellular ligand-binding portion of the human 75 kilodalton tumor necrosis factor receptor (TNFR) linked to the Fc portion of human IgGl. Etanercept is supplied in a single-use prefilled 1 mL syringe as a sterile, preservative-free solution for subcutaneous injection. Etanercept binds specifically to tumor necrosis factor (TNF) and blocks its interaction with cell surface TNF receptors. TNF is a naturally occurring cytokine that is involved in normal inflammatory and immune responses. It plays an important role in the inflammatory processes of rheumatoid arthritis (RA), polyarticular-course juvenile rheumatoid arthritis (JRA), and ankylosing spondylitis and the resulting joint pathology. It is indicated for use in various forms of arthritis, ankylosing spondylitis, and plaque psoriasis.

2. **A. Caffeine (i.e., Coffee), calcium carbonate**

   Hangover can be effectively treated with systemic analgesics (relieving headache and minor aches and pains), antacids (relieving gastric distress), and caffeine (potentially relieving fatigue and drowsiness). Caffeine is allowed in internal analgesics mainly because it boosts the potency of aspirin. However, it is irrational to choose therapy consisting only of caffeine combined with an antacid, because caffeine is a proven stimulator of gastric acid secretion.

3. **D. Take a sip of water with capsule, flex the head forward, and swallow**

   The easiest way to swallow a capsule is to sip some water, let a capsule float to the top when flexing the head forward, and swallow that way. Remember that a capsule is lighter than water and will therefore float. Although many capsules will dissolve in apple juice, the drugs may be incompatible with each other, and others have not been studied in that way. Extending the head when swallowing is ok with tables, but it increases difficulty in swallowing capsules.

4. **A. Nitrofurantoin**

   Nitrofurantoin is an antibacterial agent specific for urinary tract infections. Nitrofurantoin is bactericidal in urine at therapeutic doses. The mechanism of the antimicrobial action of nitrofurantoin is unusual among antibacterials. Nitrofurantoin is reduced by bacterial flavoproteins to reactive intermediates, which inactivate or alter bacterial ribosomal proteins and other macromolecules. As a result of such inactivations, the vital biochemical processes of protein synthesis, aerobic energy metabolism, DNA synthesis, RNA synthesis, and cell wall synthesis are inhibited. Macrobid is indicated only for the treatment of acute uncomplicated urinary tract infections (acute cystitis) caused by susceptible strains of *Escherichia coli* or *Staphylococcus saprophyticus.*

5. **E. Albuterol/Ipratropium**

   Ipratropium bromide is an anticholinergic bronchodilator, while albuterol is a relatively selective beta-2 adrenergic agonist. Combivent Inhalation Aerosol® contains a microcrystalline suspension of ipratropium bromide and albuterol sulfate in a pressurized metered-dose aerosol unit for oral inhalation administration. Albuterol/Ipratropium (Combivent®) is indicated for use in patients with COPD who require a second bronchodilator to control bronchospasm

6. C. Sulfamethoxazole/Trimethoprim

Bactrim® is an antibacterial combination product indicated for various infections including urinary tract infections and exacerbations of chronic bronchitis. It is contraindicated in infants less than 2 months of age.

7. E. Powders for Inhalation

Patients can purchase Primatene Inhalers® (epinephrine), aspirin, or acetaminophen suppositories, enteric-coated aspirin and enteric-coated bisacodyl tablets, and insulin injections, all on a nonprescription basis. However, powders for inhalation such as Foradil Capsules® (formoterol fumarate) have never been available on a nonprescription basis.

8. A. Tablet Lubricant

Magnesium stearate is used as a tablet lubricant in tablet formulation. Other common lubricants include calcium stearate, mineral oil, and zinc stearate. These substances reduce friction during tablet compression.

Tablet disintegrants are used to promote the breaking apart of solid dosage forms into smaller particles that can be more readily dispersed. Examples of tablet disintegrants are alginic acid, carboxymethylcellulose calcium, and microcrystalline cellulose.

Tablet glidants (e.g., cornstarch and talc) are used to improve the flow properties of powder mixtures.

Tablet opaquants are used to decrease the transparency of tablet coatings and may be used in combination with colorants. Titanium dioxide is an example of a tablet opaquant.

Tablet polishing agents (e.g., white wax and carnauba wax) are used to give coated tablets a pharmaceutically elegant sheen.

9. B. Gallstone formation

Estrogen/progesterone contraceptives cause several different beneficial and harmful side effects. Estrogens promote formation of bones thus decrease risk of osteoporosis, decrease vaginal dryness, slightly increase risk of stroke, decrease serum cholesterol levels (progesterone may increase), and promotes gallstone formation is susceptible women.

10. B. Nonprescription insomnia products are contraindicated with prostate enlargement

FDA-approved nonprescription products for insomnia are all antihistamines, and are contraindicated in patients with difficulty breathing, chronic lung disease, shortness of breath, emphysema, glaucoma, or trouble urinating because of an enlarged prostate gland. His insomnia is short-term and should cease when the CPA exam is completed.

11. A. Bisacodyl

Bisacodyl (Dulcolax®) and glycerin are the 2 most common rectal formulations for constipation.

Lubiprostone is a chloride channel activator taken by mouth, 24 mcg BID.

Methylcellulose is available as oral tablets or powder.

Docusate sodium is available orally as a liquid or capsule.

Sorbitol is an oral hyperosmolar agent for the treatment of constipation.

12. B. Viral

This patient has a cold sore, which is usually caused by herpes simplex 1, Herpes Simplex Labialis. The virus lies dormant between outbreaks, which are triggered by stress, sunlight (e.g., spring break), or hormones. It can occur on any mucosal surface, but usually the lips. Prodromal symptoms are burning, pruritus, and swelling. Vesicles are clustered on an erythematous base, which evolves into a crusted erosion.

13. D. 31G, 5/16 inch

Insulin syringes for home use are available with pre-attached 30 or 31 gauge needles. The lengths are 0.5 or 5/16 inch. The smaller 30 and 31 gauge needles cause less discomfort than a 25 gauge would. In any case, 25 and 33 gauges' needles are not available on insulin syringes. The shorter 5/16-inch needle is more likely to deliver an appropriate subcutaneous injection than the ½ inch needles that are also available. 1-inch needles are not available on insulin syringes.

14. C. Oxymetazoline Nasal Spray

When recommending a nonprescription product, pharmacists must consider all aspects of a patient's current medical situation including active disease states, current medical therapy, and symptoms. In this case the patient needs relief of acute nasal congestion related to a cold. The most appropriate treatment from this list of choices would be the oxymetazoline nasal spray. Topical nasal decongestants can be used for a limited time frame (2-3 days) to alleviate symptoms effectively. In this patient, diphenhydramine may improve symptoms but may cause daytime somnolence and increases risks of falls in the elderly. Pseudoephedrine may also improve symptoms but should be used only cautiously in patients with a history of hypertension. Nasal saline is less effective for moderate to severe nasal congestion. Loratadine is a poor choice because it does not treat nasal congestion.

15. E. Mild Nausea and Vomiting after a single pill use

Patient presents with vaginal candidiasis infection, which is treated with fluconazole single pill or vaginal creams. Most frequent adverse effect after single fluconazole dose in the treatment of vaginal yeast infections is mild nausea and vomiting.

Teeth discoloration may occur with doxycycline, anaphylaxis and cross reactivity may occur with cephalosporins, and disulfiram-like reaction occurs with metronidazole.

16. B. Benzocaine 20%

The patient's symptoms indicate fever blisters.

Benzocaine 20% topical is used as a topical anesthetic for pain. Benzocaine is a common ingredient, used as a local anesthetic, found in Oragel Max®, Anbesol®, and Orabase®.

Carbamide peroxide acts as a debriding agent or oral wound cleanser in the treatment of canker sores, not cold sores. Carbamide peroxide is also used as an agent to remove ear wax, as found in Murine Ear Wax Removal®.

Camphor is a topical anesthetic agent found in Anbesol® and CamphoPhenique®. However, a concentration of 20% is excessive; 3-10.8% is more commonly used.

Capsaicin is a counterirritant and is not indicated for treatment of fever blisters.

Oxybenzone is a common sunscreen agent and is not used for treatment of any condition.

17. D. Ultraviolet Radiation

This patient has a cold sore, which is usually caused by herpes simplex 1, Herpes Simplex Labialis. The virus lies dormant between outbreaks, which are triggered by stress, sunlight (e.g., spring break), or hormones. It can occur on any mucosal surface, but it is usually on the lips. Prodromal symptoms are burning, pruritus, and swelling. Vesicles are clustered on an erythematous base, which evolves into a crusted erosion.

Avobenzone is a sunscreen.

Shingles is a reactivation of chicken pox and does not trigger fever blister formation.

Chicken pox is a childhood condition and is not associated with fever blister formation.

18. D. 48 hours at controlled room temperature

According to USP <797> low-risk level products must contain no more than 3 commercially manufactured products and not more than 2 entries into any 1 sterile container. The process involves only transfer, measuring, and mixing manipulations, and it occurs under ISO Class 5 conditions. Therefore, the fentanyl citrate product meets all criteria to be considered a low-risk product. Low-risk product beyond-use dating is designated as 48 hours under controlled room temperature, 14 days under cold temperatures, or 45 days in a solid frozen state. According to the label for Fentanyl Citrate Injection, USP, the product should be stored at controlled room temperature (20-25°C). The appropriate storage conditions and dating would therefore be 48 hours at controlled room temperature.

19. A. The dose needs to be decreased by 8%

Although there is no difference in bioavailability between the 2 formulations, there is a difference in the amount of active drug. The suspension contains phenytoin as a free acid. On the other hand, phenytoin capsule contains phenytoin as a sodium salt, which is equivalent to 92% of the free phenytoin acid. Even though the difference in active drug amount between the 2 formulations is relatively small, phenytoin has a narrow therapeutic index and its concentration needs to be within a range of 10 to 20 mcg/mL for optimal efficacy and minimal toxicity. In addition, its kinetic profile is non-linear, which means that any small difference in dose can result in a disproportional change in drug concentration. Therefore, the most prudent step is to reduce the dose in small increments based on the available strength of the suspension, especially if the patient's phenytoin concentration is close to the upper end of the therapeutic range.

20. C. Take a multivitamin once daily at bedtime

The patient using Alli® must take a once-daily multivitamin, as Alli® can cause a loss of oil-soluble vitamins. Pharmacists should also counsel the patient that Alli® works best when combined with a program of physical activity to maximize weight loss results.

21. A. Monitor your blood pressure for additional decreases

Terazosin, an alpha adrenergic antagonist, is used for the treatment of benign prostatic hyperplasia and hypertension. This patient is already taking anti-hypertensives, and the addition of terazosin may provide additional blood pressure-lowering effects. Patients should be counseled to check their blood pressure and rise or sit up slowly while their body adjusts to this medication. Women of childbearing age should be counseled to avoid handling 5-alpha reductase inhibitors, another class of medications used in the treatment of benign prostatic hyperplasia. Terazosin does not lower PSA levels; however, 5-alpha reductase inhibitors do. Patients may experience common side effects upon initiation of terazosin; however, the effects are transient, mild, and do not require as much attention as blood pressure lowering.

22. C. 17%

Nonprescription salicylic acid is available in 17% and 40% concentrations. A concentration of 17% is recommended for common warts, especially in a child. A concentration of 40% is recommended for the treatment of plantar warts.

23. B. High Risk, 3 days refrigerated

Because this product is prepared using at least 1 non-sterile ingredient (thimerosal) requiring terminal sterilization by the compounder, the product must be considered a high risk product by USP <797> standards. The general beyond-use dating requirement for high risk products is 3 days at cold temperature (refrigerated), 24 hours at room temperature, or 45 days if frozen solid, unless sterility and endotoxin testing is performed. In the presence of a preservative such as thimerosal, the beyond-use date may be extended; in the case of this formulation, the USP official monograph suggests a beyond-use date of not more than 5 days refrigerated.

24. C. Doxycycline

This patient presents with signs and symptoms consistent with nongonococcal urethritis (NGU). *C. trachomatis* is the organism associated with NGU. The treatments of choice for NGU are doxycycline and azithromycin. Since this patient has an allergy to clarithromycin, doxycycline is the most appropriate treatment option.

25. A. Cool

The best option provided for storage of Latisse is a cool place. To ensure the stability of a pharmaceutical preparation for the period of its intended shelf life, the product must be stored under proper conditions. The labeling of approved pharmaceutical products includes the desired conditions of storage specifically for that product. Latisse's labeling indicates the proper storage for the solution is 2°-25°C (36°-77°F). The USP defines storage conditions as follows:

Cold - Less than 8°C; a refrigerator is a cold place in which the temperature is maintained between 2° and 8°C. A freezer is a cold place in which the temperature is maintained between -20°and -10°C.

Cool - Any temperature between 8°-15°C; a product for which storage in a cool place is directed may be stored in a refrigerator unless otherwise specified.

Room Temperature - The temperature prevailing in a working area, usually between 20°-25°C, but also allows for temperature variations between 15°-30°C.

Warm - Any temperature between 30°-40°C.

Excessive Heat - Any temperature above 40°C.

The criteria for frozen, cold, and warm conditions do not meet the specifications for storage of Latisse. This product could be stored at cooler room temperatures, but the maximum temperature it should be exposed to is 25°C. Therefore, the best option of those listed for a pharmacist to recommend is a cool place.

26. C. Escitalopram

Among the SSRIs listed, the only one that is developed and marketed as a pure isomer is escitalopram.

27. A. Compound W Freeze Off

Salicylic acid is available as an OTC agent in 17% or 40% concentrations to treat warts. Salicylic acid is available as paint-on liquid, gel, disc pads, and in an adhesive pad. Compound W Freeze Off® in a canister that contains dimethyl ether, propane, and isobutene.

28. B. Viscous vehicle

Insoluble steroids must be formulated as a suspension dosage form. Frequently, polymers are used as vehicles to enhance the viscosity of the formulation, thus decreasing the settling rate of the drug particles while also increasing residence time of administered drops on the eye.

29. C. Vancomycin

Both metronidazole and vancomycin are effective and useful for treatment of *C. difficile* infection. However, only vancomycin is approved by the FDA for this therapeutic indication. Metronidazole is likely to be less expensive, but vancomycin can achieve much higher concentration within the colon.

30. A. 10%

In general, a pharmaceutical product is considered to be not usable if more than 10% of its active ingredient, as determined by appropriate assay, is lost.

31. B. Phenytoin

Gingival hyperplasia, an overgrowth of gum tissue inside the oral cavity, predisposes a patient to loss of tooth integrity and oral infection. It is a known side effect of phenytoin and patient receiving this anticonvulsant should be advised to have good oral hygiene.

32. E. Nortriptyline 25 mg twice daily

Nortriptyline is the best option for this patient because it will assist with quitting smoking and treat signs/symptoms of depression. Although it may cause weight gain, it can also cause nausea, vomiting, and weight loss, so the patient would need to try the medication before the medication's side effects (for him specifically) could be discerned.

Bupropion is not an acceptable option for this patient because of his history of seizures.

Nicotine gum is not an acceptable option for this patient because he is a chronic gum chewer. In order for nicotine gum to be effective, the patient must not chew the gum constantly.

The nicotine 21 mg patch is not indicated for patients smoking fewer than 10 cigarettes per day (only the 7 mg patch).

Clonidine is not as effective as the other options for treatment of smoking cessation. If the nortriptyline does not work for this patient, clonidine therapy may be initiated.

33. D. Spatula and electronic balance

Crude coal tar is a highly viscous liquid that cannot be poured into a measuring device, making **liquid graduates** inappropriate. It is too viscous to be drawn into either an **oral** or **injectable syringe**. Rather, the pharmacist must use a spatula to place a specific amount in a weighing boat on the pan of a tarred electronic balance. The spatula is used to continue placing the coal tar in the weighing boat or to return excess to the mother container until the measurement is proper. The coal tar and polysorbate 80 are levigated on an ointment slab and then incorporated into the zinc oxide by spatulation and geometric dilution until the mixture is uniform. The mixture is placed in a 1-ounce ointment tube.

34. A. Henderson-Hasselbalch

The **Henderson-Hasselbalch** equation takes into account the relationship between the ionized and the unionized form of a weak electrolyte, e.g., solution of a weakly acidic compound. With all other factors being equal, it is the unionized form of the drug that will be primarily transported across the biological cell membrane.

The Arrhenius equation is useful for predicting drug product stability and shelf life.

The Cockcroft Gault equation is used to estimate a patient's creatinine clearance.

The Michaelis-Menten equation is used to calculate non-linear kinetic reactions such as enzyme kinetics or non-linear drug absorption, distribution, and elimination kinetics. Pharmacokinetic equations are used to predict drug plasma concentrations.

35. A, B, C, E

All are appropriate except intramuscular administration of heparin is painful and can cause hematomas. Heparin flush via a heparin lock is used for maintaining fluid flow through an intravenous line.

36. C. 2PAM and atropine

The presentation of a patient with organophosphate exposure shows all cholinergic symptoms: diarrhea, flushing, urination, miosis, bradycardia, emesis, lacrimation, lethargy, and salivation. Atropine and 2 PAM are used to treat organophosphate overdose. N-acetylcysteine is used in acetaminophen overdose per nomogram. Naloxone is used to reverse opioid intoxication. Physostigmine is used in anticholinergic overdose. Activated charcoal may be useful in someone who ingested a toxin orally. It is unlikely to be beneficial in this case.

37. B. DHS Tar Shampoo (Coal Tar Extract)®

The only nonprescription ingredients proven safe and effective for psoriasis are coal tar, hydrocortisone, and salicylic acid, in appropriate concentrations.

38. E. 2 to 8° C

Biological agents are readily susceptible to degradation by heat, light, or other processes such as protein aggregation, storage conditions are highly specific. Most biologicals are stored in a refrigerator at 2 to 8° C.

39. D. The formulations have same bioavailability as immediate-release formulations

Controlled-release formulations use different matrix materials to surround the active drug. The matrix slowly dissolves in the stomach and the small intestine, resulting in a sustained release of the active drug. The pharmacokinetic profiles of these formulations result in slower rate of absorption (longer Tmax) and therefore lower Cmax. However, the bioavailability is usually the same as that of immediate-release formulations, as the systemic exposure is sustained over a longer time period after drug administration. The primary site of drug absorption is usually in the small intestine as a result of its much greater absorptive surface area compared to other sites within the gastrointestinal tract.

40. E. Seborrheic dermatitis

The manifestations are those of seborrheic dermatitis. Further, the locations affected are those classically associated with seborrheic dermatitis.

41. A. Ointment Tile

To prepare this product, the pharmacist would weigh out 60 grams of Velvachol® and place it on an ointment tile. Next, the pharmacist should agitate the vials of triamcinolone suspension and measure out the appropriate amount of triamcinolone using a sterile syringe. The suspension should be squirted gently onto the Velvachol®. Using a spatula, the pharmacist should levigate the mixture until the suspension is fully and evenly incorporated into the Velvachol®. The mixture is then transferred into an ointment jar with use of the spatula. Since the triamcinolone is measured with a syringe, there is no need for a graduated cylinder or conical graduate. A stirring rod would not be appropriate for mixing the suspension and cream. Placing the Velvachol® in a mortar for mixing is possible, but doing so would be a poor choice, as it would be more difficult to remove the cream with a spatula after mixing.

42. A. Exact dose of the drug prescribed for the patient

A unit dose package contains the exact amount of a drug (single dose) to be given to the patient per the physician's order. This packaging is in contrast to bulk packaging in which multiple doses are included in the same package, to be measured out at the time of administration.

43. E. More easily penetrated by lipophilic molecules

The blood brain barrier consists of a lipid-bilayer that is more easily penetrated by lipophilic molecules, which include most of the CNS-acting drugs.

44. A. Exhale. Place inhaler in mouth. Begin inhaling slowly. Activate inhaler while continuing to inhale then hold breath for 10 seconds and exhale

The recommended technique for the proper use of a metered-dose inhaler includes: Exhale. Hold inhaler upright and place lips around mouthpiece or spacer. Inhale slowly and activate inhaler while continuing to inhale. Inhale completely and hold breath for 10 seconds or as long as possible. Repeat treatment if more than one inhalation is prescribed allowing 1 to 2 minutes between inhalations. Rinse mouth with water and expel contents when steroidal inhaler is used.

45. C. Phase III

A New Drug Application (NDA) is filed after completion of Phase III clinical testing. An Investigational New Drug Application (IND) is submitted after preclinical animal investigations have been performed. The testing then proceeds to Phases I, II, and III of human clinical trials to determine safety and efficacy. If the results of these trials are promising, the drug's sponsor may then submit an NDA to the FDA. An NDA may be over 100,000 pages in length. The FDA has 180 days to act on an NDA according to law; however, significant delays are common. An NDA is required to provide proof of safety and efficacy of any of the following before the new drug may be marketed:

1) A new molecular entity
2) A new salt of a previously approved drug
3) A new formulation of a previously approved drug
4) A new combination of 2 or more drugs
5) Duplication of an already approved drug product - i.e., new manufacturer
6) A new indication for a previously marketed drug
7) A drug product already marketed that has no previously approved NDA.

The drug is also assigned a letter to designate its review priority: *S* for standard review or *P* for priority review, indicating the new drug represents significant advances over existing treatments. If the FDA approves the NDA, the new drug then becomes available for physicians to prescribe. The FDA requires additional studies (Phase IV) on some drugs to evaluate long-term effects.

46. A. Trichomoniasis

STI	Men	Women
Gonorrhea	Mucopurulent urethral discharge. Can lead to prostatitis, epididymitis, and urethral stricture.	Often asymptomatic. Abnormal vaginal discharge or bleeding, urinary tract complaints. Can lead to pelvic inflammatory

		disease, infertility, chronic pelvic pain, and tubal pregnancy.
Trichomoniasis	Asymptomatic	Up to 50% asymptomatic. Greenish, malodorous vaginal discharge, itching, painful intercourse, postcoital bleeding.
HPV	Many asymptomatic. If symptomatic – lesions may be present on genitalia, anus, rectum, or mouth	Many asymptomatic. If symptomatic - lesions on external genitalia, anus, rectum, mouth, vagina, urethra, cervix
HSV	Many asymptomatic. Vesicular or ulcerative lesions on genitalia, thighs, buttocks.	Many asymptomatic. Vesicular or ulcerative lesions on genitalia, thighs, buttocks. Symptoms more severe in women.
Syphilis	Painless, temporary, and localized chancre Secondary – rash, generalized lymphadenopathy, hepatosplenomegaly, alopecia, oral mucous patches	Painless, temporary, and localized chancre Secondary – rash, generalized lymphadenopathy, hepatosplenomegaly, alopecia, oral mucous patches

47. E. Stomach ulcers

Nicorette gum is contraindicated in patients with heart disease, recent heart attack, irregular heartbeat, stomach ulcers, and diabetes requiring insulin. The product can delay healing of stomach ulcers.

48. A. Healthy eating habits

Drug therapy should be considered in patients with a body mass index greater than 30 kg/m^2 or greater than 27 kg/m^2 with risk factors of hypertension, dyslipidemia, coronary heart disease, type 2 diabetes, or sleep apnea. Sibutramine and phentermine are effective weight loss agents. If this patient qualified for treatment based on BMI, these agents would not be appropriate because the patient has hypertension. Orlistat 60 mg daily is helpful only if the patient is consuming a diet containing moderate to high amounts of fat. Since this patient is following a low fat eating regimen already, orlistat would not be as effective in this patient.

Asking the patient to make a drastic change in her exercise habits is unlikely to result in long term adherence to the regimen. Instead, the patient should be encouraged to gradually increase exercise as tolerated.

Based on the options, encouraging the patient to follow healthy eating habits is the most appropriate treatment at this time. The combination of health eating and increased physical activity should result in a gradual (1-2 lb/week) weight loss.

49. A. Activated Charcoal

Syrup of ipecac is contraindicated in this situation because rapid neurologic or hemodynamic deterioration may occur. Gastric lavage will not be effective in this situation because at least 2 hours have elapsed. Gastric lavage would be beneficial if initiated within 1 hour of ingestion. There is limited evidence to suggest that hemodialysis is effective in tricyclic antidepressant overdose. Administration of activated charcoal is the most appropriate treatment approach in this patient. The charcoal will adsorb the amitriptyline in the gut and prevent further absorption.

50. C. Akathisia

The newer atypical antipsychotics such as clozapine and olanzapine are less likely than the typical antipsychotic drugs to cause extrapyramidal side effects including akathisia and dystonia. On the other hand, they have been reported to cause other side effects more often, including sedation, weight gain, and agranulocytosis. Orthostatic hypotension is a common side effect of the low potency typical antipsychotic agents such as chlorpromazine.

Practice Test 2 Answers and Explanations

1. **A. Creams have a higher percentage of oil than lotions**

   Lotions, creams, and ointments are oil in water preparations. Lotions have the most water, creams, and then ointments have the most oil.

2. **B. The drug is unlikely to have any significant adverse effects**

   The therapeutic index is a measurement of the margin of safety of the drug. The greater the difference between a therapeutic dose and a toxic dose, the greater will be the therapeutic index. Therefore, a drug with a high therapeutic index is one that likely has few significant side effects and does not need close monitoring of its concentration or amount in the body. The drug interaction potential for a drug is usually influenced by its metabolism as well as its effect on the drug metabolizing enzymes in the body

3. **A. Noninferiority**

   Noninferiority trial is designed to show that a treatment is no less effective than an existing treatment. The treatment may be more effective or may have a similar effect.

   Superiority trial is designed to detect a difference between treatments and show that one treatment is more effective than the other.

   Equivalence trial is designed to show the absence of meaningful differences between treatments.

   Cohort clinical trial is a longitudinal study that begins with the gathering of 2 groups of patients, 1 which receives the exposure of interest and 1 which does not, and then following the groups over time (prospective) to measure the development of different outcomes.

   Randomized clinical trial is a trial in which the participants are assigned randomly to different treatments.

4. **B. Martindale**

   A pharmacist should have access to various resources while taking care of patients. In this example, the key reference is Martindale; this reference includes information about medications available from other countries.

   Facts & Comparisons® is a comprehensive resource for prescription and nonprescription medications available in the Unites States and Canada.

   USP contains information about the pharmacology, adverse effects, contraindications, and doses of prescriptions medications along with patient information.

   Remington is a reference for isotonicity, sterilization, and theoretical science.

   Micromedex® is a comprehensive resource for prescription and nonprescription medications available in the Unites States.

5. **C. Mode**

The most common value in data distribution is described by the mode.

The mean, or the average, is the sum of all values divided by the total number of values. The mean is most commonly used to measure central tendency.

The median is the point at which half of the observations fall below and half-life above the value.

Standard deviation applies only to data normally or near normally distributed. It uses a formula that sums the squares of the differences between each value from a sample and the mean of the sample.

6. **C. Phase 3 study is performed for evaluation of response in a large number of patients with the target disease**

A Phase 1 study primarily determines the pharmacokinetic profile of a drug in a small number of healthy volunteers. Post-marketing surveillance studies are performed after approval. There is no official designation of a Phase 4 study.

7. **E. The study is unethical**

Any new medication, regardless how good it seems to be in small Phase 1 or 2 trials, should be compared to the standard of care in Phase 3 trials. Placebo is not the standard of care in the treatment of early stage breast cancer. Tamoxifen administration should not skew results in a well-organized trial. The patients will be randomly assigned to groups based on their ER/PR positivity status; therefore, both groups should have same number of ER/PR positive patients. Most Phase 1 and 2 trials are not designed to assess clinical response or efficacy; therefore, their data should be interpreted with caution

8. **A. Remington**

A pharmacist should have access to various resources while taking care of patients. In this example, the key reference is Martindale; this reference includes information about medications available from other countries.

Facts & Comparisons® is a comprehensive resource for prescription and nonprescription medications available in the Unites States and Canada.

USP contains information about the pharmacology, adverse effects, contraindications, and doses of prescriptions medications along with patient information.

Remington is a reference for isotonicity, sterilization, and theoretical science.

Micromedex® is a comprehensive resource for prescription and nonprescription medications available in the Unites States.

9. **B. No nonprescription product can minimize or prevent hangover**

No nonprescription product can be marketed with the claim of minimizing or preventing hangover. Such products are not effective and might encourage patients to drive while under the influence.

10. E. Range

The mean, median, and mode are statistical terms used to describe the frequency distribution of the data. The prevalence usually refers to the total number of occurrences of an event (e.g., adverse reaction to a drug). The range is typically used for describing the variability for a small set of data.

11. E. Young adult Caucasian women

The WHO criteria for osteoporosis compares an individual's BMD to that of young adult Caucasian women. The T score is the number of standard deviations from the mean BMD of young Caucasian women. A T score of 0 would mean a patient's BMD is the same as the mean of young women, and a T score of -2.0 means the patient has a BMD at that site, and by that method, 2 standard deviations less than the mean. A T score of greater than -1.0 is considered normal; a T score between -1.0 and -2.5 is called osteopenia. A T score of less than -2.5 is osteoporosis.

12. B. Reduce purine-rich foods

There are many lifestyle and dietary factors that contribute to a patient's increased risk of experiencing a gouty attack. Patients should be counseled to reduce intake of purine-containing foods, for example, meats (especially organ meats), seafood, and beer. Recent information also suggests an association between consumption of fructose-containing beverages and gout. Therefore, a patient with gout should also be counseled to reduce or avoid fructose-containing beverages. Based on this patient's cardiovascular risk factors, this patient should be counseled to increase his intake of fruits and vegetables and reduce fat, cholesterol, and sodium intake.

13. C. 11 to 12 g/dL

The target range for hemoglobin levels during treatment with erythropoiesis-stimulating agent is 11 to 12 g/dL. Although labeling information suggests maintaining hemoglobin levels between 10 to 12 g/dL, the National Kidney Foundation Kidney Disease Outcome Quality Initiative recommends a target range of 11 to 12 g/dL in patients receiving erythropoiesis-stimulating agent for treatment of anemia.

14. C. Increase hemoglobin concentration from baseline

The therapeutic goal for using erythropoietic agent is an increase in hemoglobin concentration from the baseline, usually about 1 g/dL over 4 weeks, as well as a reduction in the frequency of blood transfusions

15. A. 2 weeks

This patient's INR is supratherapeutic. An INR range of 2.0 to 3.0 is recommended for patients receiving warfarin for atrial fibrillation. Knowing that this result is inconsistent with his recent values, his INR should be rechecked sooner than 1 month. The result does not require urgent attention; therefore, the 2-week time frame is the most reasonable option provided. It is unnecessary to check the INR again tomorrow because sufficient time will not have elapsed to see a significant change in the result

16. C. Serum uric acid

Since allopurinol decreases the rate of synthesis of uric acid and is used in the treatment of gout, monitoring of serum uric acid level would be appropriate to assess its therapeutic effect.

17. B. 2.0 – 3.0

According to the CHEST guidelines regarding antithrombotic therapy, post-MI patients at a high risk for left ventricular thrombosis should be maintained in a therapeutic range of 2.0 to 3.0.

18. A. Azithromycin

Azithromycin, erythromycin, and metronidazole are all classified as B category for the FDA pregnancy category. However, there are some concerns regarding the use of metronidazole and the estolate salt of erythromycin, and they should be used with caution and best avoided as there are alternatives. Doxycycline and tetracycline are Class D drugs and need to be avoided in pregnancy.

19. B. 3.5

99% of the gastric acid would be neutralized when the intragastric pH is increased from 1.0 to 3.5. Increasing the gastric pH to higher values would provide no additional therapeutic benefit.

20. A. Increased use of broad-spectrum antibiotics

Lower cost of antibiotics and increased use of broad-spectrum antibiotics are associated with higher likelihood of antimicrobial resistance, resulting in increased incidence of treatment failure.

21. C. An HDL of <40; age (men >45 yrs, women >55 yrs)

An HDL of <40 is undesirable, and so is the age factor (>45 years for men and >55 years for women). This case illustrates the rationale of pharmacotherapy in the presence of 2 or more risk factors. The specific LDL lipid level should be identified to guide the initiation and goal of pharmacotherapy. Drug therapy for patients with 2+ risk factors should be started when the LDL is >130. The LDL goal is <130.

The NCEP/ATEP has set forth explicit risk factors, as well as specific lipid goals/classifications, that clearly address what parameters dictate the initiation or cessation of pharmacotherapy. This question illustrates that in patients with a major risk factor (e.g., CHD, DM), the goal of drug therapy is to keep the level of LDL lipids <100. Likewise, drug therapy should be started when the LDL is >130. A patient with a TC of <200 is already in the desirable range and would not need drug therapy based on lipid classification alone. It should be noted that the TC is only a general marker; therefore, the individual lipid molecules need to be identified via a lipid panel/profile. The presence of 0 to 1 risk factors (HBP) mandates that drug therapy should be started when the LDL is >190; the goal of therapy is an LDL <160. Once the LDL level is identified, then the decision whether or not to initiate drug therapy can be discussed.

An HDL of >60 is very desirable; there is a direct correlation between the level of HDL and the absence of coronary plaque. It should be noted that the LDL level should still be identified in order to ascertain the true lipid picture. Cigarette smoking is only 1 risk factor; therefore, drug therapy should be initiated when the LDL is >190. The goal of therapy is an LDL level of <160. Once the LDL lipid level is identified, the option of drug therapy can be discussed.

The VLDL lipid molecule can be a separate risk factor and is usually elevated along with TG. The VLDL level becomes important (VLDL >200 - 300) when it is accompanied by elevated TG (200 - 499). As in the above explanations, the LDL lipid level should be identified due to the direct correlation between LDL and CHD. A major risk factor (e.g., diabetes) mandates that drug therapy be initiated when the LDL is >130. The LDL goal is <100. Once the LDL level is lowered to an acceptable range, the elevated VLDL and TG (especially if TG is >500) should be addressed by initiating either a combination of diet and exercise (which will lower VLDL) and/or drug therapy. The statins have a modest effect on VLDL/TG, whereas niacin and gemfibrozil have been shown to dramatically reduce these lipid levels.

22. A. Naprosyn EC is not indicated for treatment of an acute gouty attack

Naprosyn is a very effective agent in regard to relieving pain and inflammation during an acute gout attack. However, it is important to pay attention to the specific dosage form in order to insure it will be effective for the condition being treated. When acute pain relief is necessary, an immediate-release product is most appropriate. When the patient requires relief from chronic pain and the medication is scheduled around the clock, EC or enteric-coated products are appropriate to provide pain relief while preventing potential gastric complications.

23. D. Discontinue the medication in 1 year

Patients with generalized anxiety disorder who respond to medication therapy should stay on the medication for at least 1 year prior to discontinuation, assuming the patient does not relapse during that time. If the patient has experienced multiple episodes of anxiety, lifelong therapy may be considered. Of course, the pharmacist should urge the patient not to discontinue the medication without obtaining his physician's permission.

24. C. 2.5 - 3.5

According to the recent CHEST guidelines regarding antithrombotic therapy, the therapeutic range for patients with bileaflet mechanical valves in the mitral position is 2.5 to 3.5.

25. E. Noncompliance

Mycoplasma pneumonia infection commonly presents with nonproductive cough, headache, runny nose, and chest pain. Erythromycin is a good agent for atypical pneumonias, but it needs to be taken several times per day and also it is associated with bad side effects such as diarrhea. Many patients will not tolerate erythromycin due to its side effects. Noncompliance is a major issue with erythromycin prescription.

26. B. Ciprofloxacin

The best choice of those listed for treatment of this patient's acute sinusitis would be ciprofloxacin (Cipro®). Although amoxicillin (Amoxil®) is generally first-line therapy for acute sinusitis and does not interact with this patient's other medications, the patient is allergic to penicillin and therefore should not be given amoxicillin. Bactrim® (trimethoprim/sulfamethoxazole) and telithromycin (Ketek®), while appropriate alternative therapies for acute sinusitis in penicillin-allergic patients, would interact significantly with the patient's ketoconazole. Gentamicin (Gentak®) is inappropriate therapy for acute sinusitis

27. D. 7%

The ADA recommends the use of HbA1C level for monitoring glycemic control in diabetic patients. The target used by ADA is <7%, whereas the target recommended by the American College of Endocrinology and American Association of Clinical Endocrinologists is <6.5%.

28. E. Captopril

The only drugs that have been shown to improve survival in patients with heart failure are ACE inhibitors, spironolactone, and certain beta-blockers. Despite decades of use, digitalis has never been proven to have a beneficial effect on survival. Entresto® (sacubitril/valsartan) is a newer heart failure medication that is a combination of an ACEI and ARB has shown positive results for patients.

29. D. 7 days

Patients with severe generalized anxiety disorder may initially be treated with a benzodiazepine and an SSRI. It is important to counsel the patient about when they will notice the therapeutic effects of each drug. The full effects of the benzodiazepine will be evident within 1 week. The full effects of the SSRI will be evident in 8-12 weeks.

30. A. Rasagiline

Rasagiline (Azilect®) is a selective MAO-B inhibitor with recommended dosing of 1 mg given once daily. Amantadine (Symmetrel®), an antiviral medication serendipitously discovered to treat symptoms of Parkinson's disease, has a recommended dose of 100 mg given twice daily. Carbidopa/Levodopa (Sinemet®) is dosed 3 or 4 times daily. Pramipexole (Mirapex®) and ropinirole (Requip®) are dosed 3 times daily.

Caution should be exercised when administering a MAOI concomitantly with some antidepressants. Severe CNS toxicity associated with hyperpyrexia and death has been reported with the combination of tricyclic antidepressants and non-selective MAOIs (e.g., phenelzine, tranylcypromine) or the selective MAO-B inhibitor selegiline (selegiline). These adverse events have included behavioral and mental status changes, diaphoresis, muscular rigidity, hypertension, syncope, and death. Serious, sometimes fatal reactions with signs and symptoms, including hyperthermia, rigidity, myoclonus, autonomic instability with rapid vital sign fluctuations, and mental status changes progressing to extreme agitation, delirium, and coma, have been reported in patients receiving a combination of selective serotonin reuptake inhibitors (SSRIs), including fluoxetine (Prozac®), fluvoxamine (Luvox®), sertraline (Zoloft®), and paroxetine (Paxil®), and non-selective MAOIs or the selective MAO-B inhibitor selegiline. Similar reactions have been reported with serotonin-norepinephrine reuptake inhibitors (SNRIs) and non-selective MAOIs or the selective MAO-B inhibitor selegiline.

Rasagiline (Azilect®) clinical trials did not allow concomitant use of fluoxetine or fluvoxamine with rasagiline, but the following antidepressants and doses were allowed in the trials: amitriptyline ≤ 50 mg/daily, trazodone ≤ 100 mg/daily, citalopram ≤ 20 mg/daily, sertraline ≤ 100 mg/daily, and paroxetine ≤ 30 mg/daily. Although most rasagiline drug interactions are based on theoretical considerations rather than actual clinical data, the potential severity of many of the adverse outcomes dictates a conservative approach when giving rasagiline concomitantly with these drugs. Many of the potentially interacting drugs are not lifesaving and have alternatives. For other drugs that may be important for the patient, such as antidepressants, one should weigh the benefits versus the (usually small) risk of using them with rasagiline. This patient is currently taking 50 mg amitriptyline daily, which has not had any reported adverse outcomes when used with rasagiline, but theoretically may interact with rasagiline. A patient in this situation should be counseled about the possibility of adverse interactions if the physician chooses to continue antidepressant therapy.

31. D. Its teratogenic classification

While all of the mentioned characteristics should be considered (mechanism of action, smoking status, alcohol use, lactation), at this time, the most important first consideration for a pregnant woman would be the potential teratogenicity of the drug.

32. A. <130/≤80 mm Hg

This patient is a diabetic patient; her blood pressure goal is <130/≤80 according to the American College of Cardiology/American Heart Association (ACC/AHA) guidelines. Allowing the blood pressure to reach levels in excess of this target could have long-term adverse consequences (e.g., stroke or heart attack). Attempting to achieve lower levels could lead to hypotension, with dizziness or syncope upon standing.

33. B. Schedule I

Currently there is no medical reason for any practitioner to prescribe a Schedule I medication for management of patient.

34. C. <130/80 mmHg

The American College of Cardiology/American Heart Association (ACC/AHA) guidelines recommends blood pressure be treated to <130/80 mmHg in patients less than 60 years of age, even those with diabetes or chronic kidney disease.

35. E. Infliximab

Per the American College of Rheumatology Guidelines, patients with moderate disease activity and features of poor prognosis (many swollen joints, moderate disease activity, radiographic erosion) with disease duration greater than 24 months are candidates for the following oral therapies: leflunomide, methotrexate, sulfasalazine monotherapy, or methotrexate and hydroxychloroquine combination therapy. Sulfasalazine and leflunomide is not a recommended combination in the ACR guidelines. Since the patient failed methotrexate monotherapy, she is also a candidate for biologic therapy, specifically, a TNF antagonist. The patient has no contraindications to TNF antagonists; therefore, rituximab is not necessary at this time. In addition, the patient is rheumatoid factor negative so rituximab may not be the most effective option in this patient. Combination biologic therapy is not warranted due to increased adverse effects without added efficacy.

36. A. 2.0 – 3.0

According to the CHEST guidelines regarding antithrombotic therapy, the therapeutic range for treatment of deep vein thrombosis is 2.0 - 3.0.

37. B. Recommend against its use, as it is only for patients aged 12 and above

Caffeine products such as NoDoz® and Vivarin® are contraindicated for self-use in patients under the age of 12 years. For this reason, he should be advised against their use. Caffeine-containing beverages are not necessarily safe for children and should not be recommended. If his concern continues, he should be urged to consult the physician

38. C. What the body does to the drug

Pharmacokinetics is currently defined as the study of the time course of drug absorption, distribution, metabolism, and excretion.

39. D. The null hypothesis is false, but is accepted in error

A Type II error means that the null hypothesis is false, yet it is accepted in error. The study authors conclude that there's no difference but in fact there is a difference.

40. B. The value in the middle of the list

Median is the middle of the set, mode is the most common value, and mean is average of the set.

41. B. Nominal

Discrete date can be divided into four categories (gender, marital status, etc.). This is called nominal discrete value.

42. C. Continuous

Discrete data have finite values, or buckets. You can count them. Continuous data technically have an infinite number of steps, which form a continuum. The number of questions correct would be discrete--there are a finite and countable number of questions. Time to complete a task is continuous since it could take 178.8977687 seconds. Time forms an interval from 0 to infinity. You can usually tell the difference between discrete and continuous data because discrete usually can be preceded by "number of..."

Discrete:
- Number of children in a household
- Number of languages a person speaks
- Number of people sleeping in stats class

Continuous:
- Height of children
- Weight of cars
- Time to wake up in the morning
- Speed of the train

43. A, E

The specificity of a clinical test refers to the ability of the test to correctly identify those patients without the disease. A test with 100% specificity correctly identifies all patients without the disease. A test with 80% specificity correctly reports 80% of patients without the disease as test negative (true negatives) but 20% patients without the disease are incorrectly identified as test positive (false positives).

44. B. The patient cannot be dispensed abacavir

If a patient is positive for HLA-B*5701 then they cannot receive Ziagen® or abacavir either by itself or in combination due to a highly hypersensitive reaction causing multi-organ syndromes.

45. A, B, C, D

A "sulfa" allergy is most likely due to the sulfamethoxazole component in Bactrim®. If there is a reaction to this drug, then sulfasalazine and sulfisoxazole. It's rare for a reaction with zonisamide or celecoxib but they are contraindicated with a sulfa allergy and should be avoided. Sulfate is not the same as sulfa and morphine sulfate may be used.

46. A, D, E

If a patient has anaphylactic reaction, they will need to go to the ER or call 911 immediately receiving an epinephrine injection and may also receive diphenhydramine. Patients who are at risk should always carry an epinephrine pen. In Florida, pharmacists are allowed to administer epinephrine pens in emergency situations and administer to patients.

47. C. MedWatch

Use the MedWatch form to report adverse events that you observe or suspect for human medical products, including serious drug side effects, product use errors, product quality problems, and therapeutic failures for: Prescription or over-the-counter medicines, as well as medicines administered to hospital patients or at outpatient infusion centers, biologics (including blood components, blood and plasma derivatives, allergenic, human cells, tissues, and cellular and tissue-based products (HCT/Ps)), medical devices (including in vitro diagnostic products), combination products, Special nutritional products (dietary supplements, infant formulas, and medical foods), cosmetics, and foods/beverages (including reports of serious allergic reactions).

48. B. The Joint Commission

The Joint Commission is a United States-based nonprofit tax-exempt 501 organization that accredits more than 21,000 health care organizations and programs in the United States.

49. A, C, D, E

The provider only provided the route and amount of the medication, but left out many other necessary pieces of information such as frequency, child's weight and height, indication, writing for one teaspoonful instead of 5 mL, and no age.

50. C, D, E

You should always wear and use a mask that covers the nose and mouth. Placing items behind each other prevents the air to also hit that object.

Practice Test 3 Answers and Explanations

1. **B. Placing the medications in high-risk bins, with notations on the front of the bins regarding name-mixups and other relevant alerts**

   A high alert drug such as insulin should be placed in a brightly colored bin with warning on front to avoid medication errors. A medication guide and syringes or other items to be dispensed can be placed in the bin. Warning on the front should include alerts for drug name mix ups, etc.

2. **B. PCAs require an educated, coordinated health care team**

   PCA devices contain narcotics and/or anesthetics for synergy usually in hospice, post-op, and cancer settings. They require coordinated health care teams to ensure all healthcare providers such as nurses and other assistants are aware how to use. PCAs help patients administer pain medication to themselves to help lower doses required and are cost-effective

3. **E. UTIs, due to indwelling catheters**

   Indwelling catheters are the most common cause of UTIs and are sometimes due to patient non-compliance in removing and replacing catheters. Usually when the catheter is removed the infection most likely resolves

4. **A, B, C**

   Use of single vial doses are preferred since multi-dose vials should be assigned to patients and labeled. The needle/syringe should be changed after each patient use if used for multiple different patients

5. **C. Potassium chloride injection and hypertonic saline**

   These are high-alert medications per ISMP due to the high risk of potential death these may cause. Potassium fast push may stop the heart and hypertonic saline can cause pain and necrosis of the injection site if injected wrongly

6. **A. To ensure that the benefits of dangerous drugs outweigh the risks**

   The FDA requires high-risk drugs to have a Risk Evaluation and Mitigation Strategy (REMS) from the manufacturer to ensure benefits outweigh the risks. REMS drugs require specific restrictions, patient registries, and other regulations to ensure safety. An example is the iPLEDGE program for isotretinoin common among college students

7. **A. To determine safety, efficacy and dose-response relationships in the population**

   Please ensure to know the different phases of drug studies

8. **D. AB**

   The publication Approved Drug Products with Therapeutic Equivalence Evaluations (commonly known as the Orange Book) identifies drug products approved on the basis of safety and effectiveness by the Food and Drug Administration (FDA) under the Federal Food, Drug, and Cosmetic Act (the

Act) and related patent and exclusivity information. AA stands for no bioequivalence problems in conventional dosage forms, AB stands for meeting necessary bioequivalence requirements

9. C. To determine efficacy

Phase 2 studies examine the effectiveness of a compound.

10. B, C, E

Kava can be used for anxiety, but it is not recommended due to hepatotoxicity.

11. E. Vitamin B6

Pyridoxine (Vitamin B6) 25-50 mg by mouth daily is used to reduce the risk of INH-induced peripheral neuropathy.

12. A, C, E

It's important to know the names of vitamins!

13. B. To reduce the risk of serious birth defects in children born to women with low folic acid intake

Any woman of child-bearing age who is planning to conceive should take a folic acid supplement of 400 mcg or more per day to help prevent birth defects such as to the brain and spinal cord. Folic acid needs to be taken months before pregnancy.

14. B. If you take the antibiotic in the morning and at night, take the probiotic in the middle of the day

Probiotics are beneficial to take but it's important to separate out by at least a few hours from the antibiotic as the antibiotic will destroy the probiotic. Lycopene is used for prostate cancer prevention, saw palmetto prostate enlargement, and comfrey should not be recommended as hepatotoxic. Probiotics should be continued weeks after the antibiotic has stopped to prevent a rare but serious *C. diff* infection.

15. A, C, D, E

Fat-soluble vitamins should be supplemented in patients on Orlistat.

16. A, D, E

Feverfew, willow bark, butterbur, guarana (due to caffeine), fish oils, magnesium, CoQ10, and riboflavin may help prevent migraines.

17. C. Os-Cal®

Os-Cal® is oyster-shell calcium and is a more expensive form of calcium carbonate. It may be best to advise the patient to take other calcium supplements that do not require an acidic environment to help with adherence

18. C. Vitamin D

Vitamin D is essential in helping the body absorb and use calcium; in fact, the body cannot absorb calcium at all without some vitamin D. Vitamin D comes from two sources. It is made in the skin through direct exposure to sunlight, and it comes from the diet

19. E. DHEA

DHEA may help with erectile dysfunction and is a precursor to testosterone. DHEA is safe at usual doses but higher doses can cause acne, hirsutism, and increase risk for hypertension or liver damage.

20. E. Cholecalciferol is vitamin D3 and is the preferred source

Vitamin D2 is used for renal insufficiency or short-term in adults with deficiency to replenish stores. Vitamin D3 is the preferred source and is a prodrug. If the patient has severe renal impairment, they will need to use the active vitamin D3 (Calcitriol) or newer D3 analogs (doxercalciferol, paricalcitol).

21. B. Citracal

Calcium carbonate is acid-dependent absorption, so it needs to be taken with food. Calcium citrate (Citracal®) is absorbed well with food or without so it's acid independent. Most dietary calcium is carbonate and is absorbed best with an acidic gut medium; long-term use of strong acid-suppressing agents lowers calcium intake and contributes to poor bone growth. Patients on pantoprazole and other acid-reducing agents should be cautioned about overuse.

22. B. Concurrent use of birth control pills and St. John's wort

St. John's Wort is a potent inducer of hepatic enzymes. It can't be used with oral contraceptives, transplant drugs, warfarin, and other CYP450 3A4 drugs as it induces this pathway leading to rapid metabolism.

23. A, B, C, D

An SSRI plus sumatriptan has a risk of serotonin syndrome. The patient is also taking meperidine which is not effective for chronic pain and a serotoninergic agent as well. Any combination of serotonergic agents has risks and are compounded when used in combination or newer medications in same class added to regimen.

24. A. Drug A levels would stay the same, Drug B levels increase, Drug C levels increase

Drug C inhibits 2D6 and increases drug levels of B as it's a substrate. Drug A inhibits 3A4 and increases levels of Drug C as it's a substrate for 3A4. Neither Drug B or C inhibits or induces 2C9 so Drug A levels remain the same as it's a substrate for 2C9.

25. B, C, D

NSAIDs (including celecoxib) do raise blood pressure and should be avoided in patients with hypertension. Safer options for mild pain is acetaminophen (Tylenol®) use.

26. B, C, E

Inducers increase the metabolism of drugs that are substrates of the affected enzyme so if a compound is a P-gp pump inducer, it can cause the levels of P-gp substrates to decrease as it has a higher level of metabolism. Inhibitors are the opposite as the block the enzyme. Tacrolimus, cyclosporine, dabigatran, and rivaroxaban are examples of substrates of P-gp efflux pumps.

27. C. Ziprasidone

Ziprasidone can cause additive QT prolongation and must be used with caution in patients with any arrhythmia risk.

28. B, C, D, E

Potassium is renally cleared; severe renal disease causes hyperkalemia by itself, and potassium is cleared by dialysis. Additive potassium accumulation may be due to potassium retaining agents.

29. A, B, D

Grapefruit knocks out the enzymes. This is not a gut interaction problem and the effects of grapefruit last a few hours. It is best to avoid grapefruit.

30. C. Cyclosporine

Cyclosporine is CYP3A4 inhibitor and substrate, so all strong CYP3A4 inhibitors will increase digoxin level, which requires a lower dose. Examples of strong CYP3A4 inhibitors are quinidine, verapamil, erythromycin, clarithromycin, itraconazole, cyclosporine, propafenone, spironolactone, protease inhibitors (HIV regimens), amiodarone, and others.

31. C. Increased risk of bleeding and increased risk of arrhythmia

Fluoxetine and paroxetine inhibit the metabolism of warfarin. Drug inhibition results in increased drug levels and elevated INR/bleeding risk. SSRIs and SNRIs increase bleeding risk even if the INR is therapeutic (mostly 2-3 depending on what conditions). Citalopram is a QT-risk agent especially at higher doses and should not be used in this patient and two SSRIs should not be used concurrently.

32. B. Pravastatin

Pravastatin is not metabolized by CYP enzymes. When statin levels are increased due to statin enzyme inhibition, there is higher risk of muscle toxicity presenting symptoms like muscle aches, soreness, or rhabdomyolysis which may cause acute renal failure.

33. A, B, D

Triptans cannot be used with MAO inhibitors.

34. A, B, E

CNS side effects caused by lipophilic drugs entering that system and cause sedation, dizziness, confusion, and altered consciousness. Flexeril® (cyclobenzaprine) is a skeletal muscle relaxant, Restoril® (temazepam) is a benzodiazepine, Remeron® (mirtazapine) is an alpha-2 antagonist antidepressant, and Nuvigil® (armodafinil) is a CNS stimulant known to be used for narcolepsy

35. A. A value that can be life-threatening if corrective action is not taken quickly

Critical values such as lab values and diagnostic tests must be reported to providers immediately and acted quickly within a set time frame.

36. C. The patient will be at risk for serious internal bleeding

G6PD-deficiency condition causing red blood cells to break down in response to certain medications, infections, or other stressors. Patients with G6PD-defiency need to know drugs that put them at risk of hemolytic anemia.

37. D. The platelets

HIT is indicated by more than a 50% drop from baseline for patients. Usually, hospital pharmacists run a report to monitor patient levels and advanced hospitals have programs developed that would alert clinicians if platelet counts dropped significantly.

38. A. Low pH, low serum bicarbonate

Causes of metabolic acidosis are diabetic ketoacidosis, decreased renal excretion, severe diarrhea, and other conditions. It's important to quickly correct these conditions as well so for example in diabetic ketoacidosis administer insulin drips.

39. C. BiDil®

BiDil® or isosorbide dinitrate and hydralazine may cause drug-induced lupus mainly from the hydralazine portion of the drug

40. C. MCV

The volume and size will be lower (low mean corpuscular volume (MCV)) in a small cell (microcytic) anemia, and larger in a large cell (macrocytic) anemia.

41. A. Respiratory acidosis

The patient is unable to breathe out the CO_2 that he produces through respiration. Carbon dioxide, when dissolved in the blood, is an acid and causes acidosis. This is due to a problem with respiration as the patient cannot breathe out and may develop respiratory acidosis.

42. B, C, D

Severe renal insufficiency is a creatinine clearance less than 30 mL/min. CKD stage 3 is 30-59 mL/min, stage 4 is 15-29 mL/min and stage 5 is less than 15 mL/min or dialysis-dependent.

43. D. Calcium Chloride

When serum potassium is high enough to effect cardiac conduction, calcium either as chloride or gluconate should immediately be administered IV.

44. B. Higher calcium levels

PhosLo® is calcium acetate. It binds to dietary phosphate which is excreted in the feces. Calcium salts are widely used but can cause hypercalcemia.

45. B. Hyperphosphatemia causes an increase in the release of parathyroid hormone

Bone metabolism abnormalities are caused by a rise in phosphorous. The kidneys clear the excess phosphorous but cannot clear adequately if they are impaired. The rise in phosphorous causes the parathyroid gland to increase the release of parathyroid hormone (PTH). PTH elevation leads to bone disease so it's important to control phosphorous levels. Treating secondary hyperparathyroidism is aimed at restricting phosphorous levels.

46. B. This drug is a cation exchange resin that binds potassium in the gut

Sodium polystyrene sulfonate (Kayexalate®) powder comes as a premixed oral or rectal liquid or powder as mixing. This is a cation exchange resin that is taken orally and binds potassium in the gut, causing a reduction in serum potassium. Do not mix this with sorbitol. Common side effects of Kayexalate are loss of appetite, nausea, vomiting, or constipation.

47. A, C, E

Propylthiouracil (PTU) is used in the first trimester and if trying to conceive. It is preferred to treat and resolve the hyperthyroidism first as both medications are teratogenic. The medications also cause nausea and are liver-toxic.

48. C. Erythromycin, D. Estrogen-containing contraceptive, E. Verapamil

- Increase theophylline level due to 1A2 inhibition: ciprofloxacin, fluvoxamine, propranolol, zafirlukast.
- Increase theophylline level due to 3A4 inhibition: clarithromycin, erythromycin.
- Increase theophylline level due to other mechanisms: estrogen-containing contraceptive, alcohol, verapamil, allopurinol.
- Theophylline decrease concentration of lithium.

49. A. Do not swallow the capsule, D. After you close your lips around the mouthpiece, breathe in deeply and fully. Hold your breath for a few seconds, E. You must inhale twice for each capsule

Patient can clean inhaler as needed with warm water; there's no restriction to weekly cleaning. Handihaler should be air dried. It takes 24 hours to air dry it.

50. B. St. John's Wort, C. Rifampin, E. Phenytoin

Roflumilast (Daliresp®) is a subject of CYP3A4 (major) and 1A2 (minor). It is a contraindication to concomitantly use roflumilast with a strong CYP3A inducers, such as carbamazepine, oxcarbazepine, phenytoin, phenobarbital, St. John's Wort, rifabutin and rifampin.

Practice Test 4 Answers and Explanations

1. **C. Check the patient's level in 4 hours**

   Any measurement of digoxin serum concentration should take place at least 6 hours after the dose is given.

2. **C. Atorvastatin 40 mg**

   The patient is less than 75 years of age, and he has peripheral artery disease, he should be started on a high dose statin such as rosuvastatin. Coronary heart disease, stroke, and/or peripheral artery disease will dictate giving a high-intensity unless greater than or equal to the age of 75.

3. **C. Atomoxetine**

   Atomoxetine can be considered first-line therapy for children with active substance abuse problem, comorbid anxiety, or tics. Metabolized through CYP2D6.

4. **B. Switch to rosuvastatin 40 mg once daily**

   The patient still has an LDL-C of greater than 190 and is less than the age of 75, so they should be increased to a higher intensity statin such as rosuvastatin 40 mg.

5. **D. Zoledronic Acid**

   Alendronate: 10 mg/day or 70 mg/week; taken for 3 years. Alendronate (daily dose regimen) was shown to decrease vertebral fractures by 47% and hip fractures by 51% (Fracture Intervention Trial [FIT]) in women with previous fractures.

   Zoledronic acid: 5 mg intravenously annually for treatment and every 2 years for prevention (infuse over a minimum of 15 minutes); reduces non-vertebral fracture risk by 25%, hip fracture by 40%, and vertebral fracture risk by 70%. This agent has the highest decrease in vertebral fractures.

   Raloxifene reduces the risk of vertebral fractures; reduces vertebral fractures by 30%–50%; has not been shown to decrease hip fractures.

   Calcitonin-salmon (Miacalcin)
   - Inhibition of bone resorption
   - Indicated for treatment of osteoporosis in women who are more than 5 years post-menopause.
   - Not a first-line drug; useful for bone pain caused by vertebral compression fractures, no longer. Used frequently for osteoporosis therapy.
   - Efficacy: Nasal calcitonin reduces the incidence of new vertebral fractures by 36%.

6. **C. Hemorrhagic cystitis**

Hemorrhagic cystitis is characterized by diffuse bladder mucosal bleeding that develops secondary to chemotherapy (mostly cyclophosphamide or ifosfamide), radiation therapy, bone marrow transplantation (BMT), and/or opportunistic infections. Both cyclophosphamide and ifosfamide are metabolized to acrolein, which is a strong chemical irritant that is excreted in the urine. Prolonged contact or high concentrations may lead to bladder irritation and hemorrhage. Symptoms include gross hematuria, frequency, dysuria, burning, urgency, incontinence, and nocturia. The best management is prevention. Maintaining a high rate of urine flow minimizes exposure. In addition, 2-mercaptoethanesulfonate (mesna) detoxifies the metabolites and can be co-administered with the instigating drugs. Mesna usually is given three times on the day of ifosfamide administration in doses that are each 20% of the total ifosfamide dose. If hemorrhagic cystitis develops, the maintenance of a high urine flow may be sufficient supportive care. If conservative management is not effective, irrigation of the bladder with a 0.37–0.74% formalin solution for 10 min stops the bleeding in most cases. N-Acetylcysteine may also be an effective irrigant. Prostaglandin (Carboprost®) can inhibit the process. In extreme cases, ligation of the hypogastric arteries, urinary diversion, or cystectomy may be necessary.

7. **B. Acute tubular necrosis due to her CT contrast dye**

Radiographic contrast media may be directly nephrotoxic. Contrast nephropathy is the third leading cause of incident AKI in hospitalized patients and is thought to result from the synergistic combination of direct renal tubular epithelial cell toxicity and renal medullary ischemia.

8. **A. Relative Risk**

A cohort study uses relative risk and is usually prospective studies

9. **B. Odds Ratio**

Case-control studies usually use the odds ratio.

10. **D. MMWR**

The Morbidity and Mortality Weekly Report is a weekly epidemiological digest for the United States published by the Centers for Disease Control and Prevention. It is the main vehicle for publishing public health information and recommendations that have been received by the CDC from state health departments.

11. **A. Clopidogrel**

Prasugrel is contraindicated in TIA/CVA, ticagrelor is contraindicated in ICH and severe hepatic disease, and ticlopidine is an ACE inhibitor, not an antiplatelet

12. D. No treatment is needed for now

The appearance of *Candida* in the urine is an increasingly common complication of indwelling catheterization, particularly for patients in the intensive care unit, those taking broad-spectrum antimicrobial drugs, and those with underlying diabetes mellitus. In many studies, >50% of urinary *Candida* isolates have been found to be non-*albicans* species. The clinical presentation varies from a laboratory finding without symptoms to pyelonephritis and even sepsis. Removal of the urethral catheter results in resolution of candiduria in more than one-third of asymptomatic cases. Treatment of asymptomatic patients does not appear to decrease the frequency of recurrence of candiduria. Therapy is recommended for patients who have symptomatic cystitis or pyelonephritis and for those who are at high risk for disseminated disease. High-risk patients include those with neutropenia, those who are undergoing urologic manipulation, those who are clinically unstable, and low-birth-weight infants. Fluconazole (200–400 mg/d for 7–14 days) reaches high levels in urine and is the first-line regimen for *Candida* infections of the urinary tract.

13. A. Dofetilide

Non-DHP CCBs such as verapamil or diltiazem are CI in HFrEF. Adenosine is not used to cardiovert. Propafenone is useful to cardiovert if less than 7 days.

Drugs used to cardiovert (for up to 7 days):
- Proven efficacy: *DIP-AF
- dofetilide, ibutilide, propafenone, amiodarone, or flecainide
- Less effective: disopyramide, quinidine, and procainamide
- NOT effective (Class III harmful): digoxin, sotalol
- Drugs used to cardiovert (>7 days):
- Proven efficacy: dofetilide, ibutilide, amiodarone

14. B. Increased risk of respiratory tract infection

Montelukast has the common side effects of headache, upper respiratory tract infection, pharyngitis, and sinusitis. This drug may cause aggressive behavior, agitation, dream disorder, or hallucinations. Zileuton, in the same leukotriene class with montelukast, can cause dizziness.

15. C. Utibron Neohaler, D. Spiriva Handihaler, E. Arcapta Neohaler

Inhaler products, such as glycopyrrolate/indacaterol (Utibron Neohaler®), indacaterol (Arcapta Neohaler®), formoterol (Foradil®), and tiotropium (Spiriva Handihaler®), come with capsule. It is important to counsel patients that the capsule is not meant for swallowing.

16. A, B, and E
  A. Confirm HIV negative status using HIV antibody test
  B. Screen AB for hepatitis B and sexually transmitted infections (STIs)
  E. When the patient has negative HIV result, start her on Truvada® once daily and counsel on safe sex reduction practices

She has very high risk of acquiring HIV, so pre-exposure prophylaxis (PrEP) should be considered as an HIV prevention method when patient has a confirmed HIV negative result. It is also recommended to screen a patient for STIs and hepatitis B. PrEP therapy is Truvada® 1 tablet once daily (90-day supply because we want to confirm HIV status before we renew prescription). Once patient is on Truvada®, we should have follow-up appointments every 3 months.

17. D. Biktarvy®

The initial HIV regimen of one integrase strand transfer inhibitor (INSTI) and two nucleoside/nucleotide reverse transcriptase inhibitors (NRTIs). Only Biktarvy® (bictegravir, emtricitabine, and tenofovir disoproxil fumarate) contains the components that are recommended per Antiretroviral guidelines for adults and adolescents. Also, she has sulfa allergy, and Symtuza® contains darunavir, so Symtyza® is not a correct choice.

18. D. Tell him to not take Prevacid® while he is on Complera® because Prevacid® is contraindicated with Complera®. He can take Tums® 2 hours before Complera®

Complera® contains rilpivirine, emtricitabine and tenofovir disoproxil fumarate. Rilpivirine requires acidic environment for absorption. Therefore, concurrent use with PPIs is a contraindication. Tums® should be separated from Complera® (take 2 hours before or four hours after Complera®).

19. D. Gardasil®, Fluzone®, Pneumovax®, Tdap, and Menveo®

All individuals should receive influenza annually once it is available. Since he is 13 years old, he should some routine vaccines for adolescents, such as human papillomavirus vaccine (Gardasil®) for 2 doses (if he gets it before age of 15) or 3 doses (if he gets it after age of 15), Tdap (booster for every 10 years), and meningococcal vaccine (Menveo® or Menactra®) – two doses (one dose at age 11-12 and one dose at age 16 years). He is an immunocompetent patient because he has a history of type 1 diabetes and COPD, he should receive one dose of Pneumovax®.

20. B. Typhim Vi®

She is an immunocompromised patient because she has a history of kidney transplant and is on immunosuppressants (Prograf®, Cellcept®, and prednisone). Therefore, live vaccines are contraindicated in this patient. Typhim Vi® is an inactivated typhoid vaccine and safe to give the patient. There is no vaccine to prevent dengue. The other vaccines are lived attenuated ones.

21. E. Cefuroxime and Zithromax®

Patient has a history of recent antibiotic use, COPD (with current acute exacerbation), which are risk factors for drug-resistant *S. pneumoniae*. Therefore, outpatient CAP regimen should include either respiratory fluoroquinolone (monotherapy) or a combination of a beta-lactam and macrolide (preferred) or doxycycline. Cipro® does not cover *S. pneumoniae*. Cefuroxime + Zithromax® is the best option to this patient.

22. C. Fidaxomicin

Since it is the subsequent episode (3rd time *C. diff*), we have four options for TM:
1. Oral vancomycin (tapered and pulsed): Vancomycin 125 mg PO QID for 10 days, then BID for 1 week, then QD for 1 week, then every 2-3 days per week for 2-8 weeks.
2. Vancomycin 150 mg PO QID for 10 days, then rifaximin 400 mg TID for 20 days.
3. Fidaxomicin 200 mg PO BID for 10 days.
4. Fecal microbial transplant.

Therefore, fidaxomicin is the best monotherapy for him in this case.

23. D. Ceftriaxone + Vancomycin

This patient is diagnosed with bacterial meningitis (CSF labs: high WBC with predominant neutrophils, high protein, elevated opening pressure, and low glucose). Also, the preliminary gram-stain suggests that patient is more likely infected by *N. meningitis*. Since he is 34 years old, the first-line agents include: Vancomycin + ceftriaxone (or cefotaxime) for 7 days. Ampicillin and cefotaxime (or gentamicin) are recommended to neonate population (< 1 month old).

24. B. Vancomycin + tobramycin + Zosyn®

Patient has been in the hospital > 5 days and has history of IVDU and asthma. He has a high risk of multidrug-resistant (MDR) pathogens; therefore, we want to cover *MRSA* and *Pseudomonas* empirically. Vancomycin (or linezolid) covers *MRSA*. For *Pseudomonas*, we need two agents cover against it actively (both are not the same beta-lactam drug class). Aminoglycosides, Zosyn®, cefepime, ceftazidime, and carbapenems (except ertapenem) are examples of agents actively against *Pseudomonas* in the lungs. Daptomycin covers MRSA, but it is inactivated in the lungs by the lung's surfactants.

25. A. Ceftriaxone 1 gram IV QD for 5-7 days.

Common pathogens caused spontaneous bacterial peritonitis (SBP) include *E. coli, Klebsiella pneumoniae,* and *Streptococcus pneumoniae.* Ceftriaxone is the first-line gent that covers the common pathogens. Ciprofloxacin can be used; however, it is not a drug of choice in this case because of side effects and risk of drug resistant concern.

26. C. Cefazolin

Surgery often introduces skin flora into the incision site, so an antibiotic (typically, first generation cephalosporins) is given to a patient before the procedure to minimize/prevent the infection. Cefazolin is the first-line agent for perioperative antibiotic prophylaxis. Clindamycin and vancomycin are the alternatives for patients who have true allergies with penicillin. In this case, the patient has no known allergy, so cefazolin is the best choice. In general, antibiotic is given 60 minutes before the procedure. If the procedure last >3 hours, another dose of antibiotic should be given. An antibiotic can be given up to 24 hours after the incision.

27. E. Doxycycline

Doxycycline 100 mg BID for 7 days is the first-line agent to treat Rocky Mountain spotted fever (*Rickettsia ricketsii*).

28. C. Azithromycin + ceftriaxone

Drug of choice for patients with gonorrhea: Ceftriaxone 250 mg IM x 1 with either azithromycin 1 gram PO x 1 or doxycycline 100 mg PO for 7 days

29. A, B, C, D, E (All of the choices)
    A. AZO® is an OTC can help to relieve urinary pain
    B. It is not urinary antibiotic, so if you expect that you have urinary tract infection which causes the pain, you should contact your PCP
    C. It can only be used up to 2 days (no more than 2 days)
    D. It can turn your body fluids into red-orange coloring (including your urine, tears). It may also stain your clothes and contact lenses
    E. You should take it with 8 oz of water and with meal right after to minimize stomach upset

It is important to counsel patients on the adverse effects including GI upsets, red-orange coloring of the urine and body fluids, and the maximum days of use is 2 days. As understanding of the adverse effects of the drug, patients are more adherent to the medication and can prevent the adverse effects as taking it with foods to minimize the GI upset.

30. C. PO (tablet): injection = 1:1, D. PO (tablet): PO (suspension) is not 1:1

Tablets and injection forms have similar bioavailability (1:1 ratio); however, suspension (liquid form) has different bioavailability to tablet form. Therefore, it important to convert dose between forms (look at the label and packaging insert) to minimize medication errors. All oral forms (tablets and suspension) should be taken with food.

31. D. Bio-statin®

Dulera® contains mometasone and formoterol. Mometasone is an inhaled corticosteroid which requires a rinse after each dose to prevent or minimize oral candida. Thus, it is important to counsel patients to rinse with water after each dose. **Bio-statin® (nystatin) suspension,** swish and retain for several minutes then swallow, is used to treat oral candida (thrush). Also, clotrimazole (lozenges) is another option for this indication.

32. B. Dispense as written

Tamiflu® (Oseltamivir) is a neuraminidase inhibitor which was approved to treat influenza A and B. It is the most effectiveness if it (or other neuraminidase inhibitors) is taken within 48 hours of the onset. Dosing of treatment (age >12 years old): Tamiflu® 75 mg BID PO for 5 days, while dosing of prophylaxis (age >12 years old): Tamiflu® 75 mg QD PO for 10 days.

In addition to Tamiflu®, Relenza Diskhaler® is also used. However, it is not recommended to patients with history of asthma and COPD.

33. B. Dapsone

Bactrim® (single strength (SS) QD or double strength (DS) QD) is used as a PCP prophylaxis. When patient has true allergy with Bactrim® or cannot tolerate due to its adverse effects, dapsone or atovaquone is an alternative. Before initiating dapsone, we have to screen G6PD levels because dapsone increases risk of hemolytic anemia in patients with G6PD deficiency.

34. D. 3, 2, 1, 4

All C-PECs used for handling hazardous drugs must be cleaned in this order:
1. Deactivation and decontamination (2% bleach or peroxide-containing agents)
2. To prevent corrosion on the stainless-steel surfaces, sterile water or sodium thiosulfate)
3. Disinfection (using 70% isopropyl alcohol)
4. Allow the surface dry before starting compounding

The cleaning should be done before shift, every 30 minutes, or immediately after spills.

35. A, B, C, and E
A. Immediately remove the garb (gloves and gown)
B. Obtain medical attention
C. Immediately cleanse any affected skin with soap and water
E. Document the incidence in the employee's record

When a hazardous drug exposure occurs, a pharmacy technician should follow these steps:

1. Immediately remove the garb (gloves and gown)
2. Cleanse the affected skin with soap and water immediately (do NOT use bleach)
3. If the eyes get affected, flood with isotonic water for at least 15 minutes
4. Obtain medical attention
5. The incident should be documented in the employee's record

36. D. Black

Vincristine is an antineoplastic agent (hazardous drug). Any bulk antineoplastic waste (**unused or partially empty** vials, syringes, or IV bags) should be trashed in a **black** container/bin.

Do not confuse **black** bin with **yellow** bin. Yellow bin is used for trace hazardous drug waste (e.g., empty vials, syringes, or IV bags, and used PPEs that are used to prepared for hazardous drugs).

Red bin is used for bulk non-hazardous drug sharps (e.g., syringes, IV tubing, and used culture dishes.)

37. E. Sorbitan tristearate (HLB = 2.1)

Hydrophilic-lipophilic balance (HLB) scale has a range of 0-20 (10 is the midpoint value):
- Lower HLB , more lipid-soluble and are used for water-in-oil (w/o) emulsion.
- Higher HLB, more water-soluble and are used for oil-in-water (o/w) emulsion.

Since the pharmacist wants to make a water-in-oil emulsion, the most appropriate emulsifier is the one has the lowest HLB among the other options, which is sorbitan tristate (HLB = 2.1).

38. B. Flolan®

Flolan® (epoprostenol) is a prostacyclin analogue, which directly stimulates vasodilation of pulmonary and systemic arterial vascular beds and also inhibit platelet aggregation. Prostacyclin analogues (or agonists) are recommended as the first-line agent for pulmonary hypertension. In addition, since patient is pregnancy, endothelin receptor antagonists (e.g., bosentan, macitentan, ambrisentan) and riociguat are contraindicated (REMS programs are required for these drugs). Diltiazem is not used for her because she failed the vasodilatory testing.

39. E. She can take 2 inhalations of Ventolin HFA® 5-15 minutes before exercise

What TN experienced is called exercise-induced bronchospasm (EIB). Without an appropriate regimen, a patient can experience shortness of breath during exercise and can even cause exacerbation. Short-acting beta-2 agonist (SABA) is used to prevent EIB by taking 2 inhalations of her current Ventolin HFA® (Albuterol) 5-15 minutes before exercise.

40. A. 4, 2, 5, 1, 3

Ventolin® is one of the metered-dose inhalers (MDIs): **(ProAir HFA®, Ventolin®, Proventil®, Symbicort®, QVAR®, Flovent HFA®)**

Before step 1, if MDI was used before, inspect the MDI and ensure no dirt or blockage, then remove the cap. If you do not use your MDI for more than 7 days (Flovent HFA®, Symbicort®) or more than 14 days (Ventolin®), or if you dropped your MDI, it's important to prime the MDI. Priming or simply shaking the MDI and spraying it away from you should be done 4 times for Ventolin® and Flovent HFA®, or 2 times for Symbicort® before first use.

> Step 1: Shake well for 5 seconds immediately before each spray.
> Step 2: Breath out as much as possible before using.
> Step 3: Hold inhaler upright, place the mouthpiece into your mouth, ensure your teeth are not blocking MDI, and close your lips around it.
> Step 4: Press down the inhaler while breathing slowly and deeply in for 3-5 seconds.
> Step 5: Hold your breath for up to 10 seconds. If another inhalation is needed, wait at least 1 minute and repeat steps 1-5. Place cap back on the mouthpiece after use.

41. D. Dry mouth

Spiriva Respimat® is a long-acting muscarinic antagonist that causes bronchodilation by blocking the constriction of acetylcholine at M3 muscarinic receptors in bronchial smooth muscle. Common adverse effects of long-acting muscarinic antagonists include dry mouth (the most common), bitter taste, and upper respiratory tract infections.

42. E. Xopenex HFA®

All long-acting beta-2 agonist (LABA) whether they are alone or combined with corticosteroids have box warnings of risk of asthma-related death. They are Serevent Diskus®, Advair Diskus®, Symbicort®, Dulera®, Striverdi®. Typically, LABA is used as a maintenance regimen along with short-acting bronchodilator (i.e., albuterol) PRN and inhaled corticosteroids (low or high dose depending on the level of severity of asthma).

43. E. Desferal®

Although iron poisoning is on decline, it remains a serious health risk for children (especially children under 6 years old). Symptoms of iron poisoning include nausea, abdominal pain, diarrhea and dehydration initially (within 6 hours). Serious complication can develop within 48 hours such as headache, fever, shortness of breath, grayish or bluish color in skin, jaundice, and seizure. To prevent accidental poisoning in children, child-resistant (C-R) containers (i.e., screw caps that require the user to press down while turning and unit-dose packaging) are required for all prescriptions and oral OTC products. Antidotes for iron overdose is deferoxamine (Desferal®). Deferiprone and deferasirox also can be used in the case of iron overload due to blood transfusions.

44. B. Coumadin® 5 mg QD

IV Kcentra® and IV Vitamin K (Phytonadione) are used for the reversal of warfarin in life-threatening situations, which is an intracranial hemorrhage in this case, regardless of INR values.

45. B, D, and E
    B. Protect from light
    D. This drug will decrease mucus viscosity in the lungs
    E. Do not mix it with other drug(s) in the nebulizer

Pulmozyme® (Dornase alfa) is used to clear airway caused by cystic fibrosis. It degrades extracellular DNA in the lungs which results in decreasing mucus viscosity and improve pulmonary function. It is supplied in single-use ampules (2.5 mg/2.5 mL). The ampules should be stored in refrigerator (can exposure to room temperature max 24 hours) and protected from light. Do not mix it with other inhaled drugs including antibiotic inhalers and bronchodilators (e.g., albuterol).

46. D. How many cigarette(s) does he smoke per day?

There are three different strength of nicotine patches, such as 7 mg/patch, 14 mg/patch, and 21 mg/patch. It depends on how many cigarette(s) an individual take to recommend an appropriate strength to start on. The table below provides details information of the strength and duration of the nicotine replacement therapy (NRT). The most effective therapy is a combination of patch and short-acting NRT (i.e., gum and lozenge). The patch must be removed before MRI.

	Weeks 1-6	Weeks 7-8	Weeks 9-10
<10 cigarettes per day	14 mg	7 mg	None
≥ 10 cigarettes per day	21 mg	14 mg	7 mg
Duration: 10-week			

47. A. 4 hours

The allowed maximum infusion rate is 10 mEq K/hour (10 mEq/100 mL). The bag contains 40 mEq K, so it takes at least 4 hours to infuse the entire bag.

48. E. Vancomycin + ceftriaxone + ampicillin

Empiric regimen for bacterial meningitis depends on age. For neonates (<1 month old), regimen includes cefotaxime and ampicillin. Ampicillin is used for neonates and older population (>50 years old) due to high risk of *Neisseria meningitis* infection. Also, to prevent elevation of bilirubin in neonates, which can cause jaundice, cefotaxime is used instead of ceftriaxone. For older population (> 50 years old), regimen contains vancomycin, ceftriaxone (or cefotaxime), and ampicillin. Vancomycin with ceftriaxone (or cefotaxime) is recommended for patients from 2 months old to 49 years old. In this case, the patient is 57 years old, he should be on vancomycin, ceftriaxone, and ampicillin.

49. B. Add Norvasc® 5 mg PO daily to his current HTN regimen

Per ACC/AHA guidelines, because the patient is African American, the first-line agents should be calcium-channel blockers (CCBs) or thiazide diuretics. Also, patient has angioedema with lisinopril in the past, we should not challenge the patient with any renin-angiotensin-aldosterone system (RAAS) agents (e.g., ACE inhibitors, ARBs, and aliskiren). Diovan HTC® contains valsartan and hydrochlorothiazide, so we do not recommend it to the patient. Norvasc® (amlodipine), a CCB, should be recommended.

50. C. Discard the amber IV bag and verify the order

Ampicillin is one of IV medications shall be diluted in normal saline. There is no requirement on light protection (no need an amber bag), shake before using, or no leaching issue with PCV bag. Also, ampicillin is not chemotherapeutic agent. Therefore, this order can be verified once it is corrected dose, frequency, and direction. Some other common IV drugs that are diluted in NS, such as Synercid®, daptomycin, phenytoin, ertapenem, insulin, infliximab, and primaxin.

Practice Test 5 Answers and Explanations

1. **B and C**
    B. Place an auxiliary label "Do Not Refrigerate" on the bag
    C. Dilute Sulfatrim® in D5W

    Sulfatrim® (trimethoprim/sulfamethoxazole) should NOT be refrigerated and only diluted in dextrose 5%. Sulfatrim® has a short stability (about 6 hours); therefore, it is not recommended to prepare batched Sulfatrim® ahead of time.

2. **C. Contact the dentist to change drug**

    Children <12 years old or <18 years old following tonsillectomy or adenoidectomy surgery are contraindicated to take codeine. It has some evidence that these populations are being ultra-rapid metabolizers of codeine due to a CYP2D6 polymorphism, and as a result, respiratory depression and death have occurred in these populations. Therefore, a pharmacist should contact the dentist to change a different drug for severe pain.

3. **A. Nora-BE®**

    Estrogen decreases milk production and increases risk of thrombosis. Therefore, progestin-only pills (POPs) which contain no estrogen are primarily used for lactating (especially 4-6 weeks postpartum women). Examples of POPs are Errin®, Nora-BE®, and Camila®. A disadvantage of POPs is that it requires good adherence to have the most effectiveness and protection; the pill must be taken within three hours of the scheduled time.

4. **B. Switch Paxil® to Wellbutrin®**

    Common adverse effects of Paxil® (paroxetine) include sexual dysfunction, weight gain, low energy, and withdrawal symptoms (if discontinue abruptly or miss pills). Wellbutrin® (bupropion XL) can be used for patients who concern about these adverse effects. See table below (**from RxPharmacist's CPJE Guide**) for more details which antidepressants should be recommended for certain situations/adverse effect concerns.

CONDITIONS/CONCERNS	RECOMMENDED ANTIDEPRESSANTS	ANTIDEPRESSANTS SHOULD BE AVOIDED
Sexual Dysfunction	Bupropion Mirtazapine	SSRIs (especially, paroxetine and fluoxetine)
Weight Gain (obese)	Bupropion	Paroxetine Mirtazapine
Low Energy and Anhedonia	SNRIs (duloxetine and venlafaxine) Bupropion	Paroxetine Mirtazapine
Anxious and Irritable	SSRIs	SNRIs Bupropion
Additive QT Prolongation		SSRIs (citalopram, max: 20 mg/day and escitalopram, max: 10 mg/day) Venlafaxine TCAs Mirtazapine

Withdrawal Symptoms	Fluoxetine (long half-life)	Paroxetine Venlafaxine
Pregnancy	Psychotherapy (non-pharmacological treatment for mild depression)	Paroxetine (Brisdelle®)
Postpartum	**Brexanolone** (first agent approved by FDA)	
Breastfeeding	SSRIs TCAs (except of doxepin)	

Table 1: Recommended Antidepressants and Avoided Antidepressants Based on Medical Conditions and Concerns

5. A. Macrocytic anemia, folate 1 mg QD and thiamine 1 tab PO QD

Patient is diagnosed with macrocytic anemia (RBC, Hgb, Hct are low, while MCV is elevated). Low folate (2 ng/mL) and Vitamin B12 (160 mg/dL), which may be caused by a long-term intake of metformin and Prilosec® (omeprazole). To treat macrocytic anemia, folate 1 mg QD and vitamin B12 are recommended. Also, we should assess patient's GERD condition whether she needs to take it because proton-pump inhibitor is only recommended for a short period (often 2 weeks for GERD condition). If she still has it despite Prilosec®, refer to her PCP for further assessment.

6. A. 4

The maximum daily dose of sumatriptan is 200 mg in a 24-hour period. The use of more than 200 mg puts a patient at risk of developing serotonin syndrome, especially if they are using other serotonergic medications. Signs and symptoms of serotonin syndrome include hallucinations, agitation, tachycardia, nausea, vomiting, diarrhea, and loss of balance.

7. C. TSH

TSH is expected to be decreased in this patient because they are exhibiting signs of hyperthyroidism. Hyperthyroidism accelerates the body's metabolic processes because the body is producing too much thyroxine. To compensate, the body will decrease the amount of TSH. In the case of hypothyroidism, the body will create more TSH, thus making this an inverse relationship.

8. C, E

Symptoms that the patient is experiencing is consistent gonorrhea. The treatment of gonorrhea consists of a single of dose of ceftriaxone given intramuscularly plus either a single dose of 1 gram of azithromycin, or 100 mg of doxycycline taken twice a day for 7 days.

9. D. Methyldopa 250 mg PO BID up to 1000 mg PO every 8 hours

First line treatment for hypertension in pregnant women is methyldopa. Other recommended first-line agents are labetalol and nifedipine extended-release. Pregnant women should only receiver drug treatment if SBP is greater than 160 mmHg or DBP is greater than 105 mmHg. ACE inhibitors, ARBs, and aliskiren should be avoided due to a black box warning for fetal toxicity.

10. C, E

Glipizide and glimepiride are sulfonylureas and should be used with caution in patients with a sulfa allergy. Although the risk of cross reactivity is very low and often times not significant, patients should still be made aware to watch for possible adverse reactions. On the NAPLEX®, you should also watch for possible interactions.

11. A, E

Patients with pulmonary arterial hypertension are at an increased risk for developing pneumonia. Therefore, patients should be vaccinated against pneumococcal pneumonia and influenza annually.

12. E. 4 mg daily in the evening

In the treatment of asthma, montelukast is stratified according to age. In patients ages 15 years and older, the dose is one 10 mg tablet daily. For pediatric patients ages 6-14, the recommended dose is one 5 mg chewable tablet per day. For pediatric patients, ages 2-5, the recommended dose is one 4 mg chewable tablet per day or one packet 4 mg oral granules.

13. D. diarrhea

Varenicline is a partial nicotinic acetylcholine receptor agonist. Common side effects are insomnia, nausea, and abnormal dreams. Other side effects include constipation, dyspepsia, sleep disorder, vomiting, and flatulence.

14. A. 140/90 mmHg

According to ADA guidelines, the blood pressure goal for patients with hypertension, diabetes, and a ASCVD risk less than 15% is <140/80. In patients with these same comorbidities, and an ASCVD risk >15%, the blood pressure goal is <130/80.

15. B. Metformin

It is not recommended to initiate therapy with metformin if eGFR is less than 30 mL/min/1.73 m^2. Metformin is cleared from the body by tubular secretion and is excreted unchanged in the urine.

16. A. IV levothyroxine

A myxedema coma is defined by severe hypothyroidism which leads to decreased mental status, hypothermia, and other symptoms of organ failure. This is potentially fatal situation; thus, rapid treatment is required. Guidelines recommend the use of IV levothyroxine compared to IV liothyronine.

17. D. 122 mcg per day

In moderate to severe signs and symptoms of hypothyroidism, the full replacement dose Is calculated by using the formula 1.6 mcg per kilogram per day. When using this equation, the full replacement dose equals 121.6 mcg per day.

18. D. Propylthiouracil

When treating a patient experiencing a thyroid storm, consider the 5 B's: blocking synthesis with an antithyroid medication, blocking release with iodine; blocking T4 into T3 conversion with PTU, propranolol, corticosteroid, and amiodarone; beta blockade, and blocking enterohepatic circulation with an agent like cholestyramine.

19. C. Methimazole

Methimazole is contraindicated in the first trimester of pregnancy and PTU should be used instead. Birth defects include a skin disorder on the scalp of the baby and malformation of the stomach and intestines.

20. B. Hydrocortisone

Hydrocortisone is the most potent systemic that is available without a prescription. However, cortisone would be the most potent if the patient was looking for a prescription option. Remember the mnemonic "Cute Hot Pharmacists & Physicians Marry Together & Deliver Babies."

21. D. Walking barefoot

It is very important for diabetic patients to practice good foot hygiene in order to decrease their chances of obtaining a foot infection. These patients often times develop neuropathy and therefore may not feel any cuts and wounds on their feet. Therefore, wearing shoes while outdoors and maintaining a clean-living space is important.

22. B. Discard the vial

Generally, when clumps are visible in a vial of insulin, the vial should be gently rolled in to attempt to dissolve the clumps. However, in this instance, the vial is frosts and therefore no longer viable and should be discarded.

23. B. Selective alpha-1 receptor antagonist

Tamsulosin is a selective alpha-1 receptor antagonist that prefers the alpha-1A receptor in the prostate. It is there that tamsulosin can exert its effects in relaxing the smooth muscle of the bladder neck, prostate, ureter, urethra and thus reducing the size of the prostate.

24. E. Light protective container

Bactrim® is one of many antibiotics that is sensitive to light. Other antibiotics that possess similar characteristics are ciprofloxacin, levofloxacin, and clindamycin. These antibiotics should be Stored in a closed container at room temperature, away from heat, moisture, and direct light.

25. E. Fluvastatin

Patients do not have to limit grapefruit juice with fluvastatin. The other statin in which grapefruit juice does not have to be limited is pravastatin. Grapefruit juice decreases the activity of cytochrome P450 3A4 enzymes that are responsible for breaking down many drugs. Some other medications that have interactions grapefruit juice are calcium channel blockers, immunosuppressants such as cyclosporine and tacrolimus; antiarrhythmics like amiodarone and quininde; and mood stabilizing drugs such as buspirone and quetiapine.

26. A. Ketoconazole

Ketoconazole and other azole antifungals are CYP inducers and work immediately. St. John's Wort, phenytoin, carbamazepine, and rifampin are all CYP inducers and take about 2 weeks for the onset and offset of their action.

27. D. At least 72 hours

Antibiotics may interfere with the response of the typhoid vaccine. Therefore, administration of the typhoid vaccine Vivotif® should be delayed for at least 72 hours after the administration of antibiotics. Remember, this is an oral vaccine.

28. B. Varicella

Varicella is a live virus; most live attenuated vaccines are recommended to be administered by subcutaneous injection since subcutaneous injections are injected in the fatty layer of connective tissue just beneath the skin. In the subcutaneous layer, there are very few blood vessels, so their absorption is much slower.

29. A. Fecal impaction

Clozapine carries 5 black box warnings which are: neutropenia due to the risk of agranulocytosis, orthostatic hypotension, seizures, myocarditis, and increase mortality in elderly patients with dementia related psychosis.

30. A. Protamine

The reversal agent for heparin is protamine, which is a protein derived from fish sperm. Protamine binds to heparin to form a stable salt. Praxbind is the reversal agent for Pradaxa®; vitamin K is the reversal agent for warfarin, and andexanet alfa is the reversal agent for apixaban and rivaroxaban.

31. B. Colesevelam

Colesevelam has the potential to increase triglycerides which can lead to pancreatitis; therefore, frequent blood tests will be required if taking this medication. Colesevelam should be part of a complete treatment program consisting of lifestyle modifications such as dieting and exercise.

32. D. Increase atorvastatin 10 mg to 80 mg

This patient should be on a high intensity statin due to his ASCVD risk. Before switching medications or adding new medications to a patient's regimen, make sure that you use the maximum tolerated dose on their current medication.

33. D. Amlodipine

Patients on amlodipine and simvastatin should be counseled on the drug interaction between these medications. A patient on both medications should not take more than 20 mg of simvastatin per day. Concomitant use of these two medications causes liver damage and increase the risk for rhabdomyolysis.

34. C. Peripheral edema is a common adverse drug reaction

Peripheral edema is a common adverse effect of using amlodipine due to unmatched changes in vascular resistance and pressure with amlodipine therapy. Peripheral edema is the accumulation of fluid causing swelling in tissues in the peripheral vascular system.

35. C. Propranolol

Propranolol is a beta-blocker. Beta-blockers are medicines that work temporarily by lowering a person's blood pressure and preventing some of the body's natural responses. Remember, beta-blockers mask all signs of hypoglycemia of hypoglycemia except sweating.

36. C. 8am and 3pm

Isosorbide dinitrate is used for the treatment of angina and chest pain. This medication is dosed 2-3 times a day and the doses should be taken 6-7 hours apart. It is recommended to take the first dose upon waking up in the morning and then 6-7 hours later.

37. C. Chest percussion

Physical chest therapy is used as a way to help patients with cystic fibrosis breathe comfortably. This includes cuffing the patient's arms down and performing chest percussions (beating on the chest) to loosen and break up mucus in the patient's lungs.

38. D. Mannitol

Mannitol crystallizes in low temperatures and in high concentrations. To dissolve crystals, heat the solution to 70-80°F before administration.

39. A. 160 mg

Prefilled enoxaparin syringes are only available in 30, 40, 60, 80, 100, 120, and 150 mg dosages. Counsel patients on the importance of not expelling air bubbles in order to avoid loss of the drug when using the 30 mg and 40 mg syringes.

40. B. Ciprofloxacin

Requires renal dose adjustment because when creatinine clearance is less than 50 mL/min. This is because ciprofloxacin and its metabolites are excreted in the urine via glomerular filtration tubular secretion in the kidneys.

41. E. Maintain catheter patency

This heparin is not sufficient for anticoagulation prevention or therapy. In this case heparin is being used as a "heparin flush". The purpose of a heparin flush is to keep the catheter clear so that blood flows smoothly and does not clot in the catheter.

42. D. Anti Xa activity

Lovenox® (enoxaparin) is a low molecular weight heparin (LMWH). Monitoring parameters include anti Xa activity and the anticoagulation of Lovenox® cannot be accurately monitored by the aPTT. Remember, INR is only monitored in patients on warfarin.

43. D. Efavirenz

Atripla® is a combination drug consisting of efavirenz, emtricitabine, and tenofovir disoproxil fumarate used for the treatment of HIV in patients who weigh at least 88 pounds (44 kg). Atripla® can be used alone as a complete treatment regimen or in combination with other antiretroviral medications.

44. C, E

Seroquel is an atypical antipsychotic. Atypical antipsychotics have a host a many metabolic side effects, which include hyperlipidemia, hyperglycemia, sudden cardiac death, extrapyramidal symptoms, constipation, lightheadedness, and weight gain

45. B. In 6 years

According to CDC guidelines, tetanus booster shots are recommended every 10 years. Since the patient only received her last booster shot 4 years ago, she should wait another 6 years before getting another booster.

46. C. Continue the insulin drip and add dextrose

You need to add dextrose as the glucose level is going less than 250, so the glucose level does not go too low.

47. A. Ensure vitamin K is not available inpatient care areas and restrict to guideline recommendations

Vitamin K is one of the vitamins that can be overdosed in the human body due to being fat-soluble not water soluble. Vitamin K is very dangerous, so the best answer is to ensure it is not freely available in inpatient care areas and ensure proper use.

48. B. Change ritonavir and lopinavir to raltegravir and efavirenz

Most protease inhibitors inhibit the metabolism of most statins leading to increased serum levels and risk of toxicity.

49. C. Advise she may use H2 antagonist or calcium carbonate antacids

Raltegravir is better absorbed in an alkaline environment, acid suppression does not affect the INSTI drugs. Avoid mag/alum, major issue for rilpivirine and atazanavir are ones that are adversely affected with acid suppression.

50. B. The symptoms are likely due to metoclopramide and its dopamine receptor antagonism

Metoclopramide, haloperidol, and prochlorperazine should be avoided in levodopa/carbidopa as it is a centrally acting antidopaminergic drug.

Practice Test 6 Answers and Explanations

1. **A.** *Serratia spp.*, **B.** *Pseudomonas spp.*, **C.** *Acinetobacter spp.*, **D.** *Citrobacter spp.*

   The "E" in SPACE bugs stands for *Enterobacter spp.*, not *Enterococcus spp.*

2. **A. Fluoroquinolones, D. Macrolides**

   Fluoroquinolones and macrolides can cause QT prolongation.

3. **C. Carbapenems**

   KPC stands for Klebsiella pneumoniae carbapenemase, which is resistant to carbapenems.

4. **A. Ciprofloxacin, C. Amikacin, D. Moxifloxacin**

   Fluoroquinolones and aminoglycosides are concentration dependent. Aztreonam and vancomycin are time dependent.

5. **E. Cefepime**

   Cefepime needs to be renally adjusted. Ceftriaxone, clindamycin, rifampin, erythromycin do not have renally adjusted doses.

6. **B. Insulin aspart (Novolog®) vial, C. Insulin glargine (Lantus®) pen, D. Insulin lispro (Humalog®) vial**

   Insulin aspart (Novolog®) vial, insulin glargine (Lantus®) pen, and insulin lispro (Humalog®) vial can be stored at room temperature for up to 28 days.

   Insulin detemir (Levemir®) vial can be stored at room temperature for up to 42 days. NPH Novolin® pen can be stored at room temperature for up to 14 days.

7. **A. 10 days**

   A 70/30 Humulin® <u>pen</u> can be stored at room temperature for up to <u>10 days</u>. A 70/30 Humulin® <u>vial</u> can be stored at room temperature for up to <u>28 days</u>.

8. **B. 5000 units SQ q8-12h**

   Unfractionated heparin prophylactic dose is 5000 units SQ q8-12h.

9. **C. 30 mg SQ q12h**

Enoxaparin prophylactic dose is 30 mg SQ q12h. Enoxaparin treatment dose is 1 mg/kg SQ q12h or 1.5 mg/kg daily.

10. **D. 15 mg PO BID for 21 days, then 20 mg PO daily**

Rivaroxaban treatment dose for VTE is 15 mg PO BID for 21 days, then 20 mg PO daily.

11. **E. Enoxaparin and andexanet alfa**

The antidote for enoxaparin is protamine (same antidote for heparin). Andexanet alfa is the antidote for DOACs, like rivaroxaban and apixaban.

12. **D. 23-year-old person with asplenia**

Adults aged 19-64 should receive one dose of PPSV23. Adults over age 19 and who are immunocompromised or have asplenia should receive one dose of PCV13, then one dose of PPSV23 at least 8 weeks later, then another dose of PPSV23 at least 5 years later, then one more dose of PPSV23 after age 65.

13. **A. Tenofovir disoproxil fumarate + emtricitabine**

Tenofovir disoproxil fumarate + emtricitabine = Truvada®
Tenofovir alafenamide + emtricitabine = Descovy®
Tenofovir disoproxil fumarate + emtricitabine + efavirenz = Atripla®
Tenofovir alafenamide + emtricitabine + bictegravir = Biktarvy®
Tenofovir alafenamide + emtricitabine + rilpivirine = Odefsey®

14. **D. Truvada®, E. Triumeq®**

Avoid rilpivirine-based therapies in patients with a CD4+ cell count <200 cells/mm^3.

Juluca® = dolutegravir + **rilpivirine** → AVOID
Odefsey® = **rilpivirine** + tenofovir alafenamide + emtricitabine → AVOID
Complera® = **rilpivirine** + tenofovir disoproxil fumarate + emtricitabine → AVOID
Truvada® = tenofovir disoproxil fumarate + emtricitabine
Triumeq® = dolutegravir + abacavir + lamivudine

15. **A. Evotaz®, C. Kaletra®, D. Prezcobix®, E. Symtuza®**

Evotaz® = **atazanavir (PI)** + cobicistat (PK booster)
Combivir® = lamivudine (NRTI) + zidovudine (NRTI)
Kaletra® = **lopinavir (PI)** + ritonavir (PK booster)
Prezcobix® = **darunavir (PI)** + cobicistat (PK booster)
Symtuza® = **darunavir (PI)** + cobicistat (PK booster) + tenofovir alafenamide (NRTI) + emtricitabine (NRTI)

16. **B. Methotrexate + hydroxychloroquine + sulfasalazine**

Triple DMARD therapy consists of methotrexate, hydroxychloroquine, and sulfasalazine.

17. A. Hydroxychloroquine, C. NSAIDs

Hydroxychloroquine and NSAIDs can be used to treat the symptoms of drug-induced lupus. Cyclosporine and azathioprine are used to treat lupus nephritis. Procainamide can cause drug-induced lupus and should be discontinued.

18. C. Aspirin

Allopurinol, febuxostat, colchicine, prednisone, and NSAIDs (not including aspirin) can be used in the treatment of gout.

19. C. Metamucil®, E. Miralax®

Miralax® (polyethylene glycol) is a hyperosmotic that is often considered the drug of choice for constipation during pregnancy. Metamucil® (psyllium) is a bulk laxative that is ok to use in pregnancy.

Dulcolax® (bisacodyl) is a stimulant that should be avoided in the 3rd trimester. Fleet enema® is a saline laxative (osmotic) that should be avoided in pregnancy. Mineral oil is a lubricant that should be avoided in pregnancy because it decreases fetal potassium.

20. E. Kaopectate

Kaopectate is the antidiarrheal of choice in pregnancy.

Loperamide has limited human data, so it is not recommended in pregnancy. Lomotil® is not recommended for use in pregnancy due to adverse effects seen in animal studies. Pepto Bismol® has limited human data but should be avoided in the 2nd and 3rd trimesters, due to the salicylate component.

Castor oil is not an anti-diarrheal and has potential for maternal/fetal morbidity, so it should be avoided.

21. A. Naproxen

Naproxen is the only drug that would not change the INR if used together with warfarin. Naproxen is an NSAID that does not change the warfarin levels but does have a bleeding risk factor. The other medications are CYP2C9 inhibitors and since warfarin is a CYP2C9 substrate, the bleeding risk and the INR are both affected.

22. C. Microzide

Initial drug selection for hypertension in black patients is to use a thiazide or calcium channel blocker. Microzide (hydrochlorothiazide) is the only drug that fits those criteria.

23. A. Ciprofloxacin, C. procainamide, D. amitriptyline

Quinolones, class 1a antiarrhythmics (procainamide), and tricyclic antidepressants (amitriptyline) can prolong the QT interval and should be avoided with KP to prevent Torsade de Pointes (TdP).

24. A. ACE inhibitors, B. Angiotensin Receptor blockers (ARBs), C. Beta blockers, E. Aldosterone receptor antagonists

Medications that have proven mortality benefit for HF are ACE inhibitors, Angiotensin Receptor blockers (ARBs), Angiotensin receptor and neprilysin inhibitors (Entresto), Beta blockers, and Aldosterone receptor antagonists. Alpha 1 agonists are not included in the list.

25. D. Azithromycin

Azithromycin 1,000mg PO for 1 day or 500mg PO daily for 1-3 days is the preferred treatment for travelers' diarrhea if dysentery (bloody diarrhea) is present.

26. E. Nitrofurantoin 100mg PO BID

Nitrofurantoin (Macrobid) 100mg PO BID with food for 5 days or SMX/TMP DS 1 tablet PO BID for 3 days are the drugs of choice for acute uncomplicated cystitis. It is usually treated empirically.

27. C. 5-7 days

Spontaneous bacterial peritonitis (SBP) is an infection of the peritoneal space that often occurs in liver disease. The preferred treatment is ceftriaxone for 5-7 days.

28. A. Saxagliptin, C. Diltiazem, D. Naproxen

DPP4-inhibitors (Saxagliptin), non-dihydropyridine CCB (Diltiazem), and all NSAIDS (Naproxen) are select drugs that cause or worsen heart failure.

29. A. Argatroban

AJ is experiencing heparin induced thrombocytopenia and the drug of choice for HIT in the hospital setting is the injectable direct thrombin inhibitor argatroban.

30. C. Apixaban, D. Dabigatran

When switching from warfarin to another oral anticoagulant, the patient stops warfarin and depending on the INR switches to another agent. When INR <3 convert to rivoraxaban. When <2.5, Edoxaban. When <2, Apixaban or Dabigatran.

31. B. Azithromycin 1,200mg weekly

Azithromycin 1.200mg weekly is the preferred treatment for MAC infection if ART is not initiated and CD4+ count <50 cells/mm^3

32. B. Hypomagnesemia, C. Hypercalcemia

The risk of digoxin toxicity is increased with hypokalemia, hypomagnesemia, and hypercalcemia making only b and c correct. Additionally, hypothyroidism can increase digoxin levels.

33. A. Chlorthalidone, D. Sulfasalazine, E. Dapsone

Chlorthalidone, sulfasalazine, and dapsone all have a sulfa moiety and should be avoided in patients with an allergy to sulfonamide derived drugs.

34. B. Spiriva Handihaler

According to the GOLD guidelines, AM is in patient risk group C due to having a CAT score <10 and mmRC of 0-1 with at least one exacerbation leading to a hospitalization. Patient group C is treated with a LAMA over a LABA as they have been shown to have a greater effect on exacerbation rates. Spiriva Handihaler (tiotropium) is the only LAMA in the answer choices.

35. E. 7.5-20mg once weekly

7.5-20mg once weekly of methotrexate is the preferred initial therapy for most patients with rheumatoid arthritis. In patients with disease activity despite methotrexate treatment, a combination of DMARDS is used. Methotrexate should never be dosed daily for RA.

36. A. Caffeine, B. benztropine, D. pseudoephedrine

Drugs that can worsen BPH include caffeine and drugs with anticholinergic effects. Benztropine is a centrally acting anticholinergic and pseudoephedrine has anticholinergic effects. Additionally, diuretics, SNRIs and antihistamines should be avoided.

37. E. Myocardial toxicity

Myocardial toxicity (Cardiotoxicity) is a boxed warning for all anthracyclines including doxorubicin and daunorubicin.

38. A. Mirapex, B. Requip, D. Neurontin

The dopamine agonists Mirapex (Pramipexole) and Requip (ropinirole) along with the anticonvulsant Neurontin (gabapentin) are the primary treatment for restless leg syndrome.

39. A. Omeprazole, C. Lansoprazole

Omeprazole and lansoprazole are the only options listed that are available as ODTs.

40. B. PO vancomycin 125mg QID for 10 days

TM is experiencing a non-severe first episode of C. difficile which was determined using her WBC and SCr. Treatment guidelines recommend using PO vancomycin 125mg QID for 10 days in this situation. The other answers have the wrong dosage listed or is not appropriate for a non-severe first episode.

41. B. Dolutegravir / Abacavir / Lamivudine

Triumeq® is made up of 1 INSTI and 2 NRTIs

42. E. Administer calcium gluconate

In severe hyperkalemia, the most important priority for the patient is to stabilize the heart. Administering calcium gluconate should be the first step to stabilize myocardial cells and prevent arrhythmias.

43. A. Furosemide, D. Sodium polystyrene sulfonate, E. Patiromer

Insulin and dextrose move K intracellularly whereas the three correct answer choices eliminate K from the body.

44. E. Doxycycline

Doxycycline is the only drug listed that does not require renal dose adjustment.

45. A. 1 DS tablet daily

The appropriate regimen for pneumocystis pneumonia (PCP) prophylaxis is 1DS or 1 SS tablet daily

46. B. Amoxicillin

Amoxicillin, doxycycline, or a macrolide are appropriate empiric regimens for outpatient CAP.

47. A. Grapefruit, B. Ritonavir, C. Erythromycin, E. Fluconazole

Drug interactions with statins can increase the risk of muscle damage. Avoid grapefruit, protease inhibitors, azole antifungals, and macrolides when taking statins as they cause most of the CYP mediated interactions.

48. D. Fetal toxicity

Although ACE inhibitors may cause renal impairment, the boxed warning for ACE inhibitors is for injury and death to a developing fetus when used in the 2nd and 3rd trimesters.

49. A. Active internal bleeding, C. History of recent stroke, E. Severe uncontrolled hypertension

Since alteplase has a significant bleeding risk, clinicians must ensure that the patient does not fit any of the contraindications or else the drug cannot be used.

50. B. 40mg SC daily

Enoxaparin is dosed 30mg SC Q12H or 40mg SC daily for VTE prophylaxis.

Practice Test 7 Answers and Explanations

1. **D. Pacerone**
   Pacerone (amiodarone) is a strong CYP2C9 inhibitor. The S-enantiomer of warfarin, which is the more potent enantiomer, is primarily metabolized by CYP2C9.

2. **B. Neoral   C. Cartia XT   E. Amiodarone**
   Neoral (cyclosporine), Cartia XT (diltiazem), and amiodarone are all strong CYP3A4 inhibitors. Digoxin is a Pgp substrate. Modafinil is a CYP3A4 inducer.

3. **A. Flexeril   B. Wellbutrin   C. Dextromethorphan   D. Elavil   E. Prozac**
   Nardil (phenelzine) is a MAO inhibitor which increases the levels of serotonin in the brain. All of the medications listed are serotonergic which increases the risk of a hypertensive crisis when used with Nardil.

4. **A. St. John's Wort**
   St. John's Wort is a potent *inducer* of many CYPs decreasing the effective concentrations of many medications, including oral contraceptives.

5. **B. Triumeq   D. Epzicom   E. Trizivir**
   Triumeq, Epzicom, and Trizivir all contain abacavir. All patients should be tested for HLA-B*1501 prior to starting therapy to avoid serious hypersensitivity reactions.

6. **E. Sporanox**
   Sporanox (itraconzole) is the only -azole antifungal that inhibits P-glycoprotein. Diflucan (fluconazole) is a strong CYP2C9 and CYP2C19 inhibitor. Vfend (voriconazole) is a moderate CYP2C9 and CYP2C19 inhibitor. Noxafil (Posaconazole) inhibits CYP3A4. Micafungin is not a CYP inhibitor.

7. **A. Nizoral   E. Sporanox**
   Sporanox (itraconzole) and Nizoral (ketoconazole) require an acidic environment to be absorbed. Doses of these antifungals should be separated from antacids by at least 2 hours.

8. **C. Tenormin**
   Tenormin (atenolol) is a beta-blocker. Beta-blockers are no longer recommended first-line agents for hypertension in the absence of other comorbidities.

9. **A. 2**
   When switching from warfarin to Eliquis (apixaban) a patient's INR must be 2 or less to begin Eliquis. INR must be less than 3 to start Xarelto (rivaroxaban) and less than 2 to start Pradaxa (dabigatran).

10. **A. Bidil**
    Bidil (hydralazine + isosorbide dinitrate) contains a nitrate. Viagra is a phosphodiesterase inhibitor which can cause an emergent drop in blood pressure when combined with nitrates.

11. **D. Paroxysmal supraventricular tachyarrhythmias**
    Paroxysmal supraventricular tachyarrhythmias is the only cardiac arrhythmia adenosine is indicated for.

12. C. 0.9 mg/kg up to 90 mg
The dose of Activase (alteplase) for ischemic stroke is 0.9 mg/kg up to 90 mg. 10% is given as a bolus over 1 minute and the remaining 90% is administered over 1 hour.

13. A. Isoniazid   B. Levodopa   C. Carboplatin   E. Rifampin
Isoniazid, levodopa, carboplatin, and rifampin are all associated with drug induced hemolytic anemia, Penicillins, cephalosporins, methyldopa, and the other platinum-based chemotherapy drugs can also cause drug induced hemolytic anemia.

14. D. 180 days
Female patients that stop using Droxia (hydroxyurea) must avoid becoming pregnant for at least 6 months (180 days). Male patients should avoid impregnating their female partners for at least 12 months (1 year).

15. C. Vfend   E. Cialis
Vfend (voriconazole) and phosphodiesterase inhibitors such as Cialis (tadalafil) can both cause patients to experience color vision changes. Amiodarone can cause optic neuropathy. Hydroxychloroquine is associated with retinopathy. Humira is not associated with vision changes.

16. A. 1.5 to 2.5
Patients with pulmonary arterial hypertension that require anticoagulation with warfarin have an INR goal of 1.5 to 2.5.

17. D. CYP1A2
Smoking tobacco induces the CYP1A2 enzyme. Clozapine, olanzapine, and theophylline are notable CYP1A2 substrates that could have their levels impacted if a patient quits smoking.

18. A. Trulicity   D. Bydureon   E. Ozempic
Trulicity, Bydureon, and Ozempic are injected weekly. Victoza is injected once a day. Bydureon is injected twice daily.

19. A. MMR   B. Zostavax   C. Vivotif   D. YF-VAX   E. Intranasal influenza vaccine
Live vaccinations are contraindicated during pregnant. All the vaccines listed above are live vaccines and should not be given during pregnancy.

20. B. MMR   C. YF-VAX   D. Varivax
The MMR, YF-VAX (yellow fever), and Varivax (varicella) vaccines MUST be given subcutaneously.

21. C. Orbactiv
Orbactiv (oritavancin) cannot be given within 5 days of unfractionated heparin due to false elevation of aPTT.

22. A. Clostridium difficile infections   C. Bacterial vaginosis   D. Trichomoniasis
Metronidazole covers anaerobes and certain protozoal infections. This includes clostridium difficile infections, bacterial vaginosis, trichomoniasis, giardia, amebiasis, and intrabdominal infections.

23. B. 165 lbs
Plan-B and any other emergency contraception that contains 1.5 g of levonorgestrel is less effective when the patient weighs more than 165 lbs.

24. A. Depo-Provera   B. Anticonvulsants   C. Loop diuretics   E. Aromatase inhibitors
Depo-provera, anticonvulsants, loop diuretics, aromatase inhibitors, lithium, and SSRIs can all increase the risk of osteoporosis with long term use.

25. A. Fosamax   C. Evista
Bisphosphonates, including Fosamax (alendronate), and Evista (raloxifene) are indicated for prevention AND treatment of osteoporosis. Parathyroid hormone analogs such as Forteo (teriparatide) and Prolia (denosumab) are only indicated for treatment of osteoporosis in high-risk patients. Duavee (conjugated equine estrogen/bazedoxifene) is only indicated for prevention of osteoporosis.

26. A. Venlafaxine   B. Coreg   D. Catapres
SNRIs, SSRIs, beta-blockers, and Catapres (clonidine) can all worsen erectile dysfunction.

27. D. Calvert Formula
The dosing of carboplatin is based off the Calvert formula:
Total carboplatin dose= [Target AUC] x [GFR+25]
Most other chemotherapy agents are dosed off body surface area (BSA) that is calculated using a variety of equations, including the DuBois and Mosteller equations

28. C. Philadelphia chromosome positive
In order to use tyrosine kinase inhibitors for chronic myelogenous leukemia, including Gleevec (imatinib), a patient must be Philadelphia chromosome positive, also referred to as BCR-ABL positive.

Patients must be BRAF V600E positive in order to use Zelboraf (vemurafenib) and Tafinlar (dabrafenib) for melanoma.

Patients must be KRAS wildtype to receive treatment with Erbitux (cetuximab).

Patients must be EGFR mutation positive to use Gilotrif (afatinib), Tarceva (erlotinib), and Iressa (gefitinib) for non-small cell lung cancer.

Patients must be ALK mutation positive Xalkori (crizotinib), Zykadia (certinib), and Alecensa (alectinib) for non-small cell lunger cancer.

29. C. 14 days
Stimulants must be started at least 14 days after stopping MAO inhibitors

30. A. Marplan   C. Nardil   D. Emsam
Marplan (isocarboxazid), Nardil (phenelzine), and Emsam (selegiline) are all examples of common MAO inhibitors. It is important to recognize these medications in order to recognize and prevent additive serotonin toxicity. Zyban is the smoking cessation form of bupropion.
Anafranil is a tricyclic antidepressant.

31. A. FMEA
FMEA (Failure Mode and Effects Analysis) is a prospective evaluation conducted to prevent medication errors from occurring in the future.
RCA: Root Cause Analysis (retrospective evaluation)
CQI: Continuous Quality Inspection
MERP: Medication Error Reporting Form

REMS: Risk Evaluation and Mitigation Strategies

32. D. Bubble-point test

A bubble-point test is the only test to assess pore size of filter, and therefore assess the integrity of the filter. Pyrogen and visual inspection can assess the integrity of the CSP itself, and UV testing is not an appropriate testing method for CSP.

33. B. Hydromorphone 10 mg/mL vials in a cardiac telemetry unit

High concentration opioids should not be placed in an automated dispensing cabinet unless they are in unit dose packages in a unit with cancer or end-of-life care patients. Other medications that should not be placed in an automated dispensing cabinet include insulin and warfarin.

34. E. Varicella

For solid-organ transplant patients, pneumococcal, influenza, and varicella vaccinations are particularly important to be kept up to date prior to the transplant procedure.

35. B. Lower abdomen E. Upper buttocks

An important counseling point for **estradiol patches** is that they can only be placed on the abdomen and upper buttocks. This differs from contraception patches (see Question 6).

36. A. Upper arms B. Lower abdomen D. Back E. Upper buttocks

Contraception patches can be placed on a few different spots as long as there are not clothes that tightly cover the area.

37. A. Diamox®

Acetazolamide (Diamox) is the first line agent for AMS. Metoclopramide is indicated for delayed gastric emptying, while the other answer choices are indicated for other types of motion sickness.

38. A. Zostavax® E. Vaxchora®

Most vaccines need to be refrigerated, but vaccines that need to be stored in a freezer include Zostavax®, cholera vaccines, Varivax®, and MMRV. MMR vaccines can be stored in a refrigerator or a freezer.

39. B. A sore with delayed healing E. Unusually out of breath

The American Cancer Society (ACS) uses the acronym CAUTION define early warning signs of cancer:

Change in bowel or bladder habits
A sore <u>that does not heal</u>
Unusual bleeding or discharge
Thickening or lump in breast or elsewhere
Indigestion or difficulty swallowing
Obvious change in size, color, shape, or thickness of a wart or mole
Nagging cough or persistent hoarseness

Other possible warning signs include unexplained weight loss and pernicious anemia.

40. A. History of tuberculosis B. History of hepatitis D. Sexual history with multiple partners
History of SUD (substance use disorder) alone does not have high HIV risk, unless combined with other risk factors such as shared needles. The risk of HIV exposure through the exchange of bodily fluids alone is not well documented (and thus considered a negligible risk).

41. A. Glycol-encased probe D. Aluminum-encased probe E. Sand-encased probe
Proper vaccine storage required a probe buffered by either liquid (glycol), solid (aluminum) or solid (sand) to acquire accurate temperature readings. Traditional glass thermometers or electronic probes that rely on air temperature readings will not be accurate.

42. C. Increased shortness of breath   E. Increased coughing
A weight gain of greater than 5 lbs. in one week or 4 lbs. in 2 days would be a sign for heart failure patients to call their PCP. Patients with severe symptoms such as fainting, or confusion should go to the emergency room.

43. D. Blue
Refer to the chart below for the distinctive tints of certain IV preparations:

1. Color	2. Preparation
3. Red	4. Doxorubicin
5. Yellow	6. Multivitamin
7. Orange	8. Rifampin
9. Blue	10. Mitoxantrone
11. Brown/Black	12. Iron

44. C. 7-10
This is the only correct healthy APGAR score range. Any APGAR score below 7 indicates further monitoring past 5 minute and possibly further medical intervention.

45. A. Type I
The penicillin skin test can only assess for Type I (IgE mediated) immunity.
Type II = IgG or IgM mediated immunity
Type III = IgG and IgM mediated immunity
Type IV = T cell mediated immunity

46. A. Plavix®-CYP2C9
To assess Plavix® metabolism, a test specific to CYP2C19 should be conducted. A CYP2C9 test would be appropriate for warfarin.

47. B. Clorazil®-QT prolongation
While all antipsychotics have a risk for QT prolongation, only thioridazine carries a boxed warning for this adverse effect. All other boxed warning pairings are appropriate.

48. B. D2 partial agonist   C. 5-HT1A partial agonist
Aripriprazole has a slightly different mechanism of action from other second-generation drugs by acting as a partial dopamine and serotonin agonist rather than an antagonist.

49. C. NSAID use

NSAID use, as well as decreased salt intake, can result in increased lithium levels. Use of SSRIs and carbamazepine may result in increased adverse effects.

50. D. 12 lbs in 12 weeks

For patients on medications for weight loss, if they do not achieve at least a 5% weight loss over 12 weeks, then the medication should be discontinued.

Practice Test 8 Answers and Explanations

1. **E. The Diastat Acudial® syringe should be disposed of immediately after use in a garbage away from children**

   For the Acudial product, any remaining gel in the syringe must be disposed of through the removal and reinsertion of the plunger. Only after this process is complete can the remaining components be disposed of in the garbage.

2. **A. Descending Loop of Henle**

   Osmotic diuretics primary work at the descending Loop of Henle. Thiazide diuretics work at the distal convoluted tubule. Loop diuretics work at the ascending Loop of Henle. Potassium-sparing diuretics work at the distal convoluted tubule and collecting duct.

3. **B. Call PCP D. Reduce Excedrin® use to 2-3 times per week at most**

   The best recommendation for relapse headaches is to decrease the use of acute treatment, as relapse headaches often occur as a result of overconsumption of OTC products. A PCP can recommend prescription options for the patient to consider.

4. **E. CDC Pink Book**

   This publication provides the latest evidence and safety information from the CDC. The CDC Yellow Book is used for travel medicine. The other answer choices are not actual CDC publications.

5. **A. Chlorpromazine D. Thioridazine B. Loxapine C. Periphenazine E. Haloperidol**

   Chlorpromazine and thioridazine are considered low-potency, first-generation antipsychotics (FGA), while loxapine and perphenazine are considered medium-potency. Haloperidol has the high potency of all the listed antipsychotics. These potencies are significant when it comes to expected adverse effects; low-potency FGAs tend to cause more sedation, while high-potency FGAs tend to have higher rates of EPS.

6. **A. Diphenhydramine**

   The patient is elderly, so it is best to avoid first-generation antihistamines due to the increased risk of falls and dizziness. Nasal sprays are a great option to start with since they have few side effects that are more localized in nature. Second-generation antihistamines are another possible option, as they cause less dizziness and sedation.

7. **D. Dizziness**

   Combining an alpha-blocker, especially a non-selective one, with a phosphodiesterase inhibitor is dangerous and not recommended. This combination puts the patient at a higher risk of dizziness/orthostasis.

8. **D. Depo-Provera injection**

Depo-Provera is not an appropriate choice since the patient wishes for her fertility to return right away. This isn't the case with this shot, which is given every three months. In addition, this form of contraception is known to increase the risk of osteoporosis and bone fractures. Although the damage is reversible once it is discontinued, it would not be recommended to weaken the patient's bones to a greater extent.

9. **A. Aspirin, B. Furosemide, C. Hydrochlorothiazide**

It is important to recognize medications that can increase uric acid levels. Aspirin, calcineurin inhibitors (tacrolimus, cyclosporine), niacin, pyrazinamide, and diuretics (loop and thiazide) are culprits of this.

10. **B. Patient is on BiDil, which is contraindicated with Viagra.**

Since BiDil contains isosorbide dinitrate and hydralazine, the patient cannot receive Viagra due to its contraindication with nitrates. This would cause serious dizziness.

11. **A. Age ≥ 80 years**

    D. SCr ≥ 1.5 mg/dL

Eliquis (apixaban) is indicated for stroke prevention in patients with atrial fibrillation at a starting dose of 5 mg PO BID. However, patients that meet **two or more** of the following criteria are recommended a reduced dose of **2.5 mg PO BID**:
   1. 80 years or older
   2. A body weight < 60 kg (133 lbs), or
   3. A serum creatinine ≥ 1.5 mg/ dL (133 µmol/L)

12. **B. Lovenox**

It is important to recognize that a positive HCG test indicates pregnancy. The NAPLEX may not specifically state "pregnant" in case questions. Lovenox is the preferred anticoagulation treatment in pregnant women.

13. **A. Carbamazepine causes hyponatremia, monitor sodium electrolytes B. Carbamazepine decreases the effectiveness of Jolessa C. Carbamazepine is a CYP 3A4 inducer**

Most antiepileptic drugs have interactions that lower the effectiveness of combined oral contraceptives, with the exception of levetiracetam (Keppra). Other CYP 3A4 inducers include oxcarbazepine, phenytoin, phenobarbital, St. John's wort, rifampin, and smoking. Oxcarbazepine also causes hyponatremia.

14. **B. Refuse to administer the vaccine C. Inform him that he must wait for at least 3 months**

Since Zoster is the live vaccine for shingles, there is a specific spacing requirement that must be followed. If the patient received the live vaccine before IVIG, he must wait for at least 2 weeks. If he received IVIG before the live vaccine, he must wait for at least 3 months. On the NAPLEX, it is important to memorize the live vaccines and be able to distinguish them from inactivated vaccines. Live vaccines include cholera, typhoid, zoster, yellow fever, intranasal influenza, varicella, rotavirus, and MMR (measles, mumps, rubella). Remember the acronym, COZY IV RM for live vaccines.

15. B. Titrate the metformin dose down, then go up as tolerated.

Metformin may cause severe GI effects if it is not titrated appropriately. The dose should only be increased as tolerated, or the patient will most likely not adhere to therapy.

16. A. Patient is not a candidate given his increased potassium levels.
Spironolactone is a potassium sparing diuretic/ aldosterone antagonist. Thus, it cannot be initiated if potassium is >5 mEq, as hyperkalemia would put the patient at risk of arrythmias. The normal range of potassium is 3.5-5 mmol/L.

17. B. Hydrochlorothiazide, C. Valsartan, D. Diltiazem, E. Zestoretic

Hydrochlorothiazide, and any drug containing hydrochlorothiazide (Zestoretic (lisinopril/hydrochlorothiazide)) may not be used. Thiazide diuretics contain sulfa, and they must be avoided because the patient has a true sulfa allergy. Valsartan is inappropriate, as an ACE & ARB cannot be combined due to a heightened risk of toxicity. Both diltiazem and verapamil are non-DHP CCB. This class of CCB is not preferred in lowering blood pressure. DHP-CCB such as amlodipine are better options, as they are less cardio-selective and more potent vasodilators (better blood pressure lowering effects).

18. D. Buprenorphine

There are a few drugs that lower the seizure threshold. These drugs include buprenorphine, lithium, carbamazepine, carbapenems (penicillin, cephalosporin, beta-lactams), quinolones, meperidine, theophylline, clozapine, tramadol, varenicline (Chantix).

19. B. 10-20 mcg/ml

It is important to know the therapeutic range of drugs such as phenytoin (10-20 mcg/ml). Corrected phenytoin level= phenytoin observed/ [(albumin x0.2) +0.1].

20. A. 5-15 mcg/ml

It is important to know the therapeutic range of drugs such as theophylline (5-15 mcg/ml). Theophylline toxicity can cause side effects similar to those experienced with drinking too much coffee, such as rapid heartbeat, abdominal discomfort, headache, nervousness, and restlessness.

21. E. 1 mg/kg q24h

The DVT prophylaxis dose of Lovenox is either 40 mg qd SQ or 30 mg q12h SQ. It can also be 30 mg qd SQ if CrCl<30.

The DVT treatment dose is 1 mg/kg q12h SQ or 1.5 mg/kg q24h SQ. It can also be 1 mg/kg q24h SQ if CrCl<30.

22. E. 5000U q8-12h

The DVT prophylaxis dose of heparin is 5000U q8-12h subQ. The DVT treatment dose is 80 U/kg bolus IV or 18 U/kg/hr IV.

23. D. Acetaminophen

Currently, acetaminophen is the preferred analgesic choice in pregnant women.

24. D. Digoxin

Digoxin therapeutic levels in heart failure fall between 0.5-0.9 ng/ml. For atrial fibrillation, the level should be <2 ng/ml. Digoxin toxicity can cause yellow-greenish halos, nausea, vomiting, confusion, and blurry vision.

25. B. Do not fill, there is an interaction between Prilosec and clopidogrel. C. Recommend famotidine instead of Prilosec.

Prilosec and Nexium are best avoided with clopidogrel, as they may lower its effectiveness and increase the risk of a clot.

26. B. Serevent Diskus C. QVAR RediHaler D. Breo Ellipta

Dry powder inhalers (e.g. Serevent Diskus and Breo Ellipta), QVAR RediHaler, Alvesco, and Respimat products do not require shaking.

27. D. Daliresp

Roflumilast (Daliresp) is a PDE-4 inhibitor with a contraindication in moderate to severe liver impairment.

28. A. Striverdi Respimat

Respimat products follow the steps of TOP (Turn, Open, Press).

29. C. Stiolto Respimat E. Alvesco

HFA, Respimat, and products with no suffix (e.g. Alvesco) are metered-dose inhalers (MDIs).

30. C. Oral candidiasis

Formoterol (Perforomist) is a LABA with side effects that include nervousness, tremor, tachycardia, palpitations, hyperglycemia, hypokalemia, and cough. Oral candidiasis is a common side effect of inhaled corticosteroids.

31. C. Weekly

Respimat products should be cleaned with a damp cloth or tissue weekly.

32. A. Voltaren

Diclofenac (Voltaren) has increased COX-2 selectivity which results in a lower risk of GI complications. However, there is an increased risk of myocardial infarction and stroke.

33. B. Kadian, C. Oxymorphone ER, E. Zohydro ER

Extended-release opioid products such as Kadian, oxymorphone ER, Nucynta ER, and Zohydro ER cannot be consumed with alcohol due to increased drug plasma levels and the potential for fatal overdose.

34. D. Dolophine

Oxycodone (Oxycontin), morphine (Kadian), and hydromorphone (Dilaudid) are in the same chemical class as hydrocodone (Norco, Vicodin). Methadone (Dolophine) is in a different chemical class.

35. A. Ultram D. Demerol

Tramadol (Ultram) and meperidine (Demerol) have a seizure risk.

36. B. Tegaderm

Bioclusive and Tegaderm are the only adhesive film dressings permitted to cover a fentanyl patch.

37. E. Triumeq

Triumeq is an INSTI-based regimen containing dolutegravir, abacavir, and lamivudine.

38. A. Symfi

Symfi is a single tablet regimen containing efavirenz, lamivudine, and tenofovir disoproxil fumarate. Ritonavir (Norvir), darunavir (Prezista), raltegravir (Isentress), and zidovudine (Retrovir) are not single tablet HIV regimens.

39. D. Viread

Tenofovir disoproxil fumarate (Viread) is a nucleoside reverse transcriptase inhibitor (NRTI). Dolutegravir (Tivicay) and raltegravir (Isentress) are integrase strand transfer inhibitors. Atazanavir (Reyataz) is a protease inhibitor and efavirenz (Sustiva) is a non-nucleoside reverse transcriptase inhibitor.

40. A. Vincristine

A single dose of vincristine is often capped at 2 mg due to the risk of neuropathy.

41. C. Dextran

Dextran is an example of a colloid.

42. A. Exelon patch C. Aricept ODT

The rivastigmine patch (Exelon) and donepezil ODT have fewer GI side effects.

43. B. Wellbutrin C. Ultram E. Levaquin

Bupropion (Wellbutrin), tramadol (Ultram), and levofloxacin (Levaquin) can lower the seizure threshold.

44. B. Primaxin C. Invanz

Piperacillin/tazobactam (Zosyn) is a penicillin, therefore SP has a penicillin allergy. Imipenem/cilastatin (Primaxin) and ertapenem (Invanz) are carbapenems and should be avoided in patients with a penicillin allergy despite the small risk of cross-reactivity.

45. D. Mephyton

Vitamin K, or phytonadione (Mephyton), is used for warfarin reversal. Protamine sulfate is used to reverse UFH/LMWH, idarucizumab (Praxbind) is used to reverse dabigatran, and andexanet alfa (Andexxa) is used to reverse apixaban and rivaroxaban.

2023-2024 NAPLEX® Practice Exam Answers

1. D, E

Lithium is 100% renally cleared (excreted) but has important drug interactions with drugs that affect renal clearance. Salt intake is inversely related to lithium; the kidneys do not distinguish between lithium and sodium so if salt intake increases, lithium excretion increases, and lithium levels decrease. Patients need to maintain a constant salt intake

2. A, B, E

Although digoxin is largely renally cleared, a percentage of the drug is metabolized hepatically. All these agents must doses decreased 30-50% when beginning amiodarone while avoiding grapefruit juice or products with amiodarone

3. A, B, C and D

Drug 'sorption' describes the process by which the drug components themselves stick to or are absorbed into the plastic devices. Drug sorption impacts the drug's chemical make-up and results in a loss of stability. Using the acronym ACLS TIN (Amiodarone, Carmustine, Lorazepam, Sufetanil, Thiopental, Insulin, and Nitroglycerin) are the medications that have sorption issues. To prepare IV solution of these agents, non-PVC bag or glass should be used. Studies have shown a lack of sorption in antineoplastic agents shown below:

Antineoplastic Agent	Spiros Male Luer 120 Days Refrigeration, and 7 Days Room Temperature			Genie Vial Access* 30 Days Refrigeration, and 10 Days Room Temperature			Vial Access Devices* 30 Days Refrigeration, and 7 Days Room Temperature			Administration Sets* 24-Hours at Room Temperature Diluted to 3x therapeutic level		
	Functional Failure	Drug Stability 120-Days	Plastic Migration Per Device	Functional Failure	Drug Stability 30-Days	Plastic Migration Per Device	Functional Failure	Drug Stability 30-Days	Plastic Migration Per Device	Functional Failure	Drug Stability 24-Hours	Plastic Migration Per Device
Bevacizumab	0/10	NT	NT	0/10	NT	NT	0/10	NT	NT	0/10	NT	NT
Cetuximab	0/10	NT	NT	0/10	NT	NT	0/10	NT	NT	0/10	NT	NT
Cisplatin	0/10	99.60%	P= .25µg VC= <.08µg	0/10	99.60%	P= .25µg VC= <.08µg	0/10	99.96%	P= .125µg VC= <.05µg	0/10	99.93%	P= .07µg VC= <.07µg
Cyclophosphamide	0/10	NT	NT	0/10	NT	NT	0/10	NT	NT	0/10	NT	NT
Doxorubicin	0/10	NT	NT	0/10	NT	NT	0/10	NT	NT	0/10	NT	NT
Etoposide	0/10	99.60%	P= .05µg VC= <.05µg	0/10	99.20%	P= .05µg VC= <.05µg	0/10	99.66%	P= .014µg VC= <.05µg	0/10	99.73%	P= .25µg VC= .09µg
Flourouracil	0/10	99.60%	P= .58µg VC= <.07µg	0/10	99.20%	P= .58µg VC= <.07µg	0/10	99.52%	P= .014µg VC= <.05µg	0/10	99.73%	P= .60µg VC= .05µg
Methotrexate	0/10	NT	NT	0/10	NT	NT	0/10	NT	NT	0/10	NT	NT
Paclitaxol	0/10	NT	NT	0/10	NT	NT	0/10	NT	NT	0/10	NT	NT
Vincristine	0/10	NT	NT	0/10	NT	NT	0/10	NT	NT	0/10	NT	NT

*Includes CLAVE Needlefree Connector in Evaluation

4. A, B, C

He is at risk for QT prolongation due to the history of atrial fibrillation and use of amiodarone and moxifloxacin. He is also at risk for blood sugar alterations due to diabetes and the use of moxifloxacin

5. C. USP Chapter 797

This chapter contains information for Sterile Compounding standards

6. A. Zyprexa

7. C. Verapamil; Calcium Channel Blocker

8. A; Linagliptin; DPP-4 inhibitor

9. B. Saxagliptin; DPP-4 inhibitor

10. C. Sitagliptin; DPP-4 inhibitor

11. E. This medication should be refrigerated

E.E.S., Augmentin, ceftriaxone, Zostavax® (diluent is in freezer), cephalexin, Vivotif Berna® capsules, and isoniazid need to be kept refrigerated. E.E.S. is a macrolide antibiotic and is not effective for treating infections like influenza. The drug should be taken with food to minimize stomach upset and should be stored under refrigeration. Erythromycin is a major inhibitor of CYP3A4. As a macrolide antibiotic and not a penicillin, this may be an option if a penicillin allergy was present in the patient

12. E. Biaxin

Biaxin does not need to be refrigerated. Refrigeration can cause thickening and the product may crystallize

13. C, D, E

Ceftriaxone and cefazolin need to be refrigerated.

14. A, B, D

Sulfamethoxazole/trimethoprim is compatible with D5W only (not saline). Phenytoin is compatible with saline only (not dextrose).

15. E. Isosorbide dinitrate decreases preload, hydralazine decreases afterload

Isosorbide dinitrate reduces preload as a result of venous dilation. Hydralazine reduces afterload via arterial dilation. The combination, when administered orally, has the same pharmacological effect as intravenous nitroprusside

16. E. Carbamazepine

Carbamazepine is very effective in relieving and preventing the pain associated with trigeminal neuralgia and remains the drug of choice for this disorder. Phenytoin has also been reported to be helpful in some patients

17. C. Emtricitabine

Emtricitabine is a new nucleoside reverse transcriptase inhibitor approved as part of a combination therapy regimen for HIV-1 infected patients older than 3 months old.

18. E. Methacholine

Methacholine (Provocholine) is commonly used as a provocative agent in the testing of airway responsiveness. The powdered drug is reconstituted with 0.9% NaCl and delivered to the airways via nebulizer in precisely controlled concentrations to produce cholinergic stimulation of airway smooth muscle. Methacholine produces nearly pure muscarinic stimulation with virtually no nicotinic action. It is metabolized by acetylcholinesterase (more slowly than acetylcholine) but is resistant to hydrolysis by pseudocholinesterase. Neither acetylcholine nor plasma cholinesterase are employed as therapeutic or diagnostic agents. Bethanechol is a choline ester with predominantly muscarinic actions. Carbachol is a potent choline ester with both muscarinic and nicotinic actions and is used in the treatment of glaucoma. Bethanechol and carbachol, through their muscarinic actions, can produce profound bronchoconstriction, but their resistance to cholinesterases (acetyl and plasma) makes their duration of action unsuitable for diagnostic airway challenge testing

19. B. The patient cannot be dispensed *Ziagen*

If a patient is positive for this allele, they cannot receive Ziagen or abacavir by itself or in combination as they are at high risk for severe hypersensitivity reactions like multi-organ syndromes

20. B. Atazanavir; protease inhibitor

21. B. Rilpivirine/emtricitabine/tenofovir DF

Genvoya® has the same components as Stribild® (elvitegravir/cobicistat/emtricitabine/tenofovir disoproxil fumarate), but substitutes tenofovir alafenamide, or TAF, for Stribild's® tenofovir disoproxil fumarate, or TDF. TAF has been shown to be less toxic to bones and kidneys than TDF. Because TAF enters cells more efficiently than TDF, a lower dose is required and 91 percent less of the tenofovir winds up in the bloodstream, where it may lead to toxicities

22. B, C, D

A few main points to remember about renal adjustment for HIV medications:
- All NRTIs need a renal adjustment (EXCEPT abacavir)
- Combination products with cobicistat are not given below a CrCl of 70 mL/min
- All other combination products are not given below a CrCl of 50 mL/min

These are general points that should apply for most cases. In this specific case Genvoya® is not recommended for patients below a CrCl of 30 mL/min despite having cobicistat as it contains tenofovir alafenamide which is easier on the kidneys instead of tenofovir disoproxil used in Strilbild. This is also true for Truvada, Atripla, and the majority of other HIV regimens. This patient needs to be recommended for a kidney transplant depending on how well-controlled his HIV infection is controlled

23. B. Maraviroc; CCR5 on Human CD4 cells

This drug is notable because it's the only HIV medication that has a human (not viral) target. It specifically targets a binding protein on your CD4 cells, which prevents HIV from entering. But unfortunately, it only targets one binding protein: the CCR5 receptor. Some patients only have the CCR5 receptor. If that's the case, maraviroc will work. However, if the patient's CD4 cells have a

CCR4 or a CXCR4 receptor, maraviroc will not work. To prevent error in treatment, a profile test is completed if you have the appropriate binding receptor on your CD4 cells

24. A, B, D, E

Norvir® (ritonavir) is a protease inhibitor that is considered an antiretroviral booster since it can increase drug levels of protease inhibitors mainly by blocking first pass metabolism to allow higher drug levels. At low doses, ritonavir can enhance protease inhibitors by inhibiting CYP 3A4 and 2D6. It's important to avoid drugs that are highly dependent on these enzymes such as flecainide, terfenadine, and midazolam. Ritonavir does block GLUT4 insulin-regulated transporters, keeping glucose from entering fat and muscle cells causing insulin resistance and potential type II diabetes. This is why ritonavir has the side effect of hyperglycemia

25. D. Emtricitabine, efavirenz, tenofovir

26. A, C

Pre-exposure prophylaxis, or PrEP, is a way for people who do not have HIV but who are at substantial risk of getting it to prevent HIV infection by taking a pill every day. The pill (brand name Truvada) contains two medicines (tenofovir and emtricitabine) that are used in combination with other medicines to treat HIV. When someone is exposed to HIV through sex or injection drug use, these medicines can work to keep the virus from establishing a permanent infection

27. A, C, D

Fuzeon® may have the powder stored at room temperature but once mixed needs to be kept in the refrigerator and used within 24 hours. Aptivus® + Norvir should be kept refrigerated before opening; once opened it may be kept at room temperature for up to two months. Norvir capsules can be stored up to 30 days at room temperature

28. E. Patients are more easily arousable and alert when stimulated, compared to propofol

Dexmedetomidine, sold under the trade names **Precedex**® among others, is an anxiolytic, sedative, and analgesic medication. Similar to clonidine, it is an agonist of α-2-adrenergic receptors in certain parts of the brain. Dexmedetomidine is notable for its ability to provide sedation without risk of respiratory depression (unlike other commonly used sedatives such as propofol, fentanyl, and midazolam) and can provide cooperative or semi-arousable sedation.

29. A. Oil-in-water emulsion

Propofol was originally developed using a form solubilized in cremophor EL. However, due to anaphylactic reactions to cremophor, this formulation was withdrawn from the market and subsequently reformulated as an emulsion of a soya oil/propofol mixture in water. The emulsified formulation was relaunched in 1986 by ICI (now AstraZeneca®) under the brand name Diprivan®. Propofol emulsion is a highly opaque white fluid due to the scattering of light from the tiny (about 150-nm) oil droplets it contains. A water-soluble prodrug form, fospropofol, has recently been developed and tested with positive results. Fospropofol is rapidly broken down by the enzyme alkaline phosphatase to form propofol. Marketed as Lusedra®, this new formulation may not produce the pain at injection site that often occurs with the traditional form of the drug

30. D. If particles are present, the pharmacist should shake well to dissolve the particles prior to the infusion

IBW should be used to calculate the dose of IVIG. IVIG should not be shaken since this will inactivate the antibodies

31. 24.6 mL

At a concentration of 500 mg per mL, and 5 grams of drug, there would be a total volume of 10 ml. But only 9.6 mL of diluent was added, so the powder contributed 0.4 mL to the final volume. At 250 mg/mL, there would be 20 mL of volume and at 100 mg/mL there would be 50 mL of volume. In each case the amount of diluent added was 0.4 mL less than the final volume. The powder will contribute 0.4 mL to the volume.

$$5000 \ mg \times \frac{mL}{200mg} = 25 \ mL \ of \ total \ volume$$

$$25 \ mL - 0.4 \ mL = \textbf{24.6 mL} \ of \ diluent \ to \ add \ to \ make \ 200 \ mg/mL$$

32. 5.6

$$0.89 \ PPM \quad \rightarrow \quad \frac{0.89 \ mg}{L} = \frac{5 \ mg}{x \ L} \qquad x = 5.62 \ L$$

33. E. Vitamin B6

Pyridoxine (Vitamin B6) 25-50 mg PO daily is used to reduce the risk of INH-induced peripheral neuropathy

34. B & C. Macrocytic Anemia, Pernicious anemia

Vitamin B12 deficiency can cause both macrocytic anemia and pernicious anemia.

Pernicious anemia is defined as a type of vitamin B12 deficiency that results from impaired uptake of vitamin B12 due to the lack of a substance known as intrinsic factor (IF) produced by the stomach lining. Pernicious anemia is a condition caused by too little vitamin B12 in the body. It is a form of vitamin B12 deficiency anemia.

Macrocytic anemia is a disorder of the blood defined by macrocytosis. The bone marrow generates abnormally large red blood cells that lack the nutrients needed to operate normally. It is often secondary to vitamin B-12 deficiency.

35. A. Preservative

Preservation is the prevention or inhibition of microbial growth. In pharmacy, this is commonly accomplished by the addition of a preservative to a product, with the primary purpose of minimizing microbial growth (as in oral liquids, topicals, etc.), or for preventing microbial growth (as in sterile preparations such as parenterals)

36. On the exam, you will need to click and select these areas:

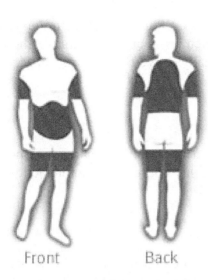

Front   Back

37. A. Administer 4900 units IV bolus, then 1100 units/hour continuous infusion

<u>DVT & PE Prophylaxis:</u> 5000 units SC q8-12hr OR 7500 units SC q12hr

<u>Treatment:</u> 80 units/kg IV bolus, THEN continuous infusion of 18 units/kg/hr, OR 5000 units IV bolus, THEN continuous infusion of 1300 units/hr, OR 250 units/kg (alternatively, 17,500 units) SC, THEN 250 units/kg q12hr

Weight based dosing is best to go by so choice a is the best answer to choose from

38. A, B, D

Lamotrigine (Lamictal®) has a risk of severe rash and needs a slow dose titration to reduce the risk. Inhibitors like valproate will increase the risk of rash

39. A, B, D

Sulfamethoxazole/trimethoprim is compatible with D5W only (not saline). Phenytoin is compatible with saline only (not dextrose). Common IV drugs which require filters are lorazepam, amphotericin, lipids, TPN, phenytoin, amiodarone, Cresemba®. Common IV drugs which do not refrigerate are Precedex®, phenytoin, Sulfatrim®, Lovenox®, moxifloxacin, and metronidazole

40. A, B, D

Phenytoin may cause all of these side effects.

41. C. Emtricitabine

About 86% of a dose of emtricitabine is eliminated unchanged by the kidneys, and dosage adjustment is necessary in patients with renal impairment.

42. D. Quinidine

Even though quinidine, paroxetine, and fluoxetine can all inhibit CYP2D6, the effect of quinidine is the most potent. A small 50 mg dose of quinidine, which is much less than usual antiarrhythmic dose of 200 to 300 mg, can potently inhibit CYP2D6 and metabolically convert an EM into a PM. Fluvoxamine is not an inhibitor of CYP2D6.

43. B. UGT1A1

Even though raltegravir is neither a substrate, inhibitor, nor inducer of the CYP family of isoenzymes, it is unique in that it is a substrate of UGT1A1, and therefore is susceptible to drug interactions with inhibitor or inducer of UGT1A1.

44. E. Linezolid

Although vancomycin has been traditionally used for treatment of Gram-positive infection when other antibiotics fail, the emergence of vancomycin resistant bacteria has diminished its role, and other agents such as linezolid has been increasingly reserved for the treatment of serious Gram-positive infection that has failed or resistant to other antibiotics.

45. B. Naloxone

Naloxone is an opioid antagonist that can be used to reverse the serious adverse effects of opiates in an overdose situation. Ketorolac is an NSAID. Pentazocine is a narcotic agonist-antagonist analgesic, whereas both codeine and methadone are narcotic analgesics.

46. C. Lamotrigine 150 to 400 mg per day

The dosage regimens are too high for lithium, risperidone, and topiramate, and too low for valproic acid.

47. A. Trimethoprim/Sulfamethoxazole and famciclovir

Patients treated with alemtuzumab are susceptible to similar infections as patients with HIV, especially *P. jiroveci* and herpes virus's reactivation; thus, they require trimethoprim/sulfamethoxazole and famciclovir prophylaxis. Ganciclovir is used for CMV with major side effect of myelosuppression. Due to this side effect, it is rarely if ever used for prophylaxis. Fluconazole is used for candida prophylaxis in bone marrow transplant recipients. Acyclovir and levofloxacin are other antibiotics used in many institutions following bone marrow transplant. Acyclovir has to be dosed 5 times per day, thus non-adherence plays a big role for this medication.

48. D. HPV vaccine

Human papillomavirus vaccine (HPV) vaccine is currently recommended for 11 to 12-year-old females. It covers most common viruses associated with cervical cancer (HPV strains 16, 18) and genital warts (HPV strains 6, 8). It is given in a 3-dose schedule with the second and third doses administered 2 and 6 months after the first dose.

49. B. Time > MIC is an appropriate measure for beta-lactams

Beta-lactams and macrolides exhibit concentration-independent bactericidal effect against susceptible bacteria. Therefore, the time or duration of concentration above the MIC is most predictive of efficacy for these antibiotics.

50. A. Magnesium 2 g IV bolus

Magnesium is the drug of choice in the setting of torsades de pointes.

51. C. Oral vancomycin 125 mg 4 times daily

Per clinical guidelines, oral vancomycin 125 mg 4 times daily up to 10 days is the preferred choice for non-fulminant (not severe or complicated) *Clostridium difficile* infections. An alternative is fidaxomicin 200 mg twice daily by mouth for 10 days. Metronidazole may be used for *Clostridium difficile* infections, but only in combination with vancomycin. This treatment combination is more for fulminant infections (severe and complicated). Studies have shown metronidazole is poorly absorbed, especially in the geriatric population. Vancomycin administered intravenously will not achieve high enough concentration within the gut. Antidiarrheal drugs would extend the toxin-related damage and worsen the course of pseudomembranous colitis caused by *Clostridium difficile*.

52. B. Orlistat

Orlistat decreases the oral absorption of vitamin D. Aspirin, lidocaine, and digoxin have not been reported to interact with vitamin D. Phenobarbital and Dilantin® (phenytoin), affect vitamin D metabolism and affect calcium absorption. So do anti-tuberculosis drugs. On the other hand, cholesterol-lowering statin drugs and thiazide diuretics increase vitamin D.

53. C. Flurazepam

The optimal drug therapy for this patient would treat anxiety and decrease sleep latency period. Flurazepam is a benzodiazepine that is rapidly absorbed; the parent drug has a relatively long half-life and is converted to an active metabolite. The rapid onset of flurazepam is useful for sleep induction and the long half-life and active metabolite will alleviate anxiety symptoms during the day after a single bedtime dose. Although triazolam has a rapid onset, it is quickly converted to inactive metabolites, thus would not alleviate anxiety symptoms during the day after a single dose. Zolpidem, ramelteon, and diphenhydramine all have hypnotic effect, but do not alleviate the symptoms of anxiety

54. A. Increase cyclosporine levels

Even though ketoconazole is well known for its potent inhibitory effect on the CYP450 enzyme, specifically CYP3A4, it is occasionally combined with cyclosporine, which is metabolized by CYP3A4, to achieve the same therapeutic effect but with a lower cyclosporine dose and drug cost.

55. B. Leucovorin should not be administered at a rate >160 mg/min

Leucovorin or folinic acid can prevent the side effects of a cancer medication called methotrexate. It can treat anemia caused by a lack of folic acid. It is also used in supportive care of patients with colon cancer and to treat overdoses of certain medicines. It should not be administered at a rate greater than 160 mg/min due to calcium content of the solution.

56. A. Ampicillin and gentamicin

Ampicillin provides appropriate empiric coverage for *Listeria monocytogenes* and *Streptococcus agalactiae* (may cover some aerobic gram-negative bacilli as well). Gentamicin provides appropriate empiric coverage against aerobic gram-negative bacilli (and some synergy with ampicillin against gram-positives, like *L. monocytogenes*). Ampicillin and cefotaxime would also be an appropriate regimen. While gentamicin is appropriate, this regimen is missing first-line empiric coverage for *L. monocytogenes* (i.e., ampicillin). Also, ceftriaxone is not a first-line agent for bacterial meningitis in neonates (≤28 days) due to risk of adverse events, for example, biliary sludging, kernicterus, and potentially life-threatening precipitation with calcium-containing products. While cefotaxime is appropriate, this regimen is missing empiric coverage for *L. monocytogenes* (i.e., ampicillin). Also, vancomycin is broader empiric Gram-positive coverage than is generally needed for neonates. While ampicillin is appropriate, cefotaxime is the preferred third-generation cephalosporin in neonates. Ceftriaxone is not a first-line agent for bacterial meningitis in neonates (≤28 days) due to risk of adverse events, for example, biliary sludging, kernicterus, and precipitation potentially life-threatening with calcium-containing products.

57. C. Water retention and osteoporosis

Water retention and osteoporosis both are adverse effects specific to corticosteroids. Water retention leads to weight gain and hypertension. It is important to ensure adequate calcium intake and screening for bone mineral density in patients taking corticosteroids chronically.

58. A. Attempt immediate IV-line placement and administer antibiotics IV for the duration of therapy

IV therapy is the preferred route for antimicrobial treatment of CNS infections in order to ensure optimal CNS penetration (including allowing for administration of high-dose regimens).

59. B. Diphenhydramine, dexamethasone, ranitidine

Paclitaxel is associated with severe hypersensitivity reactions. If a hypersensitivity reaction occurs stop the infusion and do not re-challenge if the patient experienced hypotension requiring treatment or angioedema. Premedication with dexamethasone, diphenhydramine, and ranitidine is recommended.

60. B, E

Efavirenz and nevirapine are NNRTIs. Dual NNRTI therapy is contraindicated. Truvada and Atripla are complete HIV regimens, dual therapy is also contraindicated here.

61. C. Procarbazine

Procarbazine may have a disulfiram reaction when a patient consumes alcohol. Procarbazine has a lot of unique drug/food interaction. Procarbazine possesses monoamine oxidase inhibitor activity and has the potential for severe food and drug interactions (e.g., tyramine containing foods leading to hypertensive crisis).

62. A, E

Atazanavir requires an acidic environment for optimal absorption. In treatment experienced patients, combination therapy with proton pump inhibitors is contraindicated. In treatment naïve patients, doses of omeprazole 20 mg equivalence or less, may be used *with caution*. The risk versus benefit should be weighed when combining these agents.

63. B. Cytarabine + idarubicin

The most active agents in AML are anthracyclines and the antimetabolite cytarabine. Cytarabine in combination with idarubicin is often referred to as "7+3" regimen (cytarabine 100 mg/m^2 days 1-7, idarubicin 12 mg/m^2 days 1-3). Accounting for age, other comorbidities, and patient's ejection fraction, this combination should be recommended for initial induction therapy.

64. B. Toxoplasmosis

Diagnosis of Toxoplasmosis can be made by seropositivity for IgG, diagnosis of candidiasis can be made by evaluation of risk factors and isolating a Candida species from a culture, diagnosis of MAC can be made by a positive acid fast bacilli (AFB) culture from a blood specimen, diagnosis of PCP can be made by polymerase chain reaction (PCR) procedures.

65. A. Azithromycin

Azithromycin may be utilized as MAC primary prophylaxis. Clarithromycin may be utilized as MAC primary prophylaxis; however, clarithromycin should not be administered to a patient receiving simvastatin because of a drug interaction and increased risk of rhabdomyolysis.

66. C. To provide coverage against resistant *Streptococcus pneumoniae*

While third-generation cephalosporins, for example, ceftriaxone, provide adequate coverage against most isolates of *S. pneumoniae*, some resistance has been reported. Vancomycin is added to provide empiric coverage against these resistant strains of *S. pneumonia*.

67. A. Bacterial meningitis

Elevated WBC (1000-10,000 cells/mm^3), predominance of neutrophils (80%-90%), and elevated CSF protein (>100 mg/dL) as well as low CSF glucose (<40 mg/dL, and a likely CSF:serum glucose ratio of ≤0.4) are all consistent with bacterial meningitis.

68. D. MCV4

MCV4 is the specific formulation of the meningococcal vaccine recommended as a routine vaccination for adolescents aged 11 to 12 years, with a booster dose at age 16 years. MCV4 is also recommended for children aged 2 months to 10 years, if risk factors for meningococcal disease are present, such as persistent complement deficiencies, anatomic or functional asplenia (e.g., sickle cell disease), presence during an outbreak caused by a vaccine serogroup, or travel to the African meningitis belt or to the Hajj.

69. C. Vancomycin, ceftriaxone, and ampicillin

Ceftriaxone provides appropriate empiric coverage for *N. meningitidis*, aerobic gram-negative bacilli, and most *S. pneumoniae*. Vancomycin provides additional empiric coverage for multidrug-resistant *S. pneumoniae*. Ampicillin provides additional empiric coverage for *L. monocytogenes*. Even though the patient has a penicillin allergy, he does not display any major life threatening symptoms and should be treated as meningitis is a life threatening disease.

70. B. Combination hydralazine 25 mg and isosorbide dinitrate 10 mg TID

The combination of hydralazine and isosorbide dinitrate has demonstrated a significant mortality benefit in African Americans receiving optimal HF therapy with β-blockers and ACE inhibitors.

71. B. Metoprolol succinate

Only three β-blockers have been demonstrated to reduce mortality in heart failure: carvedilol, metoprolol succinate, and bisoprolol. Metoprolol succinate is the correct answer because it has a proven mortality benefit in HFrEF and it is a cardioselective β-blocker. While metoprolol is β-1 selective, it is important to recognize that β-receptor selectivity may decrease as the dose is up titrated.

72. A, B, C, D

The brand name of Orlistat is Xenical® not Xeniteel.

73. B. Pulmonary Arterial Hypertension

ADCIRCA is a prescription medicine called a phosphodiesterase 5 inhibitor used to treat pulmonary arterial hypertension (PAH, high blood pressure in your lungs) to improve exercise ability.

74. C. Medium-dose ICS and LABA

The patient is exhibiting severe persistent asthma which requires high-dose steps 4 to 6 combination therapy.

75. B. Budesonide/Formoterol

Current 2016 list of inhaled asthma medication combinations containing both a corticosteroid and a bronchodilator:
- Fluticasone and salmeterol (Advair Diskus®)
- Budesonide and formoterol (Symbicort®)
- Mometasone and formoterol (Dulera®)
- Fluticasone and vilanterol (Breo®)

76. A, B, D

The medications used for the treatment of pinworm are either mebendazole, pyrantel pamoate, or albendazole. Any of these drugs are given in one dose initially, and then another single dose two weeks later. Pyrantel pamoate is available without prescription. The medication does not reliably kill pinworm eggs

77. A. Vitamin K1

Phytonadione or Vitamin K1 is used to reverse warfarin effects:

- INR 4.5-10, no bleeding: 2012 ACCP guidelines suggest against routine use; 2008 ACCP guidelines suggest considering vitamin K1 (phytonadione) 1-2.5 mg PO once
- INR >10, no bleeding: 2012 ACCP guidelines recommend vitamin K1 PO (dose not specified); 2008 ACCP guidelines suggest 2.5-5 mg PO once; INR reduction observed within 24-48 hr, monitor INR and give additional vitamin K if needed
- Minor bleeding, any elevated INR: Consider 2.5-5 mg PO once; may repeat if needed after 24 hr
- Major bleeding, any elevated INR: 2012 ACCP guidelines recommend prothrombin complex concentrate, human (PCC, Kcentra) plus vitamin K1 5-10 mg IV (dilute in 50 mL IV fluid and infuse over 20 min)

NOTE: High vitamin K doses (≥10 mg) may cause warfarin resistance for a week or more; consider using heparin, LMWH, or direct thrombin inhibitors to provide adequate thrombosis prophylaxis in clinical conditions requiring chronic anticoagulation therapy.

78. C. H. Pylori

PYLERA® capsules are used to treat H. Pylori infections and are a combination antimicrobial product containing bismuth subcitrate potassium, metronidazole, and tetracycline hydrochloride for oral administration. Each size 0 elongated capsule contains:
- Bismuth subcitrate potassium, 140 mg
- Metronidazole, 125 mg
- Smaller capsule (size 3) containing tetracycline hydrochloride, 125 mg

Tetracycline hydrochloride is encapsulated within a smaller capsule to create a barrier to avoid contact with bismuth subcitrate potassium

79. All of the above (A-E)

ESAs stimulate the bone marrow to make more red blood cells and are FDA approved for use in reducing the need for blood transfusions in patients with chronic kidney failure, cancer patients on chemotherapy, patients scheduled for major surgery (except heart surgery) and patients with HIV who are using AZT.

The following types of ESAs are available:
- Erythropoietin (Epo)
- Epoetin alfa (Procrit/Epogen)
- Epoetin beta (NeoRecormon)
- Darbepoetin alfa (Aranesp)
- Methoxy polyethylene glycol-epoetin beta (Mircera)

80. A, B, C

Alzheimer's disease (AD) is a progressive dementia with loss of neurons and the presence of two main microscopic neuropathological hallmarks: extracellular amyloid plaques and intracellular neurofibrillary tangles. This leads to interrupted neuron signaling and altered neurotransmitters

81. A, B, C, D

Short-intermediate acting benzodiazepine receptor agonist benzodiazepines (BzRA BZDs) are first-line therapy options for most patients and should be limited for 7-10 days for insomnia. A-D present short-intermediate acting benzodiazepines whereas choice E. Alprazolam is a short-acting benzodiazepine that may lead to dependence

82. A. Every two weeks

RISPERDAL CONSTA® is a long-acting injectable medication for Bipolar I Disorder and significantly delayed time to relapse, and is administered by a healthcare provider

83. B. Geodon, Zyprexa

Geodon® is ziprasidone, and Zyprexa® is olanzapine. Seroquel® is quetiapine.

84. A. Levonorgestrel 1.5 mg

Plan B One-Step® is levonorgestrel 1.5 mg take 1 pill within 120 hours after unprotected sex. Ella is ulipristal acetate 30 mg take 1 pill within 120 hours after unprotected sex. Plan B® is unrestricted so anyone can buy this medication.

85. All of the above (A-E)

A thyroid panel is used to evaluate thyroid function and/or help diagnose hypothyroidism and hyperthyroidism due to various thyroid disorders. The panel typically includes tests for:
- Thyroid-stimulating hormone (TSH)
- Free thyroxine (free T4)
- Total or free triiodothyronine (total or free T3)

T4 and T3 are hormones produced by the thyroid gland. They help control the rate at which the body uses energy and are regulated by a feedback system. TSH from the pituitary gland stimulates the production and release of T4 (primarily) and T3 by the thyroid. Most of the T4 and T3 circulate in the blood bound to protein. A small percentage is free (not bound) and is the biologically active form of the hormones.
The free T4 test is thought by many to be a more accurate reflection of thyroid hormone function and, in most cases, its use has replaced that of the total T4 test

86. A, C, D, E

Managing hypothyroidism requires getting a precise dose of medicine day after day. This precision is important because thyroid replacement therapy is a type of medication called a narrow therapeutic index (NTI) drug. With NTI drugs, if your dose is off even a little bit, you could experience symptoms of under-replacement (not enough medicine) or symptoms of over-replacement (too much medicine). Choice B is not correct as it allows for changes in the dose and drug levels. It's best to advise the patient to take Synthroid early in the morning 30-60 minutes before eating breakfast

87. B, C, E

Warfarin Table Identification

Tablet Strength	Tablet Color
1 mg	Pink
2 mg	Lavender (light purple)
2.5 mg	Green
3 mg	Tan
4 mg	Blue
5 mg	Peach (light orange)
6 mg	Teal (blue-green)
7.5 mg	Yellow
10 mg	White

88. A, C, D, E

Tricyclic antidepressants (TCAs) are used primarily as antidepressants. They are named after their chemical structure, which contains three rings of atoms. Tetracyclic antidepressants (TeCAs), which contain four rings of atoms.

89. A, B, D, E

All of the following are correct except C. Ibandronate should not be taken with mineral water, only plain water due to potential absorption and interaction effects.

90. A, B, D

Plavix® (clopidogrel) is a prodrug that is absorbed in the intestines. Effient® (prasugrel) is also metabolized in the intestine. Plavix® is a second-generation thienopyridine (prodrug), whereas Effient® is a third-generation thienopyridine (prodrug).

91. A. CDC Pink Book, Trissel's handbook

CDC Yellow Book is CDC's reference book on how devices and international travelers on health risk. Remington's provides compounding, manufacturing, and non-sterile compounding stability. Briggs Drugs [in Pregnancy and Lactation] provides information on pregnancy and lactation. The Sanford Guide provides antimicrobial information, and the NLM provides a database of product package inserts.

92. D. Dopamine agonist

Pramipexole is a non-ergot dopamine agonist with high relative *in vitro* specificity and full intrinsic activity at the D subfamily of dopamine receptors, binding with higher affinity to D3 than to D2 or D4 receptor subtypes.

93. A, B, E

Amantadine and modafinil are used to treat fatigue in patients with MS. Pemoline is no longer used as it has severe liver toxicity. The rest are used in MS, brand name of Fingolimod is Gilenya®.

94. A. Montelukast 4 mg, leukotriene receptor antagonist, Singulair®

The brand name of montelukast is Singulair® and the mechanism of action is a leukotriene receptor antagonist to relieve symptoms of seasonal allergies. Accolate® is another leukotriene receptor antagonist (generic is zafirlukast) and Zyflo® (generic zileuton) inhibits the 5-lipoxygenase enzyme. 15 years and older: one 10-mg tablet. 6 to 14 years: one 5-mg chewable tablet. 6 to 23 months: one packet of 4-mg oral granules. Patients with both asthma and allergic rhinitis should take only one dose daily in the evening.

95. C, D, E

Risperidone or Risperdal® is indicated based off the PI:

- Treatment of schizophrenia
- As monotherapy or adjunctive therapy with lithium or valproate, for the treatment of acute manic or mixed episodes associated with Bipolar I Disorder
- Treatment of irritability associated with autistic disorder

96. A, B, C

Based on current CDC guidelines and the patient information provided, the **influenza, Td/Tdap, and PCV20** vaccinations are recommended at this time.

- Since the patient has already received a Shingles vaccine (Zoster), he does not need to receive it again. The Zoster vaccine is only given once and recommended for adults 60 and older
- The CDC recommends either PCV15 or PCV20 for adults 65 years and older. This would be ideal for a 72-year-old patient with limited immunization history
- The CDC recommends a dose of either Td or Tdap every 10 years, or every five years in the case of a severe dirty wound or burn.
- The CDC states that persons six months and older should receive an annual flu vaccine. This season, the recommended flu vaccines are FluZone High-Dose Quadrivalent, FluBlok Quadrivalent, and the FLUAD Quadrivalent Adjuvanted influenza vaccines.

For more information about vaccine guidelines, please see the CDC website for the most up-to-date recommendations.

97. A, C, D, E

Based off the 2016 CDC vaccine guidelines, the patient should avoid live vaccines especially with a CD4 count less than 200. However, she may get the Td/Tdap vaccine. If she had a CD4 count greater than 200 then she would be okay to receive all the vaccines.

98. All the above (A-E)

All of the above are recommended based off 2016 CDC vaccine guidelines.

99. C. Flucelvax Quadrivalent vaccine

Because children younger than five years old are at a heightened risk of developing serious influenza-related complications, an annual influenza vaccine is recommended for children six months and older. **Flucelvax Quadrivalent** is a cell-based flu vaccine approved for people six months and older. It is also completely egg-free, making it the best option for **Jeffe.**

100. A, E

Sevelamer is a phosphate-binding drug used to treat hyperphosphatemia in patients with chronic kidney disease. When taken with meals, it binds to dietary phosphate and prevents its absorption. The brand name of sevelamer is Renagel® for sevelamer hydrochloride or Renvela® for sevelamer carbonate. Cinacalcet is a drug that acts as a calcimimetic (i.e., it mimics the action of calcium on tissues) by allosteric activation of the calcium-sensing receptor that is expressed in various human organ tissues to treat secondary hyperparathyroidism in CKD patients on dialysis and severe hypercalcemia in patients with primary hyperparathyroidism. The brand name is Sensipar®. Pamidronate and Fosamax® are bisphosphates to help lower calcium serum levels in the body.

101. B, D

On starting the infusion, there is no drug in the body and therefore, no elimination. The amount of drug in the body then rises, but as the drug concentration increases, so does the rate of elimination. Thus, the rate of elimination will keep rising until it matches the rate of infusion. The amount of drug in the body is then constant and is said to have reached a steady state or plateau. The factors affecting the steady state plasma drug concentration are:
- Infusion rate (R_o): The steady state drug concentration is proportional to the infusion rate. Thus, a higher infusion rate will result in a higher steady state plasma drug concentration
- Clearance: Higher clearance of the drug will result in lower plasma drug concentration at plateau

The time to reach the plateau is determined by the elimination half-life of the drug, which results from clearance and volume of distribution. Thus, the V_d does not influence the steady state concentration but merely the time required to approach the plateau. After 4 elimination half-lives the drug plasma concentration is 93,75% of the steady state plasma concentration. Likewise, when changing infusion rates, the time required to reach the new steady state also depends on the half-life of the drug.

102. B, E

JR's dose of metformin can be doubled and switching from glyburide which is considered a high risk medication due to weight gain and higher rates of hypoglycemia vs. the second generations such as glimepiride and glipizide. The FDA in April 2016 has required labeling changes that replace serum creatinine (SCr) with estimated glomerular filtration rate (eGFR) as the parameter used to determine the appropriateness of treatment with the biguanide metformin (Glucophage, and others) in patients with renal impairment.

Metformin was previously contraindicated in women with a SCr level $\geq$1.4 mg/dL and in men with a SCr level $\geq$1.5 mg/dL, but use of SCr as a surrogate indicator tends to underestimate renal function in certain populations (e.g., younger patients, men, black patients, patients with greater muscle mass). The calculation of eGFR takes into account age, race, and sex, as well as SCr level, providing a more accurate assessment of kidney function. The eGFR should be calculated before patients begin treatment with metformin and at least annually thereafter. Metformin is now contraindicated in patients with an eGFR <30 mL/min/1.73 m^2 and starting treatment with the drug in patients with an eGFR between 30 and 45 mL/min/1.73 m^2 is not recommended. If the eGFR falls below 45 mL/min/1.73 m^2 in a patient already taking metformin, the benefits and risks of continuing treatment should be assessed. Metformin should not be administered for 48 hours after an iodinated contrast imaging procedure in patients with an eGFR <60 mL/min/1.73 m^2 or a history of liver disease, alcoholism, or heart failure, or in those receiving intra-arterial contrast, and the eGFR should be re-evaluated before treatment is restarted.

103. D. Oxacillin

Penicillins such as oxacillin and nafcillin as well as cefazolin which are used more to treat MSSA infections will not be effective for MRSA infections.

104. B. Claritin®

Fexofenadine (Allegra®) is the least sedating even at higher doses but is considered a pregnancy category C. Claritin® (loratadine) is sedating at higher doses but it is less potent than Allegra® and Zyrtec®. Desloratadine (Clarinex®) is pregnancy category C, and Zyrtec® (cetirizine) may be sedating even at normally recommended doses due to the hydroxyzine analog although it is more potent as well. Pregnancy category B agents are Zyrtec®, Claritin®, and Xyzal® (levocetirizine). Chlorpheniramine is a first-generation antihistamine that causes a lot of sedative side effects.

105. C, D

Only Lantus® and Toujeo® can be left outside of the refrigerator, at room temperature, up to 28 days. Novolin R® or N® and Levemir® can be left out of the refrigerator for up to 42 days.

106. A. Glargine

Only Lantus® (insulin glargine) is a long-acting insulin that has a constant peak. Levemir has a peak at 6-8 hours, Novolin N® 4-14 hours, Novolin R® 2.5-5 hours, Apidra® 30-60 minutes.

107. A. Topiramate

Topiramate IR (immediate release) comes in sprinkle capsules as well as Depakote® that comes in a sprinkle formulation (divalproex sprinkles).

108. A. Propranolol

Propranolol, metoprolol, timolol, and nebivolol all have high lipophilicity which means it's easier for these drugs to bypass the blood brain barrier and enter the brain. This may cause suicidal thoughts. Review the pharmacist letter PL Detail Document #281201.

109. D. Daytrana

For JR, he is taking a methylphenidate long acting release medication, Concerta®, and is failing treatment and also notes he does not like taking the oral version of the medication. It may be beneficial to recommend Daytrana which is also long-acting formulation of methylphenidate but comes in a patch version. Ritalin® and Focalin® are short-acting methylphenidate derivatives, and Adderall® is an amphetamine short-acting derivative. Intuniv® is a non-stimulant guanfacine.

View: http://www.adhdmedicationguide.com/pdf/adhd_med_guide_081216.pdf

110. C. Restoring normal sinus rhythm control

Digoxin is a cardiac glycoside used in atrial fibrillation, heart failure, and atrial flutter. Digoxin is useful in controlling normal sinus rhythm response but has shown a lack of mortality benefit and may increase the risk of death. Digoxin is no longer used first line for heart failure but is useful for symptomatic relief for patients who are already on an ACE inhibitor and diuretic.

111. All of the above (A-E)

Medications in this class that do not cause QT prolongation are: Vraylar®, Rexulti® and Latuda®.

112. D. Kava is not safe due to hepatotoxicity and should be avoided

Kava has been safely used in clinical trials, short-term. But there is concern that kava extracts might not be safe. Kava has been linked to over 100 reports of hepatotoxicity, including reports of liver transplantation and death. Hepatotoxicity has been reported in some patients after as little as 3-4 weeks of use, even in normal doses. "Slow metabolizers" or those patients deficient in cytochrome P450 2D6 are theorized to be more susceptible. Due to these safety concerns, kava has been banned from the market in some countries

113. D. Feverfew

Feverfew (*Tanacetum parthenium*) is the most well-known natural medicine used to prevent migraine. Current theories are that feverfew inhibits platelet aggregation, serotonin release, leukotrienes, and prostaglandin synthesis. Most evidence suggests that feverfew can reduce the frequency of migraines, and when migraines do occur, they tend to have less severe symptoms of pain, nausea, vomiting, and sensitivity to light and noise. It might be more effective in patients who have more frequent migraine headaches.

114. C. There is no association between vaccines and autism

Between 1999 and 2001, thimerosal was removed or reduced to trace amounts in all childhood vaccines except for some flu vaccines. This was done as part of a broader national effort to reduce all types of mercury exposure in children before studies were conducted that determined that thimerosal was not harmful. It was done as a precaution. Currently, the only childhood vaccines that contain thimerosal are flu vaccines packaged in multidose vials. Thimerosal-free alternatives are also available for flu vaccine. A 2013 CDC study added to research showing that vaccines do not cause autism in children with the study population the first two years of life

115. B. Fentanyl should not be dispensed as Brock is opioid naïve and be at a high risk of respiratory depression and possibly death

Transdermal fentanyl "patches" should only be used in patients who are already receiving opioid therapy and who have demonstrated tolerance and who are not opioid naive. Giving potent, long-acting opioids like a fentanyl patch to opioid naive patients has resulted in deaths. Thus, fentanyl patches should NOT be used for acute pain

116. Click the following areas:

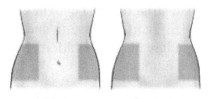

Anterior view   Posterior view
FIGURE 29-11. Sites for administration of enoxaparin.

117. E. Quetiapine

First-generation antipsychotics have a high rate of extrapyramidal side effects, including rigidity, bradykinesia, dystonias, tremor, and akathisia. Tardive dyskinesia (TD)—that is, involuntary movements in the face and extremities—is another adverse effect that can occur with first-generation antipsychotics. Second-generation (novel or atypical) antipsychotics, with the exception of aripiprazole, are dopamine D2 antagonists, but are associated with lower rates of extrapyramidal adverse effects and TD than the first-generation antipsychotics. However, they have higher rates of metabolic adverse effects and weight gain

118. D. Normal saline and hydrogen peroxide

The tracheostomy inner cannula tube should be cleaned two to three times per day or more as needed. Procedure:
1. Wash your hands.
2. Place 1/2 strength peroxide solution in one bowl and sterile salt water in second bowl.
3. Remove the inner cannula while holding the neck plate of the trach still.
4. Place inner cannula in peroxide solution and soak until crusts are softened or removed.
5. Use the brush or pipe cleaner to clean the inside, outside and creases of the tube.
6. Do not use scouring powder or Brillo® pads.
7. Look inside the inner cannula to make sure it is clean and clear of mucus.
8. Rinse tube in saline or sterile salt water.

119. A. Diarrhea

Diarrhea is a common response to high doses of sorbitol. Sorbitol can also cause: nausea, vomiting, gas, and stomach discomfort

120. D. Clopidogrel does interact with PPIs but it only applies to omeprazole

The U.S. Food and Drug Administration (FDA) is reminding the public that it continues to warn against the concomitant use of Plavix (clopidogrel) and omeprazole because the co-administration can result in significant reductions in clopidogrel's active metabolite levels and antiplatelet activity. This information was added to the drug label of Plavix in November 2009, and has been the source of continued discussion in the medical literature

121. 2.33

$$BSA = \sqrt{\frac{height\ (cm) \times weight\ (kg)}{3600}} \rightarrow \sqrt{\frac{175.26 \times 112}{3600}} = 2.33\ m^2$$

122. 1.72

$$BSA = \sqrt{\frac{height\ (cm) \times weight\ (kg)}{3600}} \rightarrow \sqrt{\frac{160 \times 66.4}{3600}} = 1.72\ m^2$$

123. C. FDA

A drug recall occurs when a prescription or over-the-counter medicine is removed from the market because it is found to be either defective or potentially harmful. Sometimes, the makers of the drug will discover a problem with their drug and voluntarily recall it. Recalls may be conducted on a firm's own initiative, by FDA request, or by FDA order under statutory authority. Class I recall: a situation in which there is a reasonable probability that the use of or exposure to a violative product will cause serious adverse health consequences or death. Class II Recall is a situation in which use of, or exposure to, a violative product may cause temporary or medically reversible adverse health consequences or where the probability of serious adverse health consequences is remote

124. A. Acute Sinusitis

The 2015 guidelines by the American Academy of Otolaryngology recommend either offer watchful waiting (without antibiotics) or prescribe initial antibiotic therapy for adults with uncomplicated acute bacterial rhinosinusitis or prescribe amoxicillin with or without clavulanate as first-line therapy for 5-10 days (if the decision is made to treat acute bacterial rhinosinusitis with an antibiotic). Nasal steroids such as fluticasone (Flonase®) or beclomethasone (Beconase®) may be added to help counter inflammation

125. C. Syphilis

Herpes is a virus and is treated by antivirals such as acyclovir. Chlamydia and urethritis are usually treated with azithromycin or doxycycline. Syphilis can be treated similarly to gonorrhea in using Penicillin G. HIV is a virus as well that is treated with antivirals such as Genvoya®.

126. B. Docusate

A surfactant is a compound that reduces the surface tension when dissolved in water and helps to increase the solubility of organic compounds. Docusate is an example of a surfactant. Psyllium is a bulk laxative used in the treatment of constipation. Senna and bisacodyl are stimulant laxatives, while milk of magnesia (magnesium hydroxide) acts as a laxative via promotion of electrolyte secretion in the gut.

127. A. Lamivudine

Because emtricitabine (FTC), lamivudine (3TC), tenofovir disoproxil fumarate (TDF) and tenofovir alafenamide (TAF) have activity against both HIV and HBV, for patients co-infected with HIV and HBV, ART should be initiated with the fixed-dose combination of TDF/FTC or TAF/FTC, or the individual drug combinations of TDF plus 3TC as the nucleoside reverse transcriptase inhibitor (NRTI) backbone of a fully suppressive antiretroviral (ARV) regimen.

128. D. Tenofovir alafenamide

Tenofovir disoproxil fumarate, tenofovir alafenamide, lamivudine, emtricitabine, abacavir, and rilpivirine are examples of medications that may be used in combination to treat Hepatitis C infections.

Daclatasvir: The NS5A inhibitor daclatasvir is a substrate of CYP3A. When daclatasvir is given with a CYP3A inhibitor, the levels of daclatasvir can increase, particularly with strong inhibitors of CYP3A. The dose of daclatasvir should therefore be reduced to 30 mg when used with either ritonavir-boosted atazanavir or lopinavir. In contrast, when used with efavirenz, a CYP3A inducer, the dose of daclatasvir should be increased to 90 mg daily.

Ledipasvir-Sofosbuvir: The NS5A inhibitor ledipasvir is not metabolized by the cytochrome P450 system but is a substrate of p-glycoprotein. Ledipasvir increases tenofovir levels by 1.3 to 2.6 fold when concomitantly given with either rilpivirine or efavirenz. Although ledipasvir administered concomitantly with tenofovir and an HIV protease inhibitor has not been studied, there is concern that tenofovir levels may increase substantially with this combination. Because of this concern and lack of data, the use of ledipasvir with ritonavir- boosted HIV protease inhibitors should, if possible, be avoided. For similar reasons, ledipasvir- sofosbuvir should not be used with cobicistat, elvitegravir, or tipranavir. Ledipasvir-sofosbuvir should not be used in HIV-infected patients on tenofovir if the baseline creatinine clearance is less than 60 mL/min.

Ombitasvir-Paritaprevir-Ritonavir: The major concern for drug interaction with this regimen is the significant P450 inhibition generated by ritonavir. This combination regimen should not be used with efavirenz, rilpivirine, darunavir, or lopinavir-ritonavir.

Ombitasvir-Paritaprevir-Ritonavir and Dasabuvir: The major concern for drug interaction with this regimen is the significant P450 inhibition generated by ritonavir. This combination regimen should not be used with efavirenz, rilpivirine, darunavir, or lopinavir- ritonavir.

Ribavirin: Significant and serious toxic drug-drug interactions and severe toxicities can occur with the simultaneous use of ribavirin and certain HIV nucleoside reverse transcriptase inhibitors. The use of ribavirin with didanosine is strictly contraindicated due to a marked increase in intracellular didanosine levels, which may cause hepatic failure, pancreatitis, and lactic acidosis. This can also occur with stavudine or zidovudine. Thus, simultaneous use of ribavirin with either didanosine, stavudine, or zidovudine should be avoided. Concurrent use of ribavirin and zidovudine should also be avoided because of additive hematologic toxicity and increased risk of severe anemia with this combination.

129. A. SQ

Interferons such as peginterferon alfa-2a is administered SQ to the following injection sites-

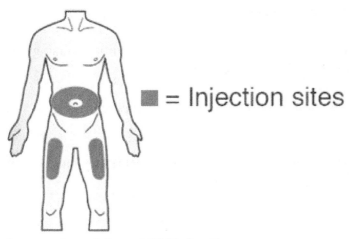

Image adapted from AIDSinfo.nih.gov

130. D. Ethambutol

Ethambutol is not typically included in a child's regimen because of the potential inability to adequately assess visual acuity. Changes in visual acuity and color vision need to be assessed during ethambutol therapy due to the drug having potential to cause retrobulbar neuritis.

131. A. Isoniazid 300 mg daily × 9 months

The patient does not have any symptoms or indications of active TB disease; so he needs treatment for latent TB infection. This is the correct first-line regimen for treatment of latent TB infection.

132. A. They retain their stained color with acid-alcohol washes

Acid-fast bacteria keep their stain color despite acid-alcohol washes. *Mycobacterium tuberculosis* is acid fast.

133. D. Immediately; do not wait for treatment

People with latent TB infection do not have symptoms, and they cannot spread TB bacteria to others. However, if TB bacteria become active in the body and multiply, the person will go from having latent TB infection to being sick with TB disease. For this reason, people with latent TB infection are often prescribed treatment to prevent them from developing TB disease. Treatment of latent TB infection is essential for controlling and eliminating TB in the United States. Treatment of latent TB infection should be initiated after the possibility of TB disease has been excluded.

People with a positive IGRA result or a TST reaction of 5 or more millimeters
- HIV-infected persons
- Recent contacts of a TB case
- Persons with fibrotic changes on chest radiograph consistent with old TB
- Organ transplant recipients
- Persons who are immunosuppressed for other reasons (e.g., taking the equivalent of >15 mg/day of prednisone for 1 month or longer, taking TNF-α antagonists)

People with a positive IGRA result or a TST reaction of 10 or more millimeters

- Recent immigrants (< 5 years) from high-prevalence countries
- Injection drug users
- Residents and employees of high-risk congregate settings (e.g., correctional facilities, nursing homes, homeless shelters, hospitals, and other health care facilities)
- Mycobacteriology laboratory personnel
- Children under 4 years of age, or children and adolescents exposed to adults in high-risk categories

Persons with no known risk factors for TB may be considered for treatment of LTBI if they have either a positive IGRA result or if their reaction to the TST is 15 mm or larger

134. C. INR 2.5

Jamie's INR target is 2.5 with a range of 2.0 – 3.0 for DVT and PE treatment. Anticoagulant therapy is recommended for 3-12 months depending on site of thrombosis and on the ongoing presence of risk factors. If DVT recurs, if a chronic hypercoagulability is identified, or if PE is life threatening, lifetime anticoagulation therapy may be recommended. This treatment protocol has a cumulative risk of bleeding complications of less than 12%.

135. A. Enoxaparin SQ 112 mg every 12 hours

Jamie is considered obese with a BMI of 43.6. Enoxaparin labeling indicates to use actual body weight when calculating for dosing, thus Jamie is 112 kg (246 lbs/2.2) and the dosing is 1 mg/kg/dose x 12 hours. Xarelto is prescribed as 15 mg twice daily with food for 21 days followed by 20 mg once daily with food for at least 3 months' duration. Pradaxa is given 150 mg twice daily after 5 to 10 days of parenteral anticoagulation.

136. D. Direct stimulation of postsynaptic dopamine receptors

Dopamine agonists bypass the nigrostriatal neurons and provide direct receptor stimulation exerting effects like dopamine.

137. E. Quetiapine

Quetiapine has a low likelihood to cause or exacerbate symptoms of Parkinson disease. The other antipsychotics are known to exacerbate movement disorders. Alprazolam is just a benzodiazepine and is not appropriate to treat psychosis.

138. A. Selegiline

Selegiline has an amphetamine metabolite and has been associated with an increased incidence of insomnia. Doses should be given no later than early afternoon to help prevent this side effect in a patient for whom it is indicated. In a patient with uncontrolled insomnia, the drug is best avoided.

139. C. Entacapone

Entacapone inhibits the action of catechol-*O*-methyltransferase in the periphery to avoid the breakdown of levodopa and dopamine before levodopa crosses the blood–brain barrier. It must be present with levodopa to achieve this outcome.

140. A. Carbidopa/levodopa, rotigotine, rasagiline

For patients with moderate to severe symptoms, carbidopa/levodopa is the preferred agent to initiate therapy. The addition of a dopamine agonist is appropriate as second-line therapy. The addition of an MAO-B inhibitor will help prolong the effects of dopamine by minimizing its metabolism by monoamine oxidase.

141. B. Sinemet is effective for many years and its loss of efficacy is due to the progression of the disease than with duration of treatment

It is a myth that Sinemet will lose its efficacy long-term. Levodopa is highly effective for many years, and its loss of efficacy has more to do with the progression of the disease than with the duration of treatment. Not all symptoms of PD respond to levodopa, and over time those symptoms become more prominent. As the disease progresses, people tend to develop more side-effects from levodopa.

142. B, C

For bare metal stents, aspirin at a dose of 162 to 325 mg per day for one month should be taken then 75 to 162 mg per day indefinitely. Plavix® (clopidogrel) 75 mg daily should be taken up to one year.

143. E, A, F, D, C, B

Garbing occurs in the ante area and should be sequenced from "dirtiest" to "cleanest":

1. Don shoe covers, hair and beard covers, and a mask.
2. Perform hand hygiene.
3. Don gown, fastened securely at the neck and wrists.
4. Sanitize hands using an ABHR and allow hands to dry.
5. Enter the buffer area (if facility layout dictates, this step may occur after the following two steps).
6. Don sterile powder-free gloves. Sanitize the gloves with application of 70% sterile IPA and allow gloves to dry.

144. D. Tylenol®

As the patient has poor renal function, it is not advisable to use NSAIDs and try Tylenol if that helps with his pain initially. Ibuprofen, naproxen, piroxicam, indomethacin, etodolac, sulindac and diclofenac are not recommended in patients with advanced renal disease (CrCl <30 mL/min)

145. B. Celebrex

For patients at risk for GI Ulceration and/or Bleeding, consider the following:

- All NSAIDs are associated with some level of increased risk for GI complications so it is best to use the lowest effective dose for the shortest duration of time
- Lowest risk for GI complications: ibuprofen and celecoxib
- Relatively low risk for GI complications: meloxicam, etodolac and nabumetone
- High (i.e., twice the risk associated with ibuprofen) for GI complications: naproxen, indomethacin and diclofenac
- Highest risk for GI complications: ketorolac and piroxicam

146. B. Use well-fitted walking shoes and inserts in addition to a pumice stone

Calluses occur more often and build up faster on the feet of people with diabetes. This is because there are high-pressure areas under the foot. Too much callus may mean that you will need therapeutic shoes and inserts. Calluses, if not trimmed, get very thick, break down, and turn into ulcers (open sores). Never try to cut calluses or corns yourself - this can lead to ulcers and infection. Let your health care provider cut your calluses. Also, do not try to remove calluses and corns with chemical agents. These products can burn your skin. Using a pumice stone every day will help keep calluses under control. It is best to use the pumice stone on wet skin. Put on lotion right after you use the pumice stone

147. A. Artificial Saliva

Treatment of dry mouth due to salivary gland hypofunction aims to alleviate symptoms and prevent complications such as dental caries, periodontal disease, halitosis, salivary gland calculi, dysphagia, and oral candidiasis. Various strategies are employed to compensate for the loss of normal salivary functions; these functions include lubricating the mucosa, helping to clear food residue that may lead to dental plaque and bacterial growth, buffering acids that favor demineralization of teeth, and providing antimicrobial effects. It's best to try artificial saliva and then if this is ineffective, move on to muscarinic agents such as pilocarpine and cevimeline. Chewing gum does help to produce saliva but in this member her salivary glands are not working. Tea and other acidic beverages due to acidity levels that affect dental enamel:

- Cola drinks – pH 2.6
- Coffee – pH 5.0
- Tea (herbal) – pH 3.2
- Tea (black) – pH 5.7 to 7.0
- Water from tap – pH 7.0 (but flavored waters are often acidic)
- Energy drinks – usually acidic

148. A. Tramadol

Cyproheptadine is an antidote to serotonin syndrome if benzodiazepines and supportive care fail to improve agitation and correct vital signs. Cyproheptadine is a histamine-1 receptor antagonist with nonspecific 5-HT1A and 5-HT2A antagonistic properties. It also has weak anticholinergic activity. Mirtazapine and bupropion have a very low risk of causing serotonin syndrome and Percocet does not have any activity on serotonin levels. Celebe is taking paroxetine- As with the other SSRIs, paroxetine is generally safe in overdose. Paroxetine ingestions had no symptoms, while common symptoms included vomiting, drowsiness, tremors, dizziness, and sinus tachycardia. Paroxetine has been associated rarely with brief, self-limited seizures and with an 18 percent incidence of developing serotonin syndrome in isolated ingestion, but rarely are cases severe. Among SSRIs, paroxetine has the highest rate of discontinuation syndrome because of its short half-life and lack of active metabolites. Symptoms are usually mild, lasting one to two weeks; they include nausea, dizziness, bad dreams, paresthesia, and a flu-like illness. Severe symptoms can occur and persist for prolonged periods, and may require restarting paroxetine.

149. E. Dopamine receptor antagonist

Risperdal® (risperidone) and Invega® are classified as prolactin-raising antipsychotics because their dopamine-blocking action can substantially increase levels of prolactin, a hormone released by the pituitary gland. In women, prolactin stimulates breast development and breast milk production. When high levels of prolactin are present in males, those excessive levels can prompt similar processes, resulting in gynecomastia, sometimes accompanied by galactorrhea (abnormal lactation). In severe cases, males have developed large, D-cup sized breasts. Risperdal® is usually prescribed to treat bipolar disorder and autism spectrum disorders.

150. C. Topical astringent and antiseptic

Aluminum acetate is produced when aluminum hydroxide reacts with acetic acid. The substance produced from this reaction is a salt that is white and water soluble. Utilized as a topical astringent and antiseptic in medicine, aluminum acetate may be prescribed by doctors for the treatment of many dermatologic conditions that can include poison ivy, rashes, athletes' foot and insect bites. Because aluminum acetate is a drying agent, it is a medication that may be beneficial for ear infections, such as external otitis.

151. A, E

HFA inhalers, more specifically their plastic actuators, need to be cleaned once weekly to ensure there is no debris or build up blocking the spray hole. CFC inhalers are no longer on the market due to ozone risk. Dry powder inhalers should not be washed and the canister should not be taken apart. Asthmanefrin is a handheld nebulizer device.

152. E. Doxazosin, alpha-1 adrenergic receptor blocker

Doxazosin, under the brand names Cardura and Carduran, is an α_1-selective alpha blocker used to treat high blood pressure and urinary retention with benign prostatic hyperplasia (BPH).

153. C. Ginger

Ginger is known to help with nausea, motion sickness, and upset stomach. Emetrol is an OTC medication that is a phosphorated sugar solution that provides a direct local effect on the GI tract in reducing smooth muscle contractions and delaying gastric emptying.

154. B. Indirect stimulation of alpha-adrenergic receptors

Cocaine causes indirect stimulation of the alpha-adrenergic receptors. Cocaine inhibits the cellular uptake of norepinephrine in the adrenergic neurons. Increased levels of norepinephrine result in enhanced sympathetic activity. Stimulation of the alpha-receptors on the coronary arteries produces vasoconstriction and myocardial ischemia.

155. D. Serotonin receptors

Ondansetron is a 5-HT3 receptor antagonist. As such, it blocks serotonin receptors in the gastrointestinal tract and central nervous system, and is useful in the management of nausea and vomiting occurring either postoperatively or induced by chemotherapeutic agents.

156. E. Hemorrhagic cystitis

Cyclophosphamide is metabolized to acrolein and this metabolite damages the bladder leading to hemorrhagic cystitis. Anthracyclines have cardiac toxicity, platinum agents have ototoxicity, and while antineoplastics cause myelosuppression the question asks about genitourinary effects.

157. C. Amifostine

Amifostine reduces the cumulative renal toxicity associated with repeated administration of cisplatin and reduces the incidence of moderate to severe xerostomia in patients undergoing postoperative radiation treatment for head and neck cancer.

158. B. Cisplatin

Cisplatin is associated with causing ototoxicity manifested by tinnitus or loss of high frequency hearing.

159. D. Metronidazole

Metronidazole and procarbazine may have a disulfiram reaction when a patient consumes alcohol. In addition, procarbazine has a lot of unique drug/food interaction. Procarbazine possesses monoamine oxidase inhibitor activity and has the potential for severe food and drug interactions (e.g., tyramine containing foods leading to hypertensive crisis).

160. View rectangle below; maraviroc is a CCR5 receptor blocker

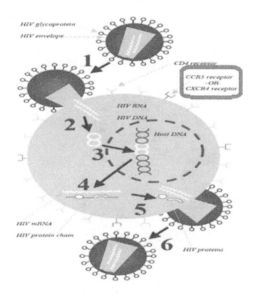

161. B. Urine may appear red, dark brown, or orange

This is a less common side effect of doxorubicin. Nail beds may turn darker, eyes watering, hair loss as chemotherapy agents destroy the fastest growing cells in body

162. View rectangle region below; efavirenz is an NNRTI

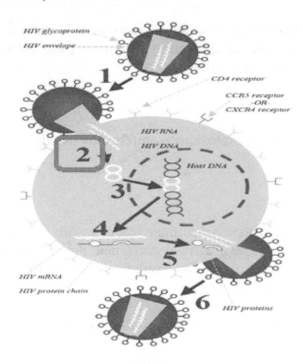

163. View rectangle below; raltegravir is an integrase inhibitor

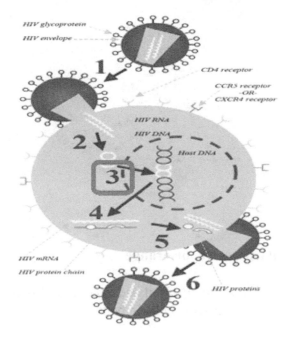

164. View rectangle below; clopidogrel irreversibly binds to P2Y₁₂, an adenosine diphosphate chemoreceptor on platelet cell membranes

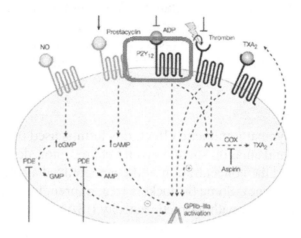

165. View rectangle below; Eptifibatide or Integrillin is an inhibitor of GPIIb/IIIa

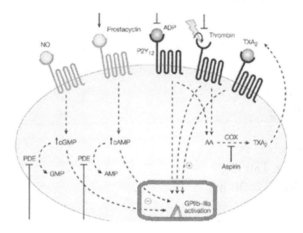

166. C. 16 mg

Tablets, capsules, and liquid:
- Initial: 4 mg orally after the first loose stool, then
- Maintenance: 2 mg after each loose stool, not to exceed 16 mg in any 24-hour period. Clinical improvement is usually observed within 48 hours

167. A. Autohaler

Pulmicort® is an example of a flexhaler, Spiriva® is a handihaler, albuterol does come in a nebulizer vial solution, and inhaler is a generic term.

168. A, B, C, D

Risperdal® comes in all of these different types of formulations except an IV injection. Injections for Risperdal® are administered IM.

169. A, D

Boniva® is available as an oral tablet and injectable. It has a monthly dosage schedule. Reclast® (zoledronic acid) is an injectable that is given yearly for treatment. Although Prolia® is a subcutaneous injection given twice yearly, it is NOT a bisphosphonate. It is a bone-modifying agent. More specifically, it is a monoclonal antibody that functions as a RANK ligand inhibitor.

170. A, C, D

Also referred to as intrinsic sympathomimetic effect, this term is used particularly with beta-blockers that can show both agonism and antagonism at a given beta receptor, depending on the concentration of the agent (beta-blocker) and the concentration of the antagonized agent (usually an endogenous compound, such as norepinephrine). Some β-blockers (e.g. oxprenolol, pindolol, penbutolol, labetalol and acebutolol) exhibit intrinsic sympathomimetic activity (ISA). These agents are capable of exerting low-level agonist activity at the β-adrenergic receptor while simultaneously acting as a receptor site antagonist. These agents, therefore, may be useful in individuals exhibiting excessive bradycardia with sustained beta-blocker therapy. Agents with ISA are not used after myocardial infarctions, as they have not been demonstrated to be beneficial

171. A, B, C

Tablet, Oral:
- Allegra Allergy®: 60 mg
- Allegra Allergy®: 180 mg

Tablet, Oral, as hydrochloride:
- Allegra Allergy®: 60 mg, 180 mg
- Allegra Allergy Children's®: 30 mg
- Allergy 24-HR®: 180 mg
- Mucinex Allergy®: 180 mg

Generic: 60 mg, 180 mg

172. A, D

Patients susceptible to fat-soluble vitamin deficiencies: Use with caution in patients susceptible to fat-soluble vitamin deficiencies. Absorption of fat-soluble vitamins A, D, E, and K may be decreased; patients should take vitamins ≥4 hours before colesevelam (Welchol®). Medications should be separated out from Welchol® by at least 4 hours due to chelation. Discontinue if triglyceride concentrations exceed 500 mg/dL or hypertriglyceridemia-induced pancreatitis occurs. The American College of Cardiology/American Heart Association recommends avoiding use in patients with baseline fasting triglyceride levels ≥300 mg/dL or type III hyperlipoproteinemia since severe triglyceride elevations may occur. Use bile acid sequestrants with caution in patients with triglyceride levels 250-299 mg/dL and evaluate a fasting lipid panel in 4-6 weeks after initiation; discontinue use if triglycerides are >400 mg/dL. A major side effect of Welchol® is constipation not diarrhea.

173. A, C, D

Allegra® is a category C; Xanax® is a category D drug. The others listed are category X.

174. B, C, D

Trexall® (methotrexate) is a chemotherapy and immunosuppressant medication. It can also be used to treat rheumatoid arthritis and psoriasis. Possible side effects include alopecia (hair loss), thrombocytopenia, stomatitis, and anemia (not bleeding).

175. C, D, E

Colyte® or PEG-3350 is used as a colon lavage to prepare for a colonoscopy. Start a clear liquid diet the day before the colonoscopy. Clear liquids are liquids that you can see through:
- Clear broth (chicken, beef, turkey, vegetable)
- Cranberry juice
- Water
- Sprite®, 7-UP®, ginger ale
- Flavored waters
- Coffee/tea with sugar or honey
- White grape juice
- Gatorade®, Kool-Aid®, Jell-O® (no red or blue)
- Apple juice
- Popsicles (no red or blue)

176. B. Commit 2 mg

IO's first cigarette is 95 minutes after waking in the morning, qualifying her to start with the 2-mg lozenge.

177. A. Nicotine transdermal patch

Because the other three options for therapy were not appropriate given the woman's medical conditions and limitations, she could be tried on the nicotine patch. The first dose would be used for approximately 6 weeks and then she would begin to step down with her therapy. If she started with the 21-mg patch, then she would follow up with 2 weeks of the 14-mg patch and 2 weeks of the 7-mg patch. If she started with the 14-mg patch, she would only need to follow up with the 7-mg patch for 2 weeks.

178. C. 21 mg/d patch

As JE has been smoking one pack per day for the past 40 years, he will need to be started on step 1 which is the 21 mg/d patch dose. A pack contains 20 cigarettes usually so you usually start with step 1 if patients smoke more than 10 cigarettes a day. If patients smoke 10 cigarettes or less per day, they may start at step 2 which is the 14 mg/d patch.

Product	Nicotine Patch
Brand Name /Generic Available	Nicoderm CQ® Habitrol Generic
Product Strength	21 mg 14 mg 7 mg
Dosing	1 patch / 24 hours **11+ cigarettes per day, use 21 mg for 4-6 wks, 14 mg for 2-4 wks, 7 mg for 2-4 wks.** **6-10 cigarettes per day, use 14 mg for 4-6 wks, 7 mg for 2-4 wks.**
Time to peak Plasma level	5-10 hours
Possible Adverse Reactions	*Mild skin reactions (rotate site, use 1% cortisone cream) *If vivid dreams or sleep disturbance, remove at night

If you smoke more than 10 cigarettes a day

If you smoke 10 cigarettes or less a day

STEP 1 21 mg · STEP 2 14 mg · STEP 3 7 mg
WEEKS 1-6 · WEEKS 7-8 · WEEKS 9-10

STEP 2 14 mg · STEP 3 7 mg
WEEKS 1-6 · WEEKS 7-8

179. E. Varenicline

In this case, varenicline is the most appropriate choice because it would have the least negative impact on his other disease states and would increase his chances of quitting over quitting without pharmacologic assistance

180. A. Vitamin B1

Thiamine or Vitamin B1 deficiency.

181. E. Doxycycline 100 mg PO BID x 14 days

Treatment of Lyme disease (Erythema migrans (early disease))

Drug	Adult dosage	Pediatric dosage
Doxycycline	100 mg PO bid x 10 to 21 d	≥8 years: 2 mg/kg PO bid (maximum 100 mg per dose) x 10 to 21 d
or Amoxicillin	500 mg PO tid x 14 to 21 d	50 mg/kg/day divided tid PO (maximum 500 mg per dose) x 14 to 21 d
or Cefuroxime	500 mg PO bid x 14 to 21 d	30 mg/kg/day divided bid PO (maximum 500 mg per dose) x 14 to 21 d

Doxycycline is the preferred regimen unless in pregnant patients and children less than the age of 8 years old should be avoided. The drugs of choice for oral therapy are doxycycline, amoxicillin, and cefuroxime axetil, although doxycycline should **not** be used in children <8 years of age or in pregnant women.

182. C. Ceftriaxone 2 grams IV once daily x 28 days

For patients with late Lyme neurologic disease, intravenous therapy with ceftriaxone, cefotaxime, or penicillin G is recommended.

183. A, C, D

Cisplatin, high dose anthracycline, high dose alkylators, anthracycline and alkylator combination, and lomustine are examples of highly emetic drugs causing nausea and vomiting. Monoclonal antibodies, vinca alkaloids, bortezomib, and bleomycin are minimal emetic risk chemotherapy drugs.

184. A-E (All of the above)

Adverse Reactions:
- Central nervous system: Neurotoxicity (peripheral neuropathy is dose/duration dependent)
- Gastrointestinal: Nausea and vomiting (76% to 100%)
- Genitourinary: Nephrotoxicity
- Hematologic & oncologic: Anemia (≤ 40%), leukopenia, thrombocytopenia
- Otic: Ototoxicity

185. B, C, D, E

Monitoring Parameters: Blood pressure, heart rate (ECG) and rhythm throughout therapy; assess patient for signs of lethargy, edema of the hands or feet, weight loss, and pulmonary toxicity (baseline pulmonary function tests and chest X-ray; continue monitoring chest X-ray annually during therapy); liver function tests (semiannually); monitor serum electrolytes, especially potassium and magnesium. Assess thyroid function tests before initiation of treatment and then periodically thereafter (some experts suggest every 3-6 months). If signs or symptoms of thyroid disease or arrhythmia breakthrough/exacerbation occur, then immediate re-evaluation is necessary. Amiodarone partially inhibits the peripheral conversion of thyroxine (T4) to triiodothyronine (T3); serum T4 and reverse triiodothyronine (rT3) concentrations may be increased and serum T3 may be decreased; most patients remain clinically euthyroid, however, clinical hypothyroidism or hyperthyroidism may occur. Ophthalmic exams should be performed.

186. D. Simvastatin 20 mg/day, lovastatin 40 mg/day

Healthcare professionals, who prescribe simvastatin or simvastatin-containing medications (Simcor, Zocor, Vytorin), should be aware that patients taking amiodarone should not take more than 20 mg per day of simvastatin. Doses higher than 20 mg each day increase the risk of rhabdomyolysis, a rare condition of muscle injury. The dose of lovastatin should not exceed 40 mg daily in patients receiving concomitant medication with amiodarone. The combined use of lovastatin at doses higher than 40 mg daily with amiodarone should be avoided unless the clinical benefit is likely to outweigh the increased risk of myopathy. The risk of myopathy/rhabdomyolysis is increased when amiodarone is used concomitantly with higher doses of a closely related member of the HMG-CoA reductase inhibitor class.

187. B. Stage B

The ACC/AHA staging system for heart failure is based on whether the patient has symptoms and structural heart disease. Stage A is reserved for patients with no symptoms and no structural heart disease. Stage B is for asymptomatic patients with structural heart disease. Stage C is for patients with symptoms as well as structural heart disease. Stage D is for patients with refractory heart failure. There is no Stage E.

188. C. Nadir

In patients receiving chemotherapy, the term nadir usually refers to the time duration it takes for the chemotherapeutic agent to produce the stage of maximum bone marrow depression characterized by low WBC and ANC, with increased susceptibility to infection.

189. A. Elevated; decreased

Cushing's syndrome has elevated cortisol levels, while Addison's disease has decreased levels of cortisol. Both conditions have elevated ACTH levels, which normally increases production of cortisol. In Cushing's disease, the elevated cortisol is often due to elevated levels of ACTH as the primary cause. In Addison's disease, there is often atrophy and dysfunction of the adrenal cortex which results in the decreased level of cortisol. Decreasing cortisol removes the feedback inhibition of ACTH; this causes the levels of ACTH to increase.

190. D. Phenytoin toxicity

Phenytoin use is not associated with renal dysfunction, increased body weight, diabetes, or infection. On the other hand, phenytoin overdose or supratherapeutic concentration can result in concentration-related toxicity.

191. B. Class II

The NYHA functional classes for heart failure are based on patient's symptoms. Class II is for patients with symptoms upon ordinary exertion. Class I is reserved for patients with no limitation in physical activity despite the heart failure. Class III is for patients with symptoms upon minimal exertion. Class IV is for patients with symptoms at rest. There is no class V.

192. E. Metabolic alkalosis

Step 1: Evaluate pH. The pH of 7.6, which is > 7.45 denotes alkalosis. The pH denotes her primary problem of alkalosis.
Step 2: Evaluate ventilation. pCO2 is normal and therefore denotes no respiratory abnormality.
Step 3: Evaluate metabolism. HCO3 of 39 mEq/L, which is > 35 mEq/L denotes metabolic alkalosis.

Therefore, the interpretation of the results is metabolic alkalosis. Mixed acidosis refers to respiratory acidosis and metabolic acidosis occurring at the same time

193. A. Gram-positive organisms

Gram positive are purple (they have a thick cell wall that absorbs crystallized violet). Gram negative are red/pink (they have a thin cell wall that absorbs the safranin counterstain).

194. 127.5

$$\frac{5\ g\ dextrose}{100\ mL} = \frac{x\ g}{750\ mL} \qquad x = 37.5\ g$$

$$\frac{3.4\ kcal}{1\ g} = \frac{x\ kcal}{37.5\ g} \qquad x = \mathbf{127.5\ kcal}$$

195. 15

$$\frac{30\ mg}{5\ mL} = \frac{x\ mg}{150\ mL} \qquad x = 900\ mg \qquad\qquad \frac{60\ mg}{1\ tab} = \frac{900\ mg}{x\ tab} \qquad x = \mathbf{15\ tablets}$$

196. 68.5

$$\frac{500\ mg}{7.3\ mL} = \frac{x\ mg}{1\ mL} \qquad x = \mathbf{68.5\ mg}$$

197. 1.25

0.025 % w/v = 0.025 g/100 mL. Convert this percent w/v to mg/mL= 25 mg/100 mL

$$\frac{25\ mg}{100\ mL} = \frac{x\ g}{5\ mL} \qquad x = \mathbf{1.25\ mg}$$

198. 322

The molecular weight of K is 39 and the molecular weight of Cl is 35; therefore, the molecular weight of KCL is 74.5

- 74.5 = 1 molecular weight for KCL
- 74.5 g = 1 equivalent weight
- 74.5 mg = 1 milliequivalent weight (0.0745 g)

$$\frac{10\ g}{100\ mL} = \frac{x\ g}{240\ mL} \qquad x = 24\ g\ KCl \qquad\qquad \frac{0.0745\ g}{1\ mEq} = \frac{24\ g}{x\ mEq} \qquad x = \mathbf{322.2\ mEq}$$

199. 356

$$MW\ of\ HCl = 36.5;\ 1\ mole = 36.5\ g$$

$$1\ millimole = \frac{36.5\ g}{1000} = 0.0365\ g \times \frac{1000\ mg}{1\ g} = 36.5\ mg$$

$$\frac{10\ g}{100\ mL} = \frac{x\ g}{130\ mL} \qquad x = 13\ g\ HCl \qquad\qquad \frac{0.0365\ g}{1\ mmol} = \frac{13\ g\ HCl}{x\ mmol} \qquad x = \mathbf{356\ mmol}$$

200. 1.69

$$31\ lb\ \times \frac{1\ kg}{2.2\ lb} \times \frac{0.6\ mg}{kg} \times \frac{1\ g}{1000\ mg} \times \frac{50}{0.25\ g} = \mathbf{1.69\ mL}$$

201. 2.75

$$\frac{1\ g}{750\ mL} = \frac{x\ g}{350\ mL} \qquad x = 0.47\ g \qquad\qquad \frac{17\ g}{100\ mL} = \frac{0.47\ g}{x\ mL} \qquad x = \mathbf{2.75\ mL}$$

202. 2.3

$$\frac{1\ mEq\ KCl}{74.5\ mg\ KCl} = \frac{2\ mEq\ KCl}{x\ mg\ KCl} \qquad x = 149\ mg\ KCl \qquad \frac{39\ mg\ KCl}{74.5\ mg\ KCl} = \frac{x\ mg\ KCl}{149\ mg\ KCl} \qquad x = 78\ mg\ KCl$$

$$\frac{78\ mg\ K}{149\ mg\ KCl} = \frac{180\ mg\ K}{x\ mg\ KCl} \qquad x = 343.85\ mg\ KCl \qquad \frac{149\ mg\ KCl}{1\ mL} = \frac{343.85\ mg\ KCl}{x\ mL\ KCl} \qquad x = \boldsymbol{2.3\ mL}$$

203. 308

Molecular weight of NaCl = 58.5 1 mole= 58.5 g
1 millimole = 58.5 mg = 2 milliosmoles, since NaCl dissociates into 2 particles

$$\frac{900\ mg}{100\ mg} = \frac{x\ mg}{1000\ mL} \qquad x = 9000\ mg\ of\ NaCl\ per\ L$$

$$\frac{58.5\ mg}{2\ mOsmol} = \frac{9000\ mg}{x\ mOsmol} \qquad x = 308\ mOsmol$$

204. 16

$$\frac{0.4\ g}{120\ mL} = \frac{x\ g}{5\ mL} \qquad x = 0.016\ g \times \frac{1000\ mg}{1\ g} = \boldsymbol{16\ mg}$$

205. 65

0.65% w/v = 0.65 g/100 L Converted to milligrams this equals 650 mg/100 mL

$$\frac{650\ mg}{100\ mL} = \frac{x\ g}{10\ mL} \qquad x = 65\ mg$$

206. 3,250,000 U

$$\frac{5,000,000\ units}{1\ mL} = \frac{x\ units}{0.65\ mL} \qquad x = 3,250,000\ units$$

207. 2.14%

- Molecular weight of NH_4Cl = is 53.5
- 1 equivalent weight = 53.5 g
- 1 mEq = 53.5 mg

$$\frac{53.5\ mg}{1\ mEq} = \frac{x\ mg}{100\ mEq} \qquad x = 5350\ mg \times \frac{1\ g}{1000\ mg} = 5.35\ g$$

$$\frac{5.35\ g}{250\ mL} = \frac{x}{100} \qquad x = \boldsymbol{2.14\%}$$

208. 1 oz

437.5 grains = 1 oz

209. D. Intangible

Intangible costs include the costs of pain, suffering, anxiety, or fatigue that occur because of an illness or the treatment of an illness. It is difficult to measure or assign values to intangible costs.

210. C. Cost-minimization

A cost minimization analysis measures cost in dollars and outcomes are assumed to be equivalent.

211. C. Cost-effectiveness analysis

Cost-effectiveness analysis (CEA) evaluates the costs that are measured in natural units (e.g., cures, years of life, blood pressure).

212. D. Cost-utility analysis

A CUA takes patient preferences into account when measuring health consequences. The most common unit used in conducting CUAs is QALYs (Quality Adjusted Life Years).

213. 7

$$16\ lb \times \frac{1\ kg}{2.2\ lb} = 7.27\ kg \qquad 0.08\frac{mg}{kg} \times 7.27\ kg = 0.58\frac{mg}{hr} \times 12\ hrs = \boldsymbol{7\ mg}\ in\ 12\ hrs$$

214. 0.01

$$\frac{0.05\ mg}{x\ mL} = \frac{500\ mg}{100\ mL} \qquad x = \boldsymbol{0.01\ mL/min}$$

215. 1

Because the time interval between preparation and administration is 6 hours, and the half-life of the radiopharmaceutical is 6 hours, approximately one-half of the original strength has decayed. Therefore, **1 mL** of the solution, which now assays at 20 mCi/mL, is needed.

216. 90%

The sensitivity of a test is determined by its ability to detect the presence of the disease. The sensitivity expressed as a percentage is determined by dividing the number of subjects with the detected disease (positive) by the total number of subjects that actually has the disease (positive + false negative): $\frac{80}{(80+10)} = 0.89 \quad \boldsymbol{\sim 90\%}$

217. 880

$$155\ lb \times \frac{1\ kg}{2.2\ lb} \times 5\ mg/kg/1\ min = 352\ mg/min$$

Because the solution concentration is 0.4 mg/mL, divide the dosage rate by the concentration:

$$352 = \mathbf{880 \; mL/min}$$

218. 1.5

Q1C1 = Q2C2

$$(1 \; mL)\left(\frac{1}{1,000}\right) = (x \; mL)\left(\frac{1}{2,500}\right) \qquad x = 2.5 \; mL$$
$$2.5 \; mL - 1mL \; (original \; volume) \; = \; \mathbf{1.5 \; mL}$$

219. 0.048

First-order half-lives relate to kinetic constant rate values by the following equation:

$$t_{\frac{1}{2}} = \frac{0.693}{k} \; \rightarrow \; 14.3 \; days = \frac{0.693}{k} \qquad k = \mathbf{0.048 \; per \; day} = 4.8\% \; per \; day$$

220. 5

The original order requested that the solution be infused over a 20-minute time span. Therefore, 100 mL divided by 20 minutes equals **5 mL/min**.

221. 7.3

The original dilution would be: $\quad \dfrac{100 \; units}{1 \; mL} = \dfrac{1,000 \; units}{x \; mL} \quad x = 10 \; mL$

The final volume is 10 mL, of which 1 mL is the volume occupied by the dissolved powder. If a 120 unit/mL concentration is requested, the new volume will be:

$$\frac{120 \; units}{1 \; mL} = \frac{1,000 units}{x \; mL} \qquad x = 8.3 \; mL$$

Since 1 mL is dissolved powder: $\quad 8.3 - 1 = \mathbf{7.3 \; mL \; diluent}$

222. 10%

The prevalence of a disease is determined by dividing the total number of subjects with the disease—(both those testing positive plus those testing negative but with the disease) by the total population tested: $\quad \dfrac{80+10}{910} = 0.099 \quad \mathbf{\sim 10\%}$

223. B. 0.2 mL

$$20 \; units \times \frac{1}{100 \; units} = \mathbf{0.2 \; mL}$$

224. B. 120 mg

$$minimum\ weighable\ quantity = \frac{sensitivity\ requirement \times 100}{\%\ error}$$

$$\frac{6\ mg \times 100}{5\%} = \boldsymbol{120\ mg}$$

225. D. 80

$$\frac{1000}{40\ mEq} \times 0.5\frac{mEq}{minute} = 12.5\frac{}{minute} \qquad \frac{1000}{12.5\ mL/min} = \boldsymbol{80\ minutes}$$

226. C. 40 mg

$$34\ in \times \frac{2.54\ cm}{in} = 86.36\ cm$$

$$BSA = \sqrt{\frac{height\ (cm) \times weight\ (kg)}{3600}} \rightarrow BSA = \sqrt{\frac{86.36 \times 12}{3600}} = 0.54\ m^2$$

$$0.54\ m^2 \times 150 = 81\frac{mg}{day} \div 2\frac{doses}{day} = \boldsymbol{40\ mg\ BID}$$

227. 68%

The standard deviation (SD) is a measure of how spread out numbers are. You will first need to calculate the mean of all values in a given set, then for each number (x) you need to subtract the mean ($\bar{x}$) from it and square these results, then divide by the total number of data points (n), and square root the result.

$$SD = \sqrt{\frac{\sum |x - \bar{x}|^2}{n}}$$

A SD is calculated mathematically for experimental data. It shows the dispersion of numbers around the mean (average value). One SD will include approximately 67% to 70% of all values, whereas two SDs will include approximately 97% to 98%. 68% is the correct answer because the question is asking for the percentage of patients that had a reduction between 5-15mm, which is one standard deviation away from the mean.

228. E. Slightly weaker than desired

There are two factors that may lead to a final concentration slightly lower than the targeted concentration. When aseptically transferring the 20 mL of concentrated dye solution, the technician should inject the dye solution and then draw up 20 mL of the normal saline solution to rinse the syringe of dye solution. Also, one must realize that LVPs of 250, 500, and 1,000 mL have volumes greater than the labeled claim. For example, the 250 mL bag of normal saline is likely to have between 260 and 270 mL. Both factors will reduce the final concentration of dye by a small amount.

229. E. Ketone

This is a ketone structure.

230. A. Cyclobenzaprine

This is a typical cyclic three ring structure and represents cyclobenzaprine.

231. C. MCV and HPV

LM has not received the MCV or HPV vaccines. College freshman should receive the MCV vaccine if they have not previously been vaccinated. The HPV vaccine is recommended at age 11 to12 years; however, it can be given in adult females up to the age of 26 who have not previously been vaccinated.

232. A. DTaP, IPV, MMR, Varicella, and Hep A

Kaly has received 4 doses in the DTaP series already and therefore needs to receive the fifth and final DTaP dose. She has also received 3 doses of IPV and should receive the fourth dose today. Kaly received her first doses of the MMR and varicella vaccines at 15 months. She needs to receive the second dose of each today. Since Kaly only received one dose of the Hep A vaccine at 15 months, she needs to complete the 2-dose series today. She only needs one dose of the Hep A vaccine.

233. E. Sofosbuvir and velpatasvir for 12 weeks

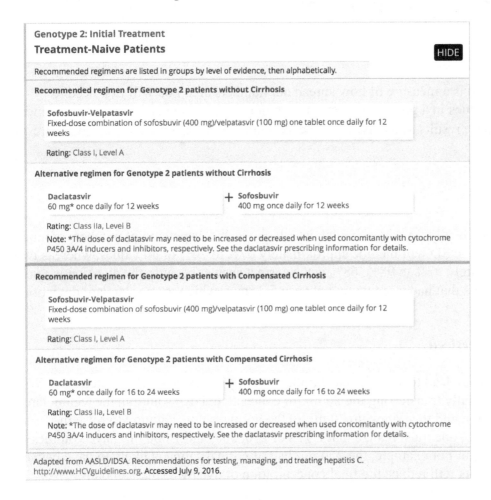

234. A. Ribavirin

The incidence of hemolytic anemia for ribavirin is 10% to 13%. The FDA requires a black box warning regarding this risk in the package insert.

235. D. Reduction in incidence of cyclophosphamide-induced hemorrhagic cystitis

Mesna binds to and inactivates the toxic oxazophosphorine metabolite (acrolein) in the urine to prevent hemorrhagic cystitis

236. B. Continue Insulin drip and add dextrose

Pharmacists need to add dextrose as the glucose level is going less than 250, so the glucose level does not go too low.

237. D. Educate the staff on appropriate vitamin K use

Pharmacists should be actively engaged daily in the education of other healthcare providers and seeking to make improvements in patient care areas.

238. B. Change ritonavir and lopinavir to raltegravir and efavirenz

Most Protease inhibitors inhibit the metabolism of most statins leading to increased serum levels and risk of toxicity.

239. C. Advise she may use H2 antagonist or calcium carbonate antacids

Raltegravir is better absorbed in an alkaline environment, acid suppression does not affect the INSTI drugs. Avoid mag/alum, major issue for rilpivirine and atazanavir are ones that are adversely affected with acid suppression.

240. B. The symptoms are likely due to metoclopramide and its dopamine receptor antagonism

Metoclopramide, haloperidol, and prochlorperazine should be avoided in levodopa/carbidopa as it is a centrally acting antidopaminergic drug.

241. C. Start her on Vitamin B12 2mg once daily

Vitamin B12 levels below 100 may cause tingling. Thiamine is vitamin B1.

242. A. Stop lisinopril and start sacubitril/valsartan 24 mg/26 mg twice daily

In patients with chronic symptomatic NYHA class II or III HFrEF who can tolerate an ACE inhibitor or ARB, replacement by sacubitril/valsartan is recommended to further reduce morbidity and mortality (Class I recommendation).

243. B. No, infliximab has a worsening effect on heart failure

The role of TNF in congestive heart failure has been commonly accepted. Elevated levels of TNF are seen in CHF patients and it is strongly correlated with the NYHA scale. In the failing heart, TNF contributes to the contractile dysfunction, provokes heart hypertrophy, and induces apoptosis of cardiac myocytes. Several potential mechanisms may be responsible for this process with beta adrenergic receptors uncoupling, oxygen species formation, and the activation of inducible nitric oxygen synthase being the most often observed ones. Moreover, chronic stimulation with TNF increases the formation of other proinflammatory cytokines such as IL-6 and IL-1 that are also involved in the pathogenesis of CHF. This is an important observation, since the combination of these cytokines exerts a more profound cardiodepressive effect than either of them alone. Loss of function of beta receptors is recognized as the most important mechanism involved in the pathogenesis of CHF.

244. C. Stop vancomycin and give a corticosteroid and fluids

The best answer here is to stop vancomycin. Drug rash with eosinophilia and systemic symptoms (DRESS) syndrome characterized by fever, rash, eosinophilia, atypical lymphocytes, and multiorgan involvement has a significant mortality. Allopurinol, antiepileptics and sulphonamides are notorious for causing the DRESS syndrome. Vancomycin is less common, but due to excessive use of vancomycin in an inpatient facility, vancomycin appears to be emerging as an important etiology of the DRESS syndrome. Treatment is mostly symptomatic, including intravenous steroids, antipyretics and topical moisturizer.

245. B. Start SnoFlow on cilostazol

Cilostazol, a phosphodiesterase type 3 (PDE3) inhibitor, may have selective antiplatelet and vasodilating effects. This drug has been shown to increase exercise tolerance in patients with severe claudication. Pentoxifylline, a xanthine derivative, is widely promoted for use in this condition but is not recommended. Both drugs are FDA approved to treat.

246. C. The newborn and children's guardian or parent

Children are defined as persons who have not attained the legal age for consent to treatments or procedures involved in clinical investigations under the applicable law of the jurisdiction in which the clinical investigation will be conducted.
Because children are unable, due to age, to give consent themselves, permission is provided by a parent or guardian on their behalf. The term informed consent under Sec. 50.20 applies to other participants in clinical investigations. FDA solicits comments on its definition of permission.
https://www.fda.gov/scienceresearch/specialtopics/runningclinicaltrials/ucm119111.htm

247. C. Increase the voriconazole dose, the levels are subtherapeutic

Voriconazole levels should be drawn 12 hours after the last dose after the patient has received at least 5-7 days of consistent voriconazole therapy. Based on relatively weak data, the optimal voriconazole trough level for both efficacy and safety appears to be between >2 and 6 mg/L.

248. D. Provide less than 50% of caloric requirements then slowly taper up to goal

Refeeding syndrome can occur in acutely (can include critically ill patients) or chronically malnourished patients when EN or PN is initiated.

- Characterized by hypophosphatemia, hypokalemia, hypomagnesemia b. Can cause cardiac dysfunction, respiratory dysfunction, and death
- Prevention of refeeding syndrome:
  - Identify patients at risk (e.g., anorexia, alcoholism, cancer, chronically ill, poor nutritional intake for 1–2 weeks, recent unintentional weight loss, malabsorption).
  - Initially, provide less than 50% of caloric requirements, and then advance over several days to desired goal.
  - Supplement vitamins before initiating PN as well as K+, phosphate, and magnesium (if needed); monitor daily for at least 1 week; and replace electrolytes as needed (many patients will need aggressive electrolyte replacement during the first week of PN).

249. A. Speak with your doctor to change your clozapine to another antipsychotic as hydroxyurea increases the effect of clozapine, potentially causing agranulocytosis

Hydroxyurea: may increase the toxicity of clozapine (specifically, agranulocytosis). Avoid combination.

250. B. CMS

Beginning in 2011, the Medicare and Medicaid EHR Incentive Programs were developed to encourage eligible professionals (EPs) and eligible hospitals to adopt, implement, upgrade (AIU), and demonstrate meaningful use of certified electronic health record technology (CEHRT).

NAPLEX® FORMULA SHEET

Conversions between units

$1 \ grain = 65 \ mg$

$1 \ mg \ aminophylline = 0.8 \times mg \ theophylline$

$°F = \left(°C \times \dfrac{9}{5}\right) + 32$

Converting mg, mEq, mmol, and mOsmol

$valence = \ of \ ions \times net \ charge$

$$MW = mmol = \frac{grams}{mol} \qquad mg = \frac{mEq}{valence} \qquad mEq = \frac{MW}{valence}$$

$$mOsmol = \frac{weight \ (g)}{MW} \times 1000 \times number \ of \ species$$

Body Mass Index (BMI)

$$BMI = \frac{weight(kg)}{\left(height \ (m)\right)^2} \qquad\qquad BMI = \frac{weight(lb)}{\left(height \ (in)\right)^2} \times 704.5$$

Ideal Body Weight (IBW)

$IBW \ (male) = 50 \ kg + (2.3 \ kg \times inches \ over \ 5 \ ft)$

$IBW \ (female) = 45.5 \ kg + (2.3 \ kg \times inches \ over \ 5 \ ft)$

Adjusted Body Weight

$AbjBW = IBW + 0.4(TBW - IBW)$

Body Surface Area

$$BSA \ (m^2) = \sqrt{\frac{height \ (cm) \times weight \ (kg)}{3600}} \qquad BSA \ (m^2) = \sqrt{\frac{height \ (in) \times weight \ (lb)}{3131}}$$

Basal Energy Expenditure (BEE) (Harris-Benedict Equation)

Using lb and in:

$males: 66 + \left(6.2 \times weight(lb)\right) + \left(12.7 \times height(in)\right) - \left(6.76 \times age(yrs)\right) = BEE$

$females: 655.1 + \left(4.35 \times weight(lb)\right) + \left(4.7 \times height(in)\right) - \left(4.7 \times age(yrs)\right) = BEE$

Using kg and cm:

$males: 66 + \left(13.7 \times weight(kg)\right) + \left(5 \times height(cm)\right) - \left(6.8 \times age(yrs)\right) = BEE$

$females: 655 + \left(9.6 \times weight(kg)\right) + \left(1.8 \times height(cm)\right) - \left(4.7 \times age(yrs)\right) = BEE$

Specific Gravity

$$specific \ gravity = \frac{weight(g)}{volume(mL)}$$

Cockcroft-Gault Equation

$$CrCl = \frac{(140 - age\ (yrs)) \times weight(kg)}{72 \times SCr} (\times 0.85\ if\ female)$$

If BUN/SCr ratio > 20, consider dehydration in the patient

Density

$$density = \frac{mass}{volume}$$

Total Energy Expenditure
Note: activity and stress factors will be given

$$TEE = BEE \times activity\ factor \times stress\ factor$$

Nitrogen Balance
1 g nitrogen = 6.25 g protein

$$nitrogen\ intake = \frac{grams\ of\ protein}{6.25}$$

Corrected Calcium
Note: use when albumin < 3.5

$$corrected\ calcium = serum\ calcium + [(4 - albumin) \times 0.8]$$

Osmolarity

$$\frac{mOsmol}{L} = \frac{concentration\left(\frac{g}{L}\right)}{MW\left(\frac{g}{mol}\right)} \times of\ species \times 1000$$

Sodium Chloride Equivalent (E Value)
Note: i = dissociation factor

$$E = \frac{58.5 \times i}{MW \times 1.8} \qquad mole = \frac{g}{MW} \frac{mg}{mmol} = \frac{mg}{MW} \qquad mEq = \frac{mg \times valence}{MW} = \frac{mmol}{valence}$$

Absolute Neutrophil Count (ANC)
Note: Normal limits 2200-8000

$$ANC = WBC \times neutrophils(\%)$$

$$neutrophils = segs + bands$$

Anion Gap (AG)
Note: High is >12mEq/L = gap acidosis

$$anion\ gap = Na^+ - (Cl^- + HCO_3^-)$$

Henderson Hasselbach equation

<u>Weak Acid:</u>

$$pH = pKa + \log\left(\frac{salt}{acid}\right)$$

<u>Weak Base (pKw IS ALWAYS 14):</u>

$$pH = pKa + \log\left(\frac{base}{salt}\right)$$

<u>Aliquot Measurement</u>

$$mean\ weighable\ quantity\ (MWQ) = \frac{sensitivity\ requirement\ (SR)}{\%\ of\ error}$$

<u>Relative Risk (RR)</u>

$$relative\ risk\ (RR) = \frac{exposed\ or\ treated\ group\ event}{nonexposed\ or\ placebo\ group\ event}$$

RR <1 reduces risk of event occurrence with treatment
RR = 1 no reduction of risk between treatment vs. nontreatment group
RR > 1 increases risk of event occurrence with treatment

<u>Relative Risk Reduction (RRR)</u>

relative risk reduction (RRR)

$$= \frac{(\%\ event\ occurrence\ of\ control\ or\ placebo) \times (\%\ event\ occurrence\ of\ treatment)}{\%\ event\ occurrence\ control\ or\ placebo}$$

$$relative\ risk\ reduction\ (RRR) = 1 - relative\ risk\ (RR)$$

<u>Flow Rate</u>

$$flow\ rate\ \left(\frac{ml}{hr}\right) = \frac{total\ volume\ (mL)}{infusion\ time\ (hr)}$$

<u>Ke</u>

$$\frac{Cl}{V_d} = \frac{\ln\left(\frac{C_1}{C_2}\right)}{(t_2 - t_1)} = \frac{\ln(C_1) - \ln(C_2)}{(t_2 - t_1)}$$

<u>Bioavailability</u>

$$Bioavailability\ (F\%) = 100 \times \frac{AUC\ extravascular}{AUC\ intravenous} \times \frac{dose\ intravenous}{dose\ extravascular}$$

<u>Clearance</u>

$$Cl = \frac{dose \times F}{AUC}$$

$$Cl = k_e \times V_d$$

<u>Half Life</u>

$$t_{\frac{1}{2}} = \frac{0.693}{k} = \frac{0.693 \times V_d}{Cl}$$

<u>Elimination rate constant</u>

$$k_e = \frac{Cl}{V_d} = \frac{\ln\left(\frac{C_1}{C_2}\right)}{(t_2 - t_1)} = \frac{\ln(C_1) - \ln(C_2)}{(t_2 - t_1)}$$

<u>Minimum weighable quantity</u>

$$minimum\ weighable\ quantity = \frac{sensitivity\ requirement \times 100}{\%\ error}$$

<u>TPN kcal:</u>
Dextrose = 3.4 kcal/g
Amino acids = 4 kcal/g
Lipids = 9 kcal/g
10% lipid emulsion = 1.1 kcal/g
20% lipid emulsion = 2 kcal/g
Glucose = 4 kcal/g

Like the book? Help us help you more!

- Please help positively rate this book (5 stars) on Amazon.com, search title "2023-2024 NAPLEX", find our book and rate us under customer reviews

- Access our website for more guides at: www.rxpharmacist.com

- Want to share feedback to improve this guide? Please contact us directly at help@rxpharmacist.com!

- Don't have a guide there you need? Send us a recommendation and any comments/suggestions to: help@rxpharmacist.com